Baby and Child Health

Carolyn Meggitt

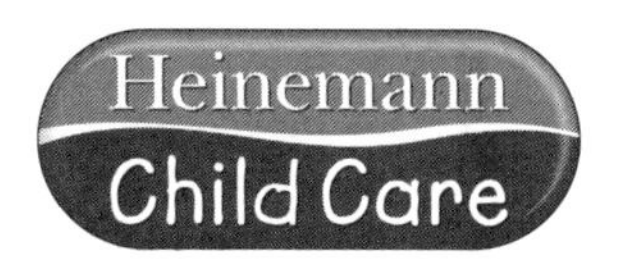

Heinemann Educational Publishers,
Halley Court, Jordan Hill, Oxford OX2 8EJ
A division of Reed Educational & Professional Publishing Ltd

Heinemann is a registered trademark of Reed Educational & Professional Publishing Limited

OXFORD MELBOURNE AUCKLAND JOHANNESBURG BLANTYRE GABORONE IBADAN
PORTSMOUTH NH (USA) CHICAGO

First published 2001
2005 2004 2003 2002 2001
10 9 8 7 6 5 4 3 2 1

A catalogue record for this book is available from the British Library on request.

ISBN 0 435 40151 3

Typeset by Tek-Art, Croydon, Surrey

Printed and bound in Great Britain by The Bath Press, Bath

Acknowledgements

I gratefully acknowledge contributions from Carolyn Lees, Health Visitor; the Hospital Play Staff Association; Gerald Sunderland for the photographs on pages 5-8 and for the specially commissioned photographs in the nutrition and first-aid colour sections of this book.

Thanks as always to my family, Dave, Jon, Leo and Laura for their patience and support.

The author and publisher would like to thank the following organisations and individuals for permission to reproduce photographs and copyright material:

British Heart Foundation/French & Ribbans – page 31
Haddon Davies – page 21
Meningitis Research Trust – page 104
Peter Morris – page 46
S.P.L. – pages 4, 12, 18, 79, 248 (right), 278
Tony Stone – page 248 (left)
Gerald Sunderland – colour photographs in inserts after page 40 and after page 236;
and pages 5–8, 19, 56, 57
Wellcome Trust – page 97
Mike Wyndham – colour photographs in insert after page 220 and pages 128, 182.

Tel: 01865 888058 www.heinemann.co.uk

Contents

Author's note

The main aim of this book is to help students to learn about children's **health needs** and how they can be provided for in the context of child care and early years education. I have written this guide to baby and child health using a **holistic** framework. This means that, although much of the book's focus is on *physical health* and how children can be kept healthy, it also recognises the needs of children to be healthy in other equally important ways – emotionally, mentally and socially. There is also an emphasis on child safety and first-aid measures which will help the student to feel confident in dealing with accidents and sudden illness.

This book will be equally useful for students following child care courses and for managers and teachers already qualified and working in early years settings. The text is supported by a variety of student activities – case studies, revision questions and short quizzes.

For additional information on the various organisations mentioned in this book, you can access their websites.

PART 1

Promoting and maintaining health

Chapter 1: What is child health?

◆ *A holistic approach to understanding health* ◆ *A child's rights to health* ◆ *The needs of children* ◆ *Providing for children's needs*

A holistic approach to understanding health

The concept of good health or 'being healthy' means different things to different people. It is often easier to determine whether or not a person is healthy by looking at possible diseases or conditions they may or may not have, or by assessing their lifestyle. Being healthy is really a mixture of all the following factors:

- **Being fit**: for example being able to run for a bus without getting out of breath; or taking part in sports.
- **Not being ill**: for example hardly ever going to the doctor; or never suffering from anything more serious than a mild cold or the occasional tummy upset.
- **Being able to adapt**: for example enjoying your studies or job and being able to do it without too much stress and strain; or adapting easily to changes in life, such as getting married or becoming a parent.
- **Living to an old age**: for example reducing your chances of dying young, by never smoking, eating the 'right' foods and being the ideal weight for your height.
- **Being happy**: for example feeling glad to be alive when you wake up in the morning; enjoying being with your family and friends, or enjoying some form of relaxation and leisure time.

The **World Health Organisation (WHO)** defines health as 'a state of complete physical, mental and social well-being and not merely the absence of disease or infirmity'. A more useful definition of health includes three other very important aspects of health: emotional, environmental and spiritual.

A child's rights to health

Children are entitled to basic human rights such as food, health care, a safe home and protection from abuse. However, children are a *special* case because they cannot

The six aspects of health

Environmental health
Environmental health refers to the general health of the society in which we live. In areas of famine – where the first priority for health is to obtain enough food – people may be denied access to health. Poverty and overcrowded living conditions are all negative aspects of environmental health.

Physical health
This is the easiest aspect of health to measure. It involves the physical functioning of the body and includes the **growth** and **physical development** of the baby and child.

Emotional health
Emotional health involves how we express emotions such as joy, grief, frustration, hurt and fear. This ability to express our own emotions and to react to other people's emotions leads on to coping strategies for anxiety and stress.

Spiritual health
Spiritual health involves personal, moral codes of conduct – as well as religious beliefs and practices.

Mental health
Mental health involves our ability to organise our thoughts logically, and is closely linked to emotional and social health.

Social health
Social health involves the way we relate to other people and form relationships.

always stand up for themselves. They need a *special* set of rights which take account of their vulnerability and ensure that adults take responsibility for their protection and development.

The United Nations (UN) drew up a legally binding treaty – **The United Nations Convention on the Rights of the Child (UNCRC)** – setting out the full range of rights for all children and young people up to the age of 18. It has been signed by almost every country in the world.

The rights which particularly relate to child health are:

- Children have the right to **be with their family** or with those who will care for them best.
- Children have the right to **enough food and clean water** for their needs.
- Children have the right to an **adequate standard of living**.
- Children have the right to **health care**.
- Children have the right to **play**.
- Children have the right to **be kept safe and not hurt or neglected**.
- **Disabled children** have the right to special care and training.
- Children must **not be used as cheap workers or as soldiers**.
- Children have the right to **free education**.

ACTIVITY

Understanding health

Read the 'profiles' below and then discuss the questions below in groups:

Samantha is 17. She lives at home with her mother and stepfather and two younger brothers. She is studying Advanced VCE in Business Studies at her local sixth form college, and would like to work in the retail industry. Samantha enjoys clubbing and going to the cinema. She used to be very anti-smoking but took up the habit when her steady boyfriend left home to go to university. They are still in touch, but Samantha often feels lonely. She also says she feels overwhelmed by the amount of work at college, but is keen to do well.

Jack is 21. He lives at home with his parents and younger sister. Jack uses a wheelchair because he had an accident on holiday two years ago, which resulted in a broken spine. Jack works in a computer sales and service office; he likes socialising with friends and enjoys watching his local rugby team and taking part in archery contests. He sometimes feels frustrated when he has to rely on friends and family to take him to different places; he is saving up for a specially adapted car which will give him more freedom of movement.

Atiya is six years old and lives at home with her parents and her four-year-old brother. Atiya has severe asthma. She has daily **steroid** treatment and has to carry her reliever inhaler with her at all times. She enjoys playing computer games and swimming. Atiya would like to try tap dancing with her best friend, Hayley, but her parents are worried that she will have a severe asthma attack, so are reluctant to let her go.

George is 44. He lives with his wife, Pat, and works as a driving instructor. George is overweight and smokes heavily. Recently Pat had to go into hospital for a hysterectomy and at about the same time a good friend of theirs had a sudden heart attack and died. George enjoys his job, but is worried about the stress it causes. He has begun to feel rather low and to worry about the future.

Questions

Consider each person in turn and answer the following questions:

1. Are they healthy?
2. Why might they want to be healthier?
3. What could they – or their families – do to help them to better health?

The needs of children

From the moment they are born, all children depend completely on an adult to meet all their needs, but the *way* in which these needs are met will vary considerably according to family circumstances, culture and the personalities of the child and the caring adult.

Maslow's hierarchy of needs

Abraham Maslow (1908–1970) devised a hierarchy of needs, which proposes that basic physical needs, such as hunger and thirst, must be satisfied before the higher needs (such as **self-esteem** and self-actualisation) can be achieved. This hierarchy of needs is usually presented as a pyramid. It is important that each level of need is satisfied before moving on to the next level; otherwise energy has to be directed at fulfilling the lower needs at the expense of moving on to the next level – and eventually to self-fulfilment. The highest need – **self-actualisation** – varies from one person to another. For example, it might involve becoming a top athlete, creating a masterpiece or perhaps being a good parent. It can be described as reaching one's potential or finding self-fulfilment.

Self-actualisation needs (achieving full potential)

Self-esteem needs (respect, including self-respect)

Love and emotional needs (affection from others, being with others)

Safety and security needs (freedom from anxiety and chaos; stability; predictability)

Basic physical needs (food, drink, oxygen, sleep, warmth)

Maslow's hierarchy of needs

To achieve and maintain healthy growth and development (that is, physical, intellectual, emotional and social), certain basic needs must be fulfilled:

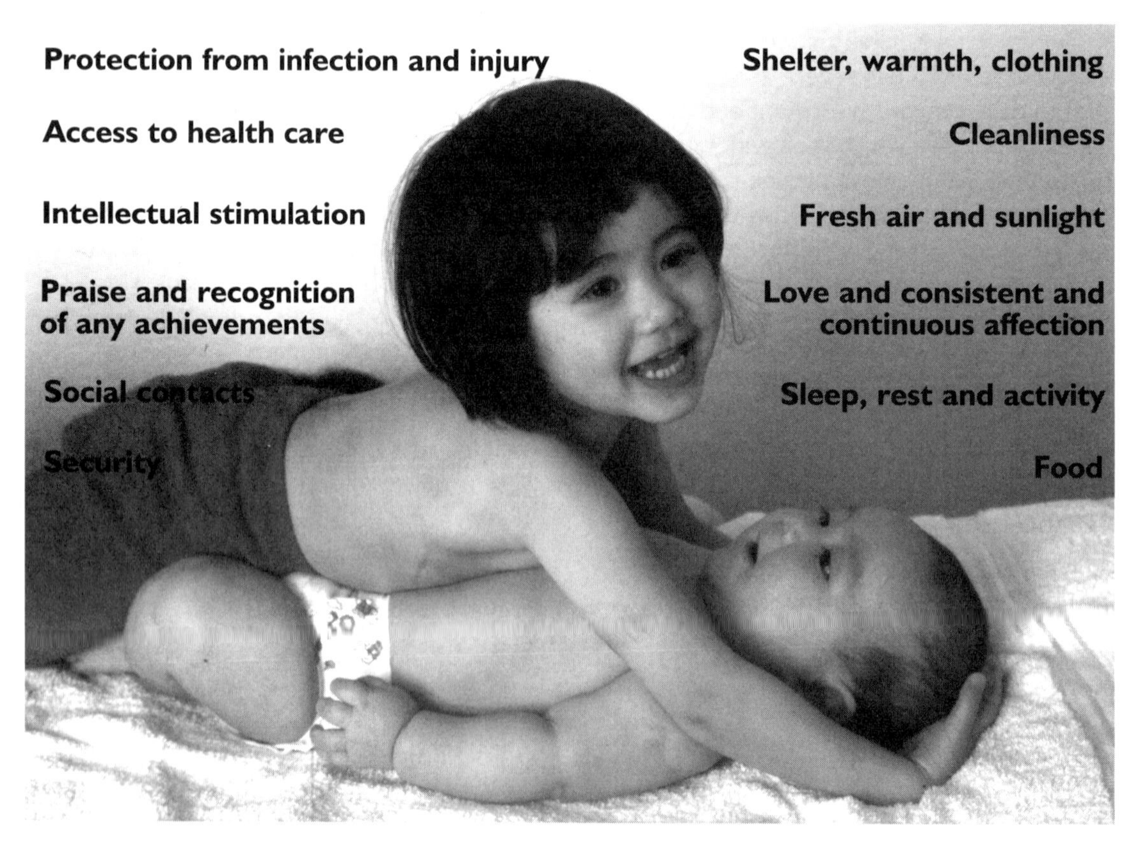

The needs of babies and children

It is difficult to separate these basic needs in practical care, as they all contribute to the **holistic** development of a healthy child.

Providing for children's needs

All those who care for young children need a thorough knowledge of child development, so that provision of care can be planned to match each child's needs at each stage of development. The following gives a brief outline of the stages of development for babies and children.

Holistic development during the first year

New-born babies explore their new environment through their senses – of sight, smell, touch and taste. When not asleep, they are alert and already learning to cope with a huge amount of new information. They can focus their eyes on objects less than one metre away and show a definite preference for looking at human faces.

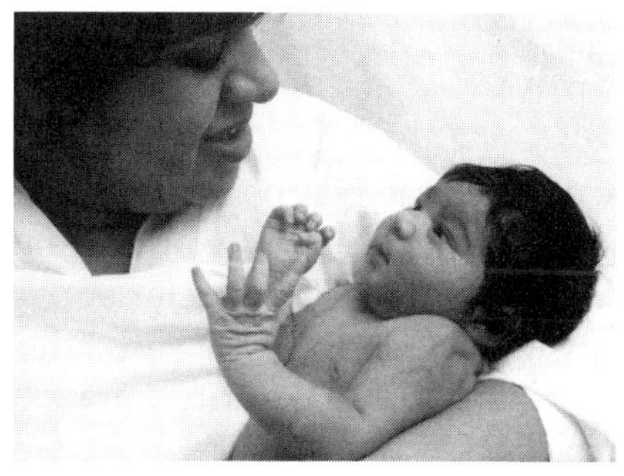

A new-born baby

By 3 months babies are showing more interest in playthings – e.g. rattles. They like to kick vigorously and to clasp their hands together. They respond to familiar situations by a combination of excited movements, smiles and a variety of sounds, such as cries, cooing sounds and chuckles.

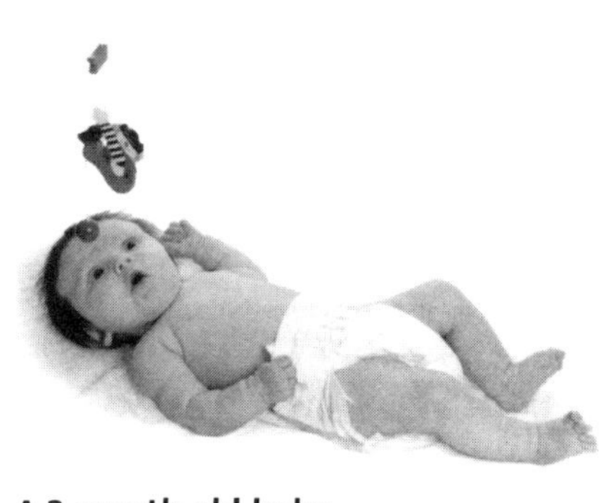

A 3-month-old baby

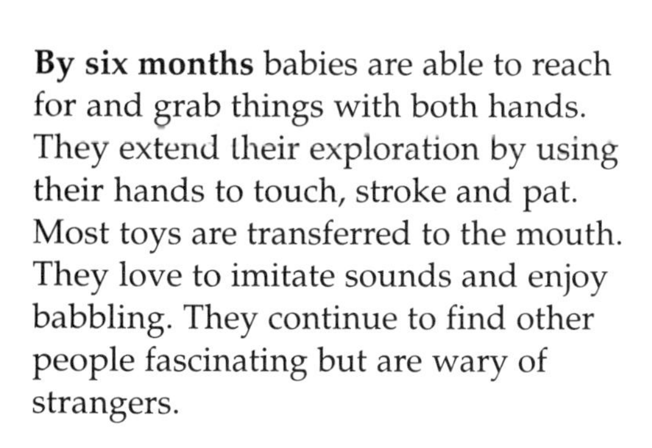

By six months babies are able to reach for and grab things with both hands. They extend their exploration by using their hands to touch, stroke and pat. Most toys are transferred to the mouth. They love to imitate sounds and enjoy babbling. They continue to find other people fascinating but are wary of strangers.

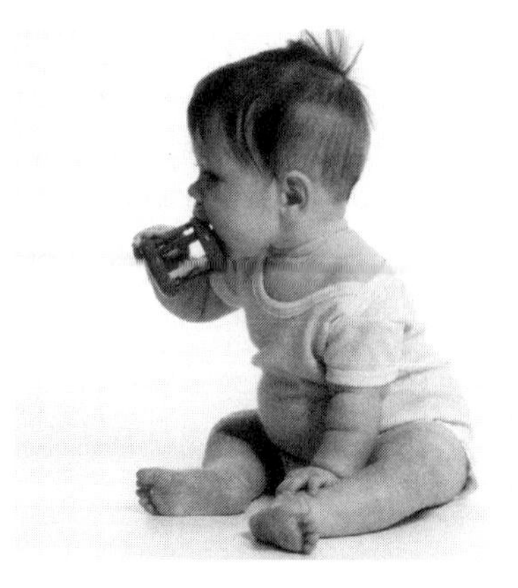

A 6-month-old baby

By nine months babies enjoy exploring their environment by crawling or shuffling on their bottoms. They often bounce in time to music and take pleasure from songs and action rhymes. They can sit, lean forward and pull objects towards them. Babies understand their daily routine and like to imitate adult speech and gestures.

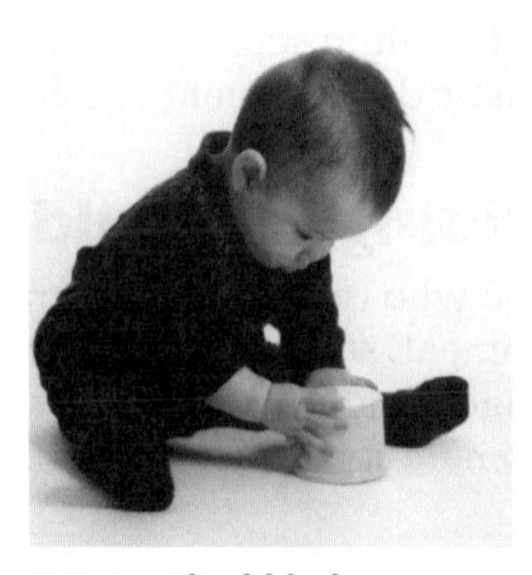

A 9-month-old baby

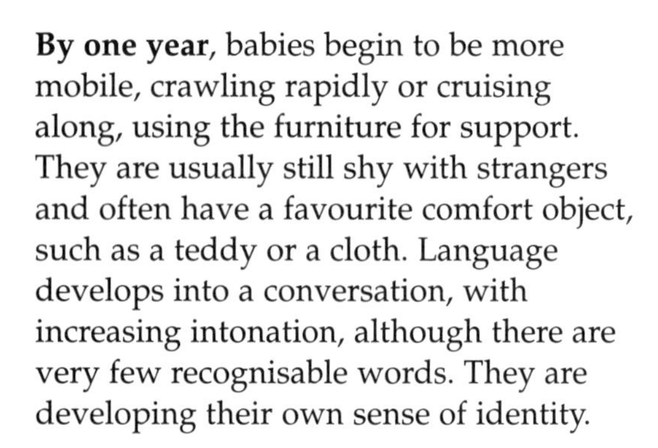

By one year, babies begin to be more mobile, crawling rapidly or cruising along, using the furniture for support. They are usually still shy with strangers and often have a favourite comfort object, such as a teddy or a cloth. Language develops into a conversation, with increasing intonation, although there are very few recognisable words. They are developing their own sense of identity.

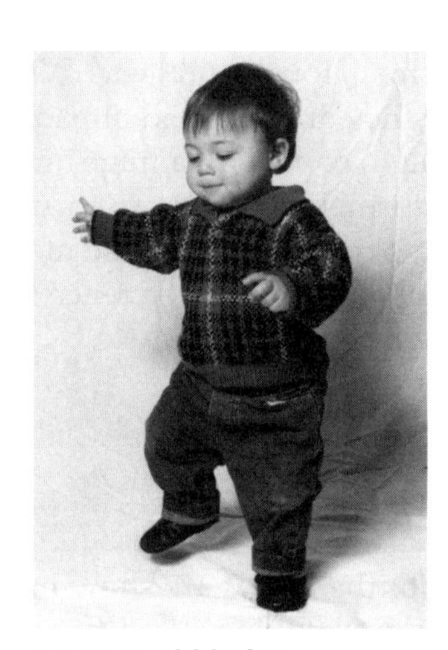

A 1-year-old baby

Holistic development from 18 months to 4 years

By eighteen months children enjoy being able to walk well and to climb up and down stairs with help. They can pick up small objects with a delicate pincer grasp and are beginning to show a preference for using one hand. They enjoy simple picture books and can understand and obey simple commands. They have an increasing desire for independence and are developing a strong sense of personal identity.

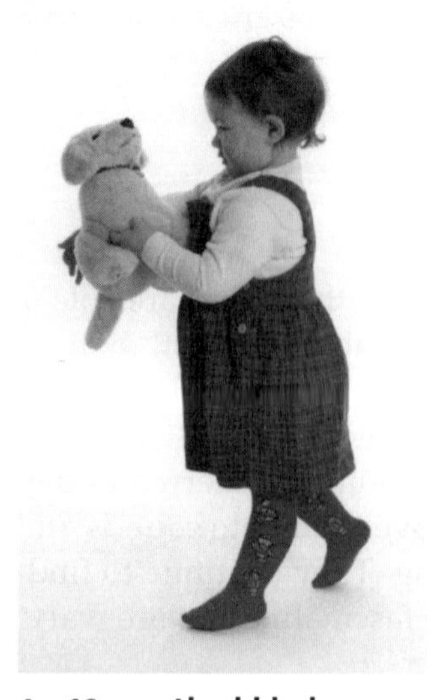

An 18-month-old baby

By two years children can run, jump, kick, and use words as well as actions to express themselves. They are eager explorers of their environment and want to be as independent as possible. They become easily frustrated when they cannot express themselves or are prevented from doing something they want to do. They may show strong emotions in 'temper tantrums' or bursting into tears.

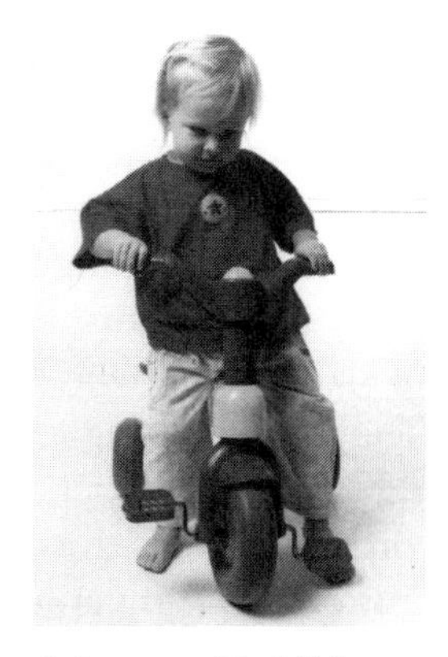

A 2-year-old child

By three years children can jump and stand on one foot; they now demonstrate that they have an inner world of thinking and they can also talk about it. They now play *with* other children rather than just around them and are making their first friends.

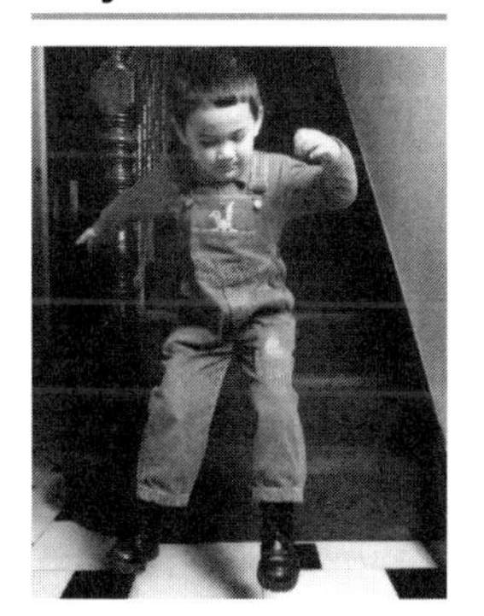

A 3-year-old child

By four years children are quite capable and independent. They walk with swinging steps, almost like an adult's, and like to hop and jump. They are fascinated by cause and effect and their increasing mastery of language prompts them to ask questions about the way things work in the world.

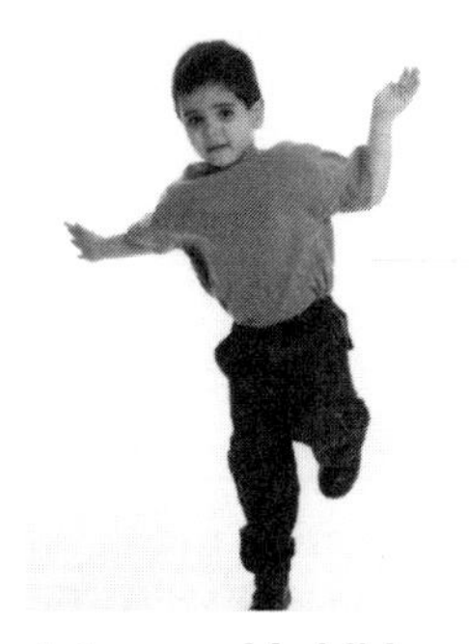

A 4-year-old child

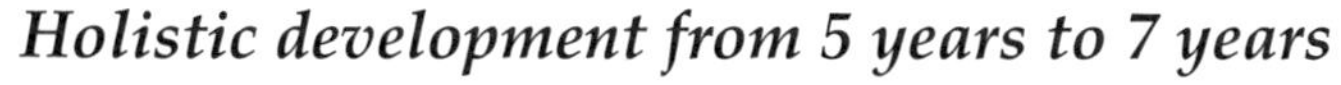

Holistic development from 5 years to 7 years

By five years children enjoy showing what they can do – hopping, skipping, dancing and playing group ball games. They have a growing awareness of the world and their language shows this understanding. Children are learning self-control, how to wait, and how to take turns. They are completely independent in everyday skills, such as washing, dressing and eating.

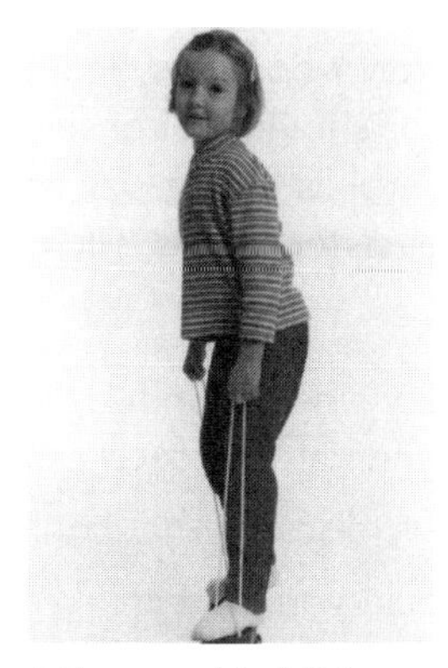

A 5-year-old child

By six years children have increased agility, muscle co-ordination and balance; they can hop easily and jump off apparatus at school. They are full of curiosity and are developing their own interests. They are also forming new concepts of size, shape, weight and distance. They are growing towards reading and writing independently, putting words and ideas down on paper and often using invented spelling.

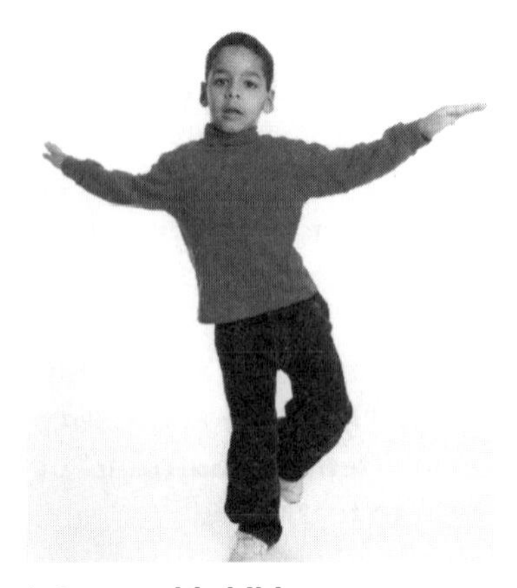

A 6-year-old child

By seven years children have a well-developed sense of balance and enjoy activities that involve precise movements, such as hopscotch or skipping games. They are completely independent in washing, dressing and toileting skills. They are interested in talking, listening, reading and writing and enjoy games with rules. They have a clear sense of right and wrong and see friendships as very important.

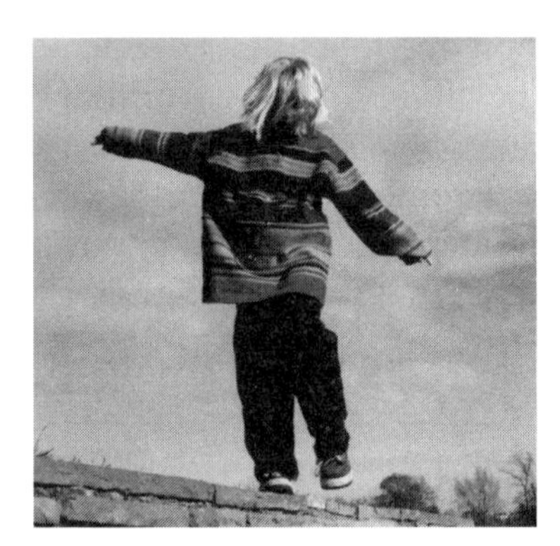

A 7-year-old child

CASE STUDY

Harry is three years old. He lives with his parents and his five-year-old sister, Katie. Harry has often been described by his parents as a 'problem' child. He has never slept through the night and is very 'picky' about what he will eat. Recently, he has started to refuse to go to nursery school, preferring to sit at home watching cartoons on TV. His mother took him to the doctor, who could find nothing physically wrong with Harry, but suggested that the health visitor should be consulted. The health visitor advised the parents to persevere with nursery school as Harry was becoming increasingly isolated and showing signs of behavioural disturbances, such as rocking backwards and forwards and pulling at his hair.

Questions

1 List Harry's needs under the headings physical, emotional, mental, social, spiritual, environmental. For each category decide whether these needs are being met.
2 In groups, discuss what could happen if each of these needs are not met.
3 How could you, as a child care worker at Harry's nursery school, help Harry to settle in and to enjoy his time in the nursery?

Chapter 2: The factors affecting health in children

◆ *Factors affecting child health* ◆ *Factors affecting health before and around birth* ◆ *Factors affecting health in the perinatal period* ◆ *Factors affecting health during infancy and early childhood*

Factors affecting child health

Every aspect of our lives can have an effect on our health and well-being. Health is not just a personal matter. It is affected by the *people around us*, by *where* we live and *how* we live. The following factors – see Table 2.1 – all have a direct bearing on child health, and are discussed in more detail below.

Table 2.1 Factors affecting child health

□ **Genetic factors** Certain illnesses and conditions are inherited through the **genes**, e.g. **sickle cell disease** or a tendency to heart disease or asthma. **Down's syndrome** results from a **chromosomal** abnormality and may be associated with health problems, such as heart defects and a tendency to chest infections.	□ **Pre-conceptual factors** It is now thought to be best to begin pre-conceptual care several months before trying to conceive. By taking care of her body, the woman is ensuring that her own health is at the optimum level by the time she becomes pregnant.
□ **Antenatal factors** A child's health is affected by parental choices regarding both diet and lifestyle habits both *before* conception and *during* the woman's pregnancy. Certain infections can also pass through from the mother to the foetus and have an adverse effect on health, e.g. **rubella**, **cytomegalovirus** and **toxoplasmosis**.	□ **Perinatal factors** Any risks associated with the actual birth – or delivery – of the baby may affect their health and development; these risks include long and complicated labours, lack of oxygen to the baby during labour, and the use of analgesic (pain-killing) drugs during labour.
□ **Nutrition** Children should be offered a diet that contains all the necessary **nutrients** for healthy living. Babies and children who do not receive a healthy diet are at risk from delayed physical and intellectual development as well as poor growth and health problems such as **anaemia** and **rickets**.	□ **Infectious diseases** Certain illnesses such as rheumatic heart disease or **pneumonia** can have a lasting effect on later health, e.g. weakness in the heart or chest. Several childhood infections can also affect growth and development. Some of these, e.g. polio, measles, meningitis and diphtheria, are controlled by childhood **immunisation**.

▶

□ **Housing** Overcrowding encourages the spread of infectious diseases. Cold, damp housing can aggravate conditions such as **bronchitis** or **asthma**. Poor housing and overcrowded conditions can have an adverse and lasting effect on the physical, emotional and social well-being of the child and their family.	□ **Income** Generally, people with a high level of earnings enjoy a better lifestyle, with better housing, better food, warm clothes and own transport. Poorer people tend to make less use of NHS care even though they have worse health; this is known as the **inverse care law**.
□ **Accidents** Accidents – or unintentional injuries – are the chief cause of death in children under the age of 14. The type of accident is directly related to the age and developmental stage of each child. Many accidents are preventable with good care and knowledge of safety procedures.	□ **Emotional and social factors** Children need a stable, continuous, reliable and loving relationship with their parents (or permanent parent-substitutes); Bowlby calls this **attachment.** All children need a secure framework within which to develop, and when deprived of continuous affection, their emotional and social well-being may be affected.
□ **Lifestyle – social and personal habits** Children are deeply influenced by the lifestyle factors of their families and carers; these include smoking, alcohol use, diet and exercise. A happy and relaxing social life can counteract many of the stresses and strains in both family life and the workplace.	□ **Environmental factors** Polluted air, whether from smoke or from chemicals, causes a variety of different respiratory illnesses. Some chemicals and radioactive pollution have been linked with childhood cancers. Damp climates also aggravate conditions such as asthma and respiratory disorders.
□ **Government policy** Government policies determine priorities for spending on specific health issues. For example, life-threatening illnesses such as cancer tend to attract more research and money than do chronic diseases such as **juvenile arthritis** or heart disease.	

Factors affecting health before and around birth

Genetic factors

Growth and development of the embryo and foetus are controlled by **genes**. The influence of our genes is almost too great to comprehend. They determine everything from eye colour to body shape and even affect intelligence and personality.

Each of us inherits two copies of all our genes – one from each parent. Abnormalities of these genes (or of whole **chromosomes**) may cause **birth defects**, or symptoms that may not appear until later (see also pages 152–154 on genetics and inheritance).

Preconceptual factors

Preconceptual care involves both partners cutting known risks *before* trying to conceive, so that they can create the best conditions for an **embryo** to grow and develop into a healthy baby. The first twelve weeks of life in the womb (or **uterus**) are the most crucial as it is the period in which all the essential organs are being formed. The guidelines in Table 2.2 should be considered by a couple *at least* three months, and preferably several months, *before* trying to become pregnant.

Table 2.2 Preconceptual care and care during pregnancy: guidelines

Stop smoking As smoking cuts the amount of oxygen supplied to the baby through the placenta, women should try to stop smoking before planning a pregnancy. Smoking during pregnancy can result in miscarriage or low birth weight. Some men who smoke are less fertile because they produce less sperm.	**Use barrier methods of contraception** It is advisable to discontinue the contraceptive pill so that the woman's natural hormonal pattern can be re-established. Use a condom or diaphragm for three months before trying to conceive. This makes it easier to calculate the exact dates of the last menstrual period and so the length of the pregnancy.
Genetic counselling If there is a fairly high risk that a child may carry a genetic fault, such as cystic fibrosis or sickle cell disease, then **genetic counselling** may be offered. Tests may be carried out to diagnose any problem during pregnancy, but all involve some element of risk in themselves.	**Avoid hazards at work** Some gases and chemicals may increase the risk of miscarriage and birth defects. Women should be aware of the risks and take precautions after discussion with an environmental health officer or a workplace health and safety professional.
Eat a sensible diet A balanced diet helps a woman to build up reserves of the nutrients vital to the unborn baby during the first three months in the womb: ✓ **Eat something from the four main food groups every day**: potato and cereals, vegetables and fruit, milk and milk products, high protein foods – e.g. fish, meat. ✓ **Cut down on sugary foods** and eat fresh foods where possible. ✓ **Do not go on a slimming or reducing diet**; instead follow your appetite and try not to eat more than you really need. ✓ **Avoid pre-packed foods and highly-processed foods;** avoid any foods that carry the risk of **salmonella** or **listeria**. ✓ **Vegetarian diets** which include milk, fish, cheese and eggs provide the vital proteins needed by the unborn baby. ✓ **Vegans** should eat soya products, nuts and pulses to provide essential proteins; vitamin B12 may need to be taken as a supplement. ✓ **Folic acid tablets** and a **diet rich in folic acid** both help the development of the unborn baby's brain and spinal cord.	

▶

Substance use and misuse Do not take any drugs unless they are prescribed by a doctor. Existing conditions such as epilepsy or diabetes will need to be monitored and controlled before, during and after pregnancy. Many addictive drugs cross the placental barrier and can harm the unborn baby.	**Radiation – X-rays** Avoid X-rays during the first three months of pregnancy – although the risks to the foetus are thought to be very slight.
Cut down on alcohol The best current health advice is to cut out alcohol completely. Moderate drinking (1–2 glasses of beer or wine a day) increases the risk of miscarriage and babies are born smaller and more vulnerable. Heavy drinking, particularly in the first few weeks of pregnancy, can cause **foetal alcohol syndrome** in which the baby is severely damaged.	**Sexually transmitted diseases (STDs)** Sexually transmitted diseases should be treated – if either partner thinks there may be any risk of syphilis, gonorrhoea, genital herpes or HIV infection, then both partners should attend a special **GUM** clinic for advice and tests. STDs can cause miscarriage, stillbirth or birth defects.

Antenatal (Prenatal) factors

During pregnancy there are many factors which can have an effect on the health of the unborn child. These include:

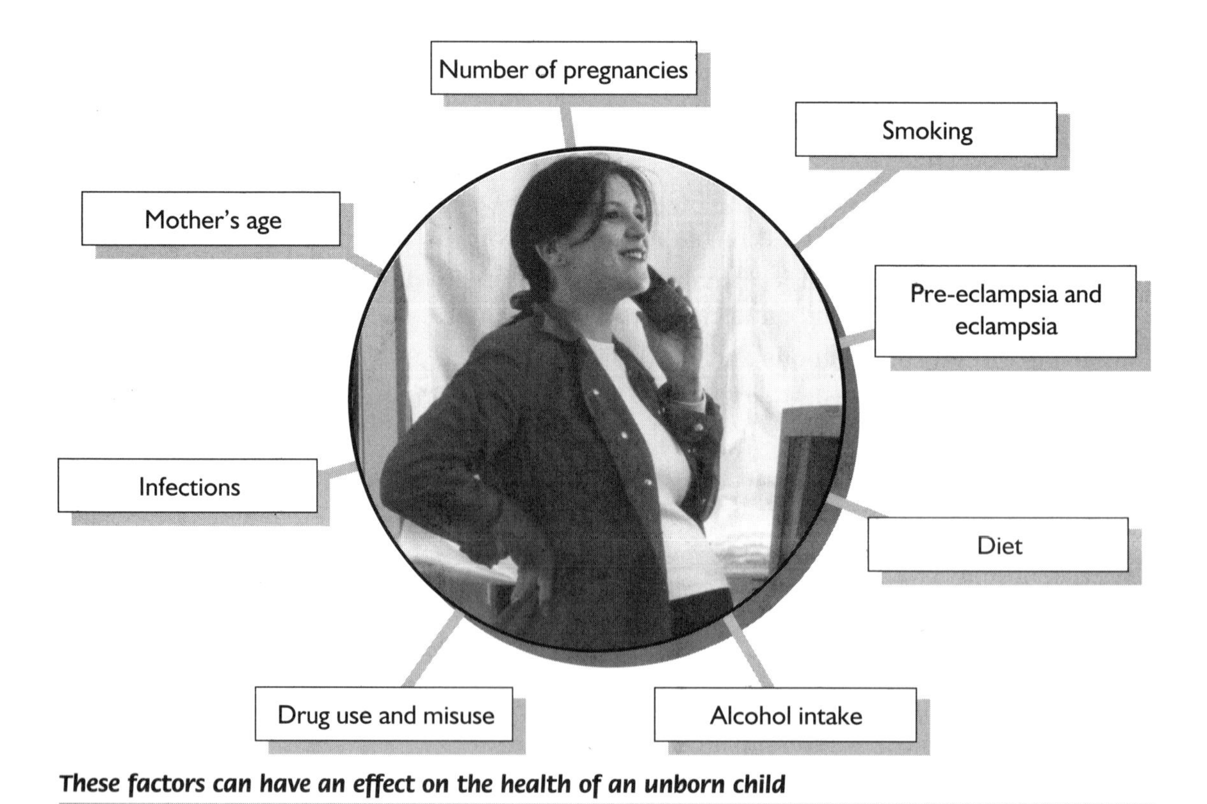

These factors can have an effect on the health of an unborn child

The mother's age

From a purely *physical* point of view, the best age for a woman to have a baby is probably between 18 and 30 years. There are more likely to be complications during pregnancy and labour for women who are above and below these ages.

Younger mothers: Under the age of 16 there is a higher risk of having a small or premature baby, of becoming **anaemic** and suffering from high blood pressure. Emotionally and socially, very young teenagers are likely to find pregnancy and motherhood much harder to cope with and they will need a great deal of support.

Older first-time mothers: First-time mothers over the age of 35 run a risk of having a baby with a **chromosomal** abnormality. The most common abnormality associated with age is **Down's syndrome**. The older the woman has her first child, the greater the risk; for example, at the age of 40 the incidence of Down's syndrome is about 1 in every 110 births, and at age 45 the risk rises to about 1 in every 30. A test called **amniocentesis** (in which fluid is taken from the amniotic sac around the foetus in early pregnancy) can detect the extra chromosome which results in Down's syndrome, and this screening test is usually offered routinely to women who are thirty-seven or over.

Number of pregnancies

Some problems occur more frequently in the *first* pregnancy than in later ones. For example, there is a greater incidence of **breech presentation**, **pre-eclampsia**, **low birth weight** and **neural tube defects**. First babies represent a slightly higher risk than second and third babies do. The risks begin to rise again with a fourth and successive pregnancies; this is partly because the uterine muscles are less efficient, but it also depends to a certain extent on age and social factors associated with larger families.

Pre-eclampsia and eclampsia

Pre-eclampsia is a complication of later pregnancy, which can have serious implications for the well-being of both mother and baby as the oxygen supply to the baby may be reduced and early delivery may be necessary. Careful checks are made to ensure that the signs of pre-eclampsia are not present during the antenatal period. These signs include:

- a rise in blood pressure
- swelling of hands, feet, body or face due to fluid accumulating in the tissues – this is known by the medical term **oedema**
- protein in the urine.

In severe cases, pre-eclampsia may lead to **eclampsia**, in which convulsions (seizures) can occur. This can occasionally threaten the life of both mother and baby, as there is a lack of oxygen supply during such seizures. If pre-eclampsia is diagnosed during antenatal checks, the woman is admitted to hospital for rest and further tests.

Infections

Infection – in the form of viruses or small bacteria – can cross the placenta from the mother to the **foetus** and may interfere with normal growth and development. The first three months (the first **trimester**) of a pregnancy are when the foetus is particularly vulnerable. The most common examples are detailed in the table below:

Table 2.3 Infections during pregnancy

Infection and *cause*	**Effect on the unborn child**
Rubella (German measles) *Virus*	Can cause congenital defects such as blindness, deafness and mental retardation. The most dangerous time to contract rubella is during the first 12 weeks of pregnancy. All girls in the UK are now immunised against rubella before they reach child-bearing age, and this measure has drastically reduced the incidence of rubella-damaged babies.
Toxoplasmosis *Parasite*	Can be caught from eating anything infected with the parasite. This could be: □ raw or undercooked meat, including raw cured meat such as Parma ham or salami □ unwashed, uncooked fruit and vegetables □ cat and dog faeces and soil contaminated with cat faeces □ unpasteurised goat's milk and dairy products made from it. In about one-third of cases, toxoplasmosis is transmitted to the foetus and may cause blindness, **hydrocephalus** or mental retardation. Infection in late pregnancy usually has no ill-effects.
Syphilis *Bacteria*	Syphilis is a rare sexually transmitted disease (STD). It can only be transmitted across the placenta *after* the 20th week of pregnancy. It will cause the baby to develop congenital syphilis, or can even lead to the death of the foetus. If the woman is diagnosed as having the disease at the beginning of pregnancy it can be satisfactorily treated before the 20th week.
HIV (human immuno-deficiency virus) *Virus*	Mothers who are HIV positive run a 50% chance of their new-born baby being infected. Recent research shows that babies known to be infected during their time in the womb may sometimes clear the infection spontaneously.
Listeria *Bacteria*	A rare cause of serious problems in a new-born baby, and can also cause stillbirth. It is caused by the organism found in soft ripened cheeses such as brie and camembert and in pâtés.
Cytomegalovirus (CMV) *Virus*	Causes vague aches and pains and possibly fevers, and poses similar risks to the rubella virus, i.e. blindness, deafness and mental retardation, but as yet there is no preventive vaccine. It is thought to infect as many as 1% of unborn babies, and of those infected babies, about 10% may suffer permanent damage.

Smoking

Smoking during pregnancy reduces placental blood flow and therefore cuts the amount of oxygen the foetus receives. A pregnant woman who smokes is more likely to produce a low birth weight baby unless she stopped smoking before the 20th week. Smokers also tend to have more complications during pregnancy and labour, and there is a greater risk of the baby dying during labour and the first week of life. Smoking during pregnancy has also been found to have a detrimental effect on the physical growth and development of the child up to the age of 11 years.

Drug use and misuse

Most drugs taken by the mother during pregnancy will cross the placenta and enter the foetal circulation. Some of these may cause harm, particularly during the first three months after conception. Drugs that adversely affect the development of the foetus are known as **teratogenic**.

- **Prescription drugs** are those drugs sometimes prescribed by the woman's doctor to safeguard her health during pregnancy, for example antibiotics or anti-epilepsy treatment. Any drugs prescribed must be very carefully monitored to minimise any possible effects on the unborn child.
- **Non-prescription drugs**, such as aspirin and other painkillers, should be checked for safety during pregnancy.
- **Illegal drugs**, such as cocaine, crack and heroin, are teratogenic and may cause the foetus to grow more slowly. Babies born to heroin addicts are usually addicted to heroin themselves and may suffer painful withdrawal symptoms. They are also likely to be underweight and may even die. Research indicates that babies who have been exposed to **ecstasy** while in the womb are more likely to be born with abnormalities; however, many women who have taken ecstasy have *also* taken alcohol and other drugs, so it is very difficult to decide which drug is responsible for any defects. The particular abnormalities found were heart defects and problems with the muscles and bones, such as club foot (**talipes**).

ACTIVITY

1. Research the effects of drug misuse during pregnancy and produce a booklet that clearly explains the risks of each drug to the health of the unborn child. Include the following drugs: tobacco, alcohol, heroin, and cocaine.
2. Design a poster to inform pregnant women (and their partners) of the dangers of smoking during pregnancy and in the perinatal period.

Alcohol intake

Alcohol can harm the foetus if taken in excess. Babies born to mothers who drank *large* amounts of alcohol throughout the pregnancy may be born with **foetal alcohol syndrome**. These babies have characteristic facial deformities, stunted growth and mental retardation. More moderate drinking may increase the risk of miscarriage, but many women continue to drink small amounts of alcohol throughout their pregnancy with no ill-effects.

Nutrition during pregnancy

A balanced diet

Research shows that that the quality of a baby's nutrition before birth may also lay the foundation for good health in later life. During pregnancy women should eat a well-balanced diet using the following guidelines:

Table 2.4 A healthy diet in pregnancy

✓ Lean meat, fish, eggs, cheese, beans and lentils are all good sources of **nutrients**. Eat some every day.	✓ Eat plenty of fruit and vegetables that provide vitamins, minerals, and fibre. Eat them lightly cooked or raw.
✓ Starchy foods, like bread, potatoes, rice, pasta and breakfast cereals, should – with vegetables – form the main part of any meal.	✓ Green, leafy vegetables, lean meat, dried fruit and nuts contain iron, which is important for preventing **anaemia**.
✓ Dairy products, like milk, cheese and yoghurt, are important as they contain **calcium** and other nutrients needed for the baby's development.	✓ Dairy products, fish with edible bones (e.g. sardines), bread, nuts and green vegetables are rich in calcium, which is vital for making bones and teeth.
✓ Citrus fruit, tomatoes, broccoli, blackcurrants and potatoes are good sources of **vitamin C**, which is needed to help the absorption of iron from non-meat sources.	✓ Margarine or oily fish (e.g. tinned sardines) contain **vitamin D** to keep bones healthy.
✓ Cut down on sugar and sugary foods like sweets, biscuits and cakes and sugary drinks like cola. ✓ Cut down on fat and fatty foods as well.	✓ Include plenty of **fibre** in the daily diet; this will prevent constipation, and help to keep the calorie intake down
✓ **Folic acid** is a B vitamin, which is very important throughout pregnancy, but especially in the first twelve weeks when the baby's systems are being formed. (Most doctors recommend that pregnant women take a **folic acid supplement** every day, as more folic acid is required than is available from a normal diet.)	
Department of Health advice is to eat according to appetite, with only a small increase in energy intake for the last three months of the pregnancy (200 kcal a day).	

Food safety in pregnancy

Food safety issues cause pregnant women a great deal of anxiety. The following guidelines should be followed in pregnancy.

Table 2.5 Food safety in pregnancy

□ Cook all meat and poultry thoroughly so that there is no trace of pink or blood and wash all surfaces and utensils after preparing raw meat. This will help to avoid infection with **toxoplasma**.	□ Wash fruit, vegetables and salads to remove all traces of soil which may contain **toxoplasma**.

▶

☐ Make sure eggs are thoroughly cooked until the whites and yolks are solid, to prevent the risk of **salmonella** food poisoning. ☐ Drink only pasteurised or UHT milk, which have had the harmful germs destroyed.	☐ Avoid eating peanuts and foods containing peanut products (e.g. peanut butter, unrefined groundnut oil and some snacks, etc.) if there is a family history on either side of hay fever, asthma, eczema or other allergies. This may reduce the risk of the baby developing a potentially serious allergy to peanuts. Read food labels carefully and if still in doubt about the contents, avoid these products.
☐ Avoid eating all types of pâté and mould-ripened soft cheese, like brie and camembert, and similar blue-veined varieties, because of the risk of **listeria** infection.	☐ If using cooked/chilled ready meals or ready-to-eat poultry, always re-heat thoroughly to destroy listeria infection.
☐ Don't eat liver or liver products, like liver pâté or liver sausage, as they may contain a lot of vitamin A. Too much **vitamin A** could harm the unborn baby.	☐ Drink coffee, tea and cola drinks in moderation, as there may be a slight risk that too much caffeine may affect the baby's birth weight.
☐ Take sensible food hygiene precautions when preparing and storing food, like washing your hands before and after handling food; using separate chopping boards for raw meat and other food; storing foods at the correct temperature and cooking them thoroughly.	☐ Always wash hands and wear gloves when in contact with cats, cat litter, soil and sheep, because of the risk of **toxoplasmosis**.

Factors affecting health in the perinatal period

There are various factors which affect the health of the baby in the period surrounding the actual birth. These include the following:

- **Babies who are born early – pre-term** or **premature** babies. Babies born earlier than 34 weeks may need extra help breathing, feeding and keeping warm. The earlier they are born the more help they are likely to need in the following areas:
  - **Breathing**: Their respiratory system is immature and the baby may have difficulty breathing by themself because of **respiratory distress syndrome (RDS)**. This is caused by a deficiency in **surfactant**, a fatty substance which coats the baby's lungs and is only produced from about 22 weeks of pregnancy.
  - **Control of their body temperature**: Heat production is low and heat loss is high, because the surface area is large in proportion to the baby's weight and there is little insulation from subcutaneous fat (which has not had a chance to be formed).

- **Infection**: Resistance to infection is lowered; this is because they have not had enough time in the uterus to acquire **antibodies** from the mother to protect them against infection.
- **Jaundice**: This is a yellowness of the skin due to excessive **bilirubin** in the blood; it is caused by immaturity of the liver function.

◆ **Babies who are very small** or who have **life-threatening conditions**, usually affecting their breathing, heart and circulation.

◆ **Post-term babies**: Babies born after the expected date of delivery – i.e. after 40 weeks of pregnancy – may also experience feeding and breathing problems during the first few weeks. These occur because the placenta stops functioning after about 42 weeks and so fails to provide the larger baby with enough oxygenated blood. Most doctors will intervene by artificially inducing labour and monitoring the labour very carefully.

◆ **Difficult births**: Although most births are straightforward, leading to the delivery of a healthy baby, there are various risks associated with the labour process. These include:

- **Multiple births**. Twins, triplets and more carry extra risk to both babies and their mother during pregnancy and labour.
- **Foetal distress**. This is usually caused by a lack of oxygen to the baby's brain (**anoxia**). During labour, midwives and doctors look out for signs of distress and will often accelerate the delivery by using special **forceps**.
- **The effects of analgesia**. Analgesics – or painkillers – and anaesthetics given to the mother immediately before delivery can pass through to the baby and cause him or her to be 'floppy' and to need resuscitation.
- **Prolonged labour**. Any prolonged labour can cause the baby to be tired and short of oxygen. This may be because there is an abnormal presentation, such as **breech presentation**, which slows down the labour process.

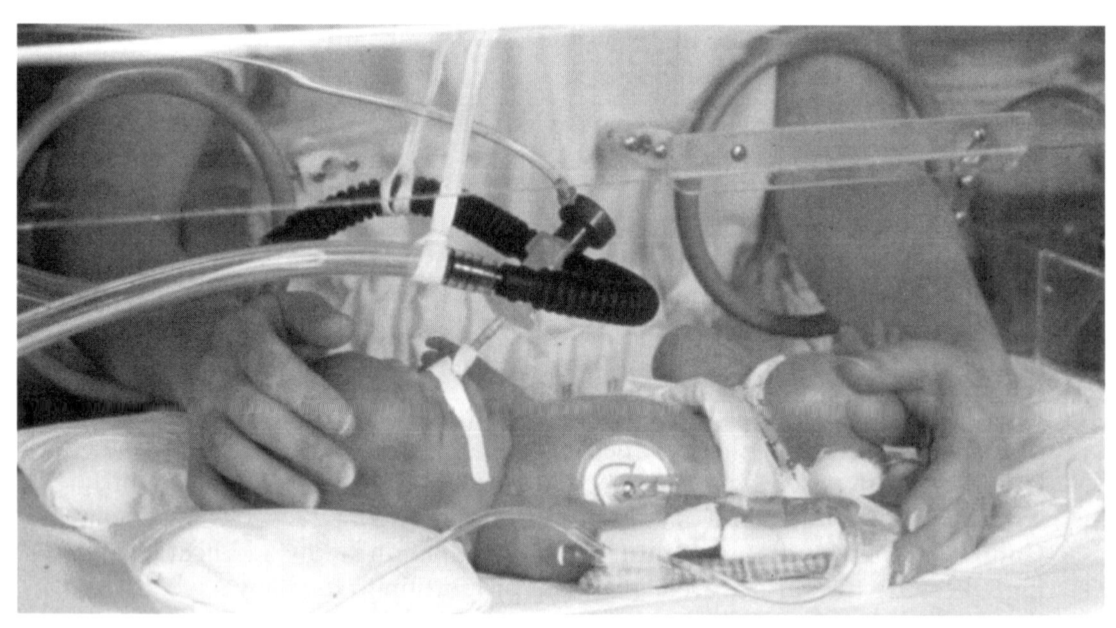

Caring for a baby in an incubator

ACTIVITY

Arrange to visit a Special Care Baby Unit (SCBU) in your local hospital, or ask a midwife to come in and talk to you about the special care of new-born babies. Compile a list of questions that will help you to understand the special needs of these babies and their families. For example, you could ask:

1. What is the most common reason for a baby being in need of special care?
2. How do members of staff cope with the needs of parents when their baby is very ill?
3. How long do babies stay in the SCBU?
4. What is the ratio of staff to patients? What training do you need to work in an SCBU?
5. What are the ups and downs of a career looking after very small babies?

When preparing for the visit or talk, make sure that the professional you contact is fully briefed about the session. You could compile a fact-file of useful information for other students.

Factors affecting health during infancy and early childhood

There are very many factors which affect the healthy growth and development of children. These factors work in combination and so it is often difficult to estimate the impact of any single factor on child health.

Many of the factors which *adversely* affect child health are closely interrelated, and can be seen as a cycle of deprivation. For example, poor families will tend to live in poorer housing conditions and may also have an inadequate diet. Lack of adequate minerals and vitamins as a result of poor diet leads to an increased susceptibility to infectious diseases, and so on.

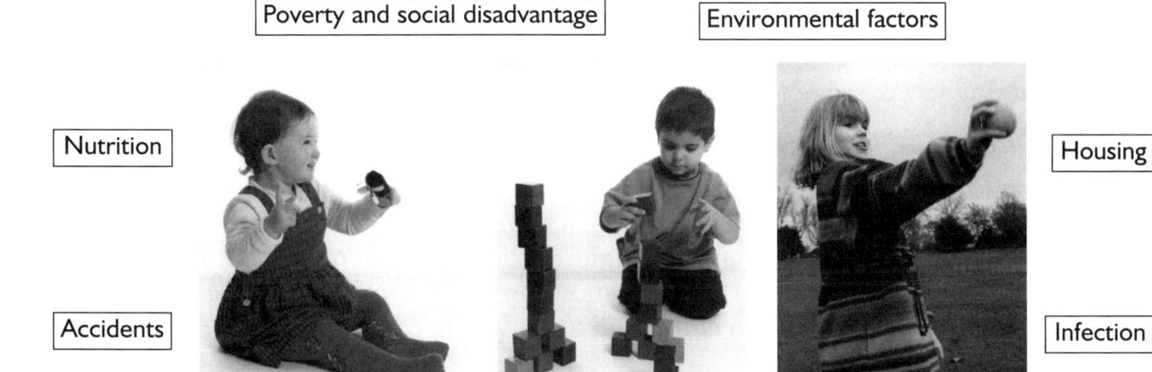

Factors affecting child health

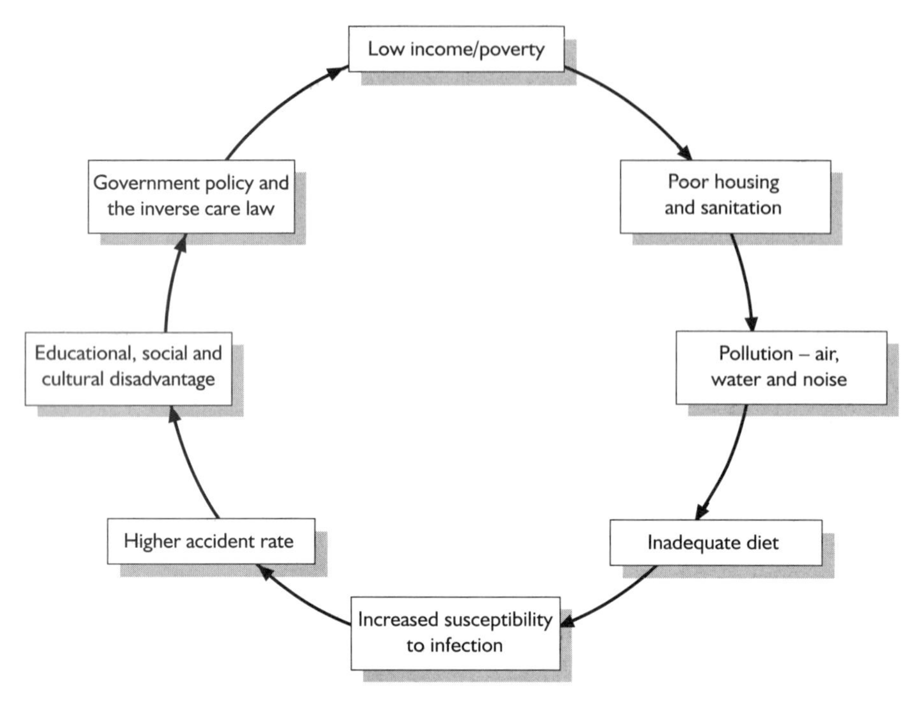

The cycle of deprivation

Nutrition

Milk, whether human or formula, is the fuel that makes babies grow more rapidly during the first year than at any other time. Both human and formula milk provide the right nutrients for the first months of life, with just the right balance of carbohydrates, proteins, fats, vitamins and minerals.

Breastfeeding

Human milk provides the perfect balance of nutrients. It also contains **antibodies** from the mother; these are special proteins that protect the baby against gastrointestinal and respiratory infections. The physical contact between mother and baby also encourages bonding. Breastfed babies are also less likely to become overweight due to excessive feeding

Bottle feeding

Commercial formula milk contains all the right nutrients in the right proportions and has the advantage of reassuring parents and carers about how much feed their baby is taking. Mothers should have the right to choose which method of infant feeding is right for them, and not feel pressured by health professionals or others.

Guidelines for a healthy diet in childhood are given in Chapter 3.

How nutrition in childhood affects health

Eating habits that are developed in childhood are likely to be continued in adult life. This means that children who eat mainly processed, convenience foods will tend to rely on these when they leave home. There are various conditions which may occur in childhood that are directly related to poor or unbalanced nutrition:

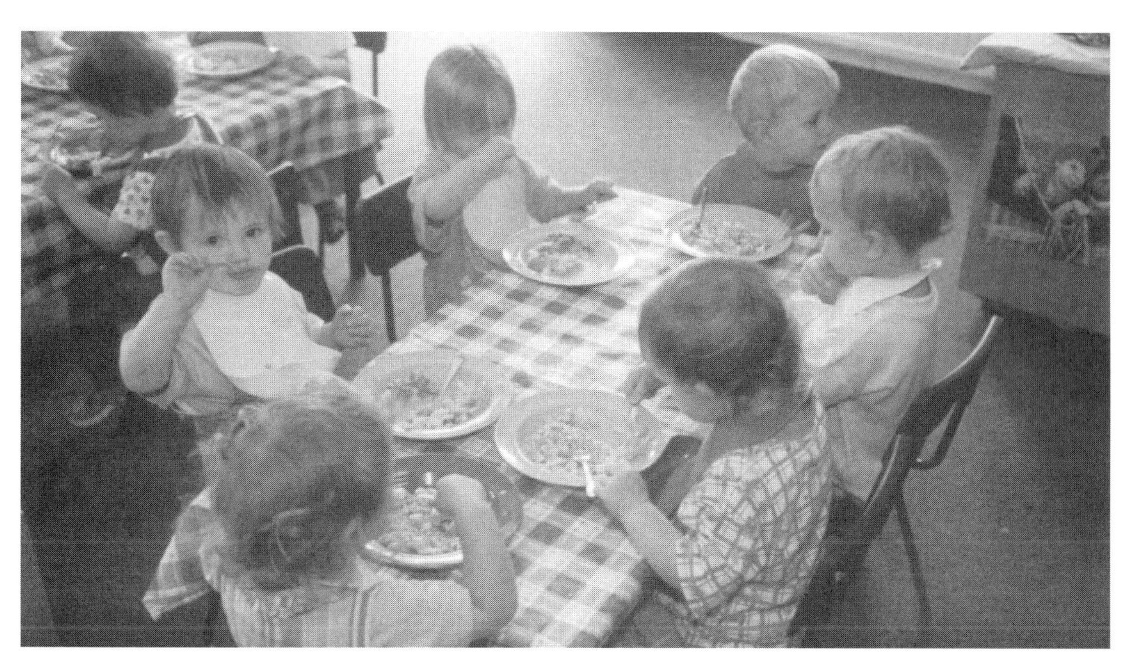

Enjoying a healthy meal

- **Failure to thrive**: poor growth and physical development.
- **Dental caries or tooth decay**: associated with a high consumption of sugar in snacks and fizzy drinks.
- **Obesity**: children who are overweight are more likely to become obese adults.
- **Nutritional anaemia**: due to an insufficient intake of iron, folic acid and vitamin B12.
- **Increased susceptibility to infections**, particularly upper respiratory infections, such as colds and bronchitis.

CASE STUDY

Recently an inquest revealed that a baby died from salt poisoning after being fed an adult diet.

Curtis Andrews was just three months old when he died. His parents were devastated because they didn't think they were doing anything wrong. Cathy and Darren Andrews did just what they thought the baby books suggested. They fed their baby on 'family foods', but they started far too soon. (Experts recommend that babies should not be introduced to solids until they are at least four months old.) They didn't realise that the 'family foods' referred to in most baby care manuals are not the sort of meals that include instant cereals, instant potato mash and instant gravy. Lots of parents decide to use baby foods well before the recommended time – there is always someone around to advise new parents to try thickening feeds to help babies sleep through the night.

Curtis's parents tried baby rice as a feed thickener; then they moved on to Ready Brek and instant mashed potato and gravy, because it was cheaper. In fact, cereals such as Ready Brek are more than *six times* cheaper than prepared and labelled commercial baby rice.

▶

So, in addition to thickening their baby's feed with baby rice, Cathy and Darren were giving Curtis an adult salted cereal. This caused baby Curtis to become thirsty and to cry again. As he was then fed even more thick feeds, not only was he taking in too much salt, he was also getting an even lower proportion of liquid to calories and was bound to suffer **dehydration**. When he died, Curtis's body contained *18 times* the recommended amount of salt for a baby – but only slightly more than the average adult daily intake.

Questions

1 What did Cathy and Darren feed Curtis with – and why?
2 What is wrong with using adult meals for very young babies?
3 What is the recommended age for starting to feed solids to a baby?
4 What sort of family foods *could* have been given to a baby just starting on solids?
5 How could parents be made aware of the problems involved in feeding babies the wrong foods at the wrong time?

Infection

During childhood there are many infectious illnesses that can affect children's health and development. Some of these infections are controlled by childhood immunisations; these are diphtheria, tetanus, polio, whooping cough, measles, meningitis, mumps and rubella. Other infections can have long-lasting effects on children's health. See Chapter 6.

Poverty and social disadvantage

There is no official definition of poverty, but the two that are often used are:

- Claiming the benefit of income support (usually because of unemployment).
- Having an income of less than 50% of the national average income after housing costs are met.

It is estimated that about 2½ million children live in poverty in the UK today. Poverty is linked with the health of children because of the following:

  - It costs more to provide a nutritionally balanced diet than one which is based on convenience foods that tend to be high in sugar and fats.
  - Low income families tend to live in poorer housing and overcrowded conditions than those who are better off.
  - Parents who are unemployed have a larger incidence of mental health problems, long-term physical illness, disability and higher mortality rates.

All these factors can have a lasting impact on the physical, emotional and social well-being of the child and family. Poverty is closely linked with **social disadvantage**; this means that families who have low incomes are likely to have fewer physical and personal resources to cope with illness and so will be at a disadvantage socially. They are also less likely to attend health clinics and therefore to receive adequate medical care.

The inverse care law

The inverse care law is a term used to describe the fact that the amount of health care available to the individual is in an *inverse* proportion to the level of need.

In other words, the people who have most need of health care are the very people who are least likely to receive it. There are various reasons why this happens:

- The health service is not geared to the individuals' needs: there may be a lack of awareness about the health services available; for example, children from poor families are less likely to attend for routine screening services.
- Parents who have not experienced positive health care themselves are often unaware of its importance for their children.
- People who have had previous bad experiences of professional services may be suspicious of the health professionals who are seen as interfering and authoritarian.
- Those whose first language is not English may find accessing health services difficult.
- Those from cultural backgrounds other than the white middle classes can find that the services offered do not meet their needs: for example, screening for conditions such as sickle cell anaemia, which affects African-Caribbean people.

Housing

Poor housing is another factor which puts people at a social disadvantage. Low-income families are more likely to live in the following conditions:

- Homes which are damp and/or unheated: this increases the risk of infection, particularly respiratory illnesses.
- Neighbourhoods that are unattractive and densely populated, with few communal areas and amenities: children without access to a safe garden or play area may suffer emotional and social problems.
- Overcrowded conditions: homeless families who are housed in 'hotels' or bed and breakfast accommodation often have poor access to cooking facilities and have to share bathrooms with several other families. Often children's education is badly disrupted when families are moved from one place to another.

Homelessness

It is estimated that about 180,000 children become homeless in England each year. Most of them will be living in temporary hostel accommodation or 'bed and breakfast' housing. The vast majority – 90% – of these are single-parent families, with very little financial and family support. Most of these families had become homeless to escape from violence from a male partner or ex-partner, or from neighbours. The experience of homelessness causes many health problems for the children in such families:

- Mental health problems, including delays in social or language development.
- Behavioural problems.
- Disruption of social relationships and difficulty in forming new friendships.
- Experience of marital conflict and domestic violence.

Accidents

Accidents are the most common cause of death in children between the ages of 3 and 14.

- More children are killed or injured in road accidents than in any other sort of accident.
- Three children in the UK are killed in accidents every day.
- 10,000 children are permanently disabled each year as a result of accidents.
- Each year 1 in 4 children attend accident and emergency hospital departments.

Many childhood accidents are preventable. See Chapter 7 on preventing accidents.

Emotional and social factors

A child who is miserable and unhappy is also not healthy, although he or she may appear *physically* healthy. Children need to feel secure and to receive unconditional love from their primary carers. Child abuse, although not common, is bound to affect a child's health and well-being, and can have long-lasting health implications. It is a sad fact that there are, and will always be, children who are victims of abuse in one way or another. The categories of child abuse are:

- **Physical abuse**
- **Emotional abuse**
- **Neglect**
- **Sexual abuse**

Physical abuse

Non-accidental injury (NAI) involves someone deliberately harming a child. This may take the form of:

- **Bruising**: from being slapped, punched, shaken or squeezed.
- **Cuts**: scratches, bite marks, a torn frenulum (the web of skin inside the upper lip).
- **Fractures**: skull and limb fractures from being thrown against hard objects.
- **Burns and scalds**: from cigarettes, irons, baths and kettles.

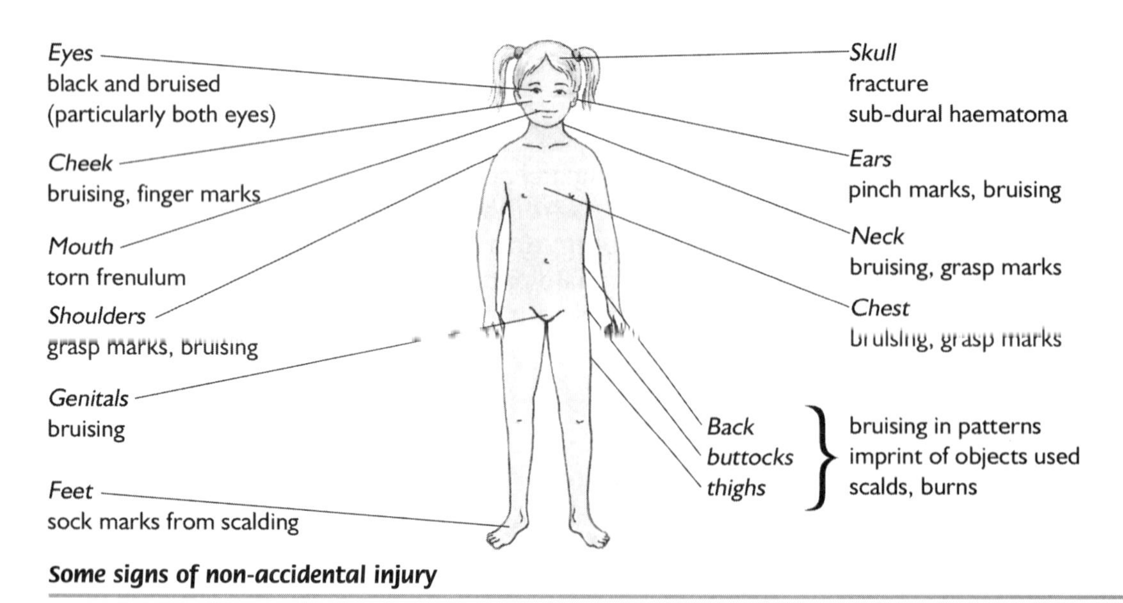

Some signs of non-accidental injury

Often particular injuries can be easily explained, but you should always be suspicious if a child has any bruise or mark which shows the particular pattern of an object, for example a belt strap mark, teeth marks or the imprint of an iron. Also look out for **behavioural** disturbances in the child, such as aggressiveness towards others or a withdrawn attitude.

Emotional abuse

Emotional abuse occurs when a child consistently faces threatening ill-treatment from an adult. This can take the form of **verbal abuse**, for example ridiculing, mocking and insulting the child. It is difficult to find out how common this form of abuse is, because it is hard to detect. Signs of emotional abuse include:

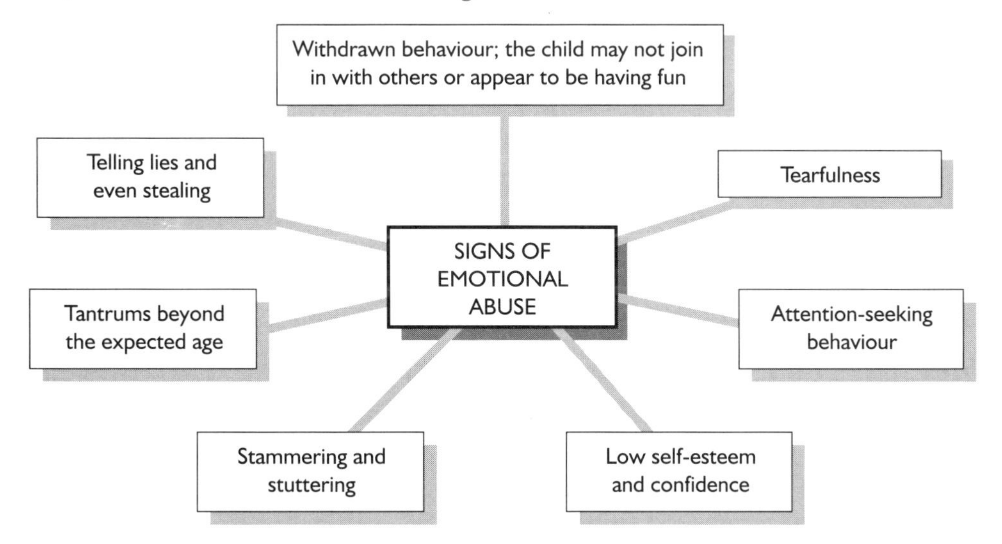

Emotional neglect means that children do not receive love and affection from the adult. They may often be left alone without the company and support of someone who loves them.

Neglect

Physical neglect occurs when the adult fails to give their child what they need to develop physically. They often leave children alone and unattended. Signs of physical neglect include:

- Being underweight for their age and not **thriving**.
- Unwashed clothes which are often dirty and smelly.
- The child may have poor skin tone, dull matted hair and bad breath; a baby may have a persistent rash from infrequent nappy changing.
- Being constantly tired, hungry and listless or lacking in energy.
- Frequent health problems, and prone to accidents.
- Low self-esteem and poor social relationships. Delay in all areas of development is likely because of lack of stimulation.

Sexual abuse

There is much more awareness today about the existence of sexual abuse. Sexual abuse means that an adult uses a child to gratify their sexual needs. This could involve sexual intercourse or anal intercourse. It may involve watching pornographic material with the child. Sexual abuse might also mean children being encouraged in sexually explicit behaviour or oral sex, masturbation or the fondling of sexual parts. Signs of sexual abuse include the following:

- Bruises or scratches as in a non-accidental injury or physical injury
- Wetting or soiling themselves
- Poor self-esteem and lack of confidence
- Poor sleeping and eating patterns
- Itching or pain in the genital area
- Discharge from the penis or vagina
- May regress and want to be treated like a baby
- Withdrawn and solitary behaviour

Your role in reporting suspected abuse

You need to be aware of the indicators of child abuse as outlined above. However, it is important not to jump to conclusions. If you have any cause for concern, you should always talk to your immediate superior or to the head of the nursery or school. Every child care setting has a policy for dealing with suspected child abuse.

If you suspect child abuse in the *home setting*, then you should contact your local social services or the NSPCC (The National Society for the Protection of Children).

If a child tells you that they have been abused

If a child tells you that they have been abused, you should:

- reassure the child, saying that you are glad that they have told you about this
- always *believe* the child; tell the child that you will do your best to protect them, but don't *promise* that you can do that, because you may not be able to
- remember that the child is not to blame; it is important that you make the child understand this
- do a lot of listening; don't ask a lot of questions
- report your conversation with the child to your immediate superior
- write down what was said by the child as soon as possible after the conversation.

Environmental factors

Pollution of the environment can have a marked effect on children's health and development. The three main threats to health are water pollution, air pollution and noise pollution:

1 Water pollution

We all need clean, non-polluted water to prevent the spread of infectious diseases and poisoning. Many harmful germs are carried in water, including cholera, typhoid and the polio virus. In developing countries, over 4 million children die each year from drinking unclean water, mainly because it is contaminated with harmful organisms. Toxic chemicals in industrial, agricultural and domestic waste are common pollutants of water. In the UK water is purified before we use it, but although the treatment can remove bacterial contamination, it cannot cope with heavy chemical pollution. Examples of chemical pollutants in water which can affect children include:

- **Lead**: lead is taken into our bodies via air, food and water. It concentrates in the liver, kidney and bones and can cause mental retardation.
- **Nitrates**: these enter water from fertilisers which are leached out of the soil; too much nitrate in drinking water has been found to cause a serious blood disorder in babies under three months, called blue-baby syndrome.

2 Air pollution

Children are particularly vulnerable to air pollution. This is partly because they have a large lung surface area in relation to their small body size; this means that they absorb toxic substances quicker than adults do and are slower to get rid of them. The effects of air pollution from factory chimneys, the use of chemical insecticides and car exhausts include:

- **Lead poisoning**. Children are particularly susceptible to lead poisoning, mostly caused by vehicle exhaust fumes. Even very low levels of lead in the blood can affect children's ability to learn and higher levels are associated with damage to the kidneys, liver and reproductive system.
- **Asthma**. Air pollution can act as a trigger for asthma and can make an existing condition worse. The incidence of asthma is much higher in traffic-polluted areas.
- **Cancer**. The use of insecticides and fertilisers by farmers has been linked with various childhood cancers. Radioactivity from nuclear power stations has also been found to cause cancer.

3 Noise pollution

Noise pollution can also be a hazard to child health. There is much evidence for higher levels of noise, mostly caused by heavy traffic, being responsible for medical and social problems. For example, it has been found that children living on noisy main roads had far fewer friends than those in quiet suburbs, and that traffic noise adversely affects children's progress at school.

Lifestyle factors

1 Smoking

Children who live in a smoky atmosphere are more likely to develop:

- coughs and colds
- chest infections (temperature with a bad cough)
- asthma
- ear infections and glue ear.

Every year 17,000 children are admitted to hospital with respiratory infections; research has found that many of these children are exposed daily to cigarette smoke. There is also an increased risk of children taking up the smoking habit themselves if one or both of their parents smoke.

2 Exercise

There are many enjoyable activities for children which do not involve taking physical exercise – watching TV, playing computer games, etc. Some children take no regular physical exercise apart from at school, and this is often because of the family's attitude and habits. Taking regular exercise allows children to develop their motor skills and to 'run off' any pent-up feelings of frustration and aggression. Coronary heart disease is the greatest single risk to health in the UK.

Generally, these are the risks of not taking enough exercise:

- Adults who are physically inactive have about double the chance of suffering from coronary heart disease.
- Children who do not take much exercise tend to become inactive adults.
- Obesity is more common in children who take little exercise.

CASE STUDY

Patrick's story

Patrick is three and a half years old and has already lived in five different homes. His mother, Maggie, also has a 10-month-old baby called Holly. The problems all started when Patrick's father started beating Maggie up on a regular basis just after Patrick was born. Maggie went to a women's refuge for a while but then met an old boyfriend, Peter, who had just come out of prison and they rented a small flat together. Money was always tight and Peter ended up in prison once more after being caught breaking into a neighbour's house. Now Maggie, Patrick and Holly were officially homeless as they couldn't afford to pay the rent any more. The social services have provided temporary bed and breakfast accommodation, but they have had to move from one hostel to another. Maggie has very few friends and is becoming increasingly depressed about the future and the effect her living conditions are having on Patrick and Holly. Patrick used to attend a day nursery close to home, but after the last move, they were unable to get there on public transport and Maggie is trying to find a local nursery with spare places for both children so that she can get some sort of job. Patrick has become withdrawn and has started to wet the bed every night. He has started to hit out at Maggie, and once even bit his little sister Holly when his mother was busy cooking. Maggie rarely sees her parents as they have retired and moved to the coast. She feels completely alone and overwhelmed by her situation.

Questions

1. List the problems which each family member has.
2. How is the health of each family member likely to be affected by their circumstances?
3. How would you support Maggie and the children if they were to come to your day nursery?
4. What organisations and support services could help Maggie and her family?

Revision questions

1. List the factors affecting the health of the unborn child during pregnancy.
2. List two effects of severe malnutrition on the unborn child during pregnancy.
3. What problems might occur when a baby is born prematurely – e.g. several weeks before the expected date of delivery?
4. What is the inverse care law? Give three possible reasons for its occurrence.
5. List six health problems which may result from poverty and inadequate housing.

Chapter 3: Keeping children healthy

◆ *How children's bodies work: Hormones – Skin – Blood and circulation – Skeletal system – Digestive system – Respiratory system – Eye – Ear – Urinary system – Brain and nervous system* ◆ *Maintaining health in childhood: Hygiene – Nutrition – Exercise – Rest and sleep – Preventing infection – Immunisation – Providing a safe, hygienic environment*

How children's bodies work

Anyone looking after children should have a basic understanding of how children's bodies work. The following sections of this chapter describe the different body systems and provide the underpinning knowledge for a sound understanding of child health and of what can go wrong.

How hormones work

Hormones are made in a set of glands called the **endocrine glands**. Endocrine glands:

- ◆ release tiny amounts of hormones into the blood
- ◆ are carried by the blood all over the body, but only certain parts called **target organs** respond to them
- ◆ produce responses that may last a few minutes, e.g. the response to adrenaline, or continue for years, e.g. thyroxine.

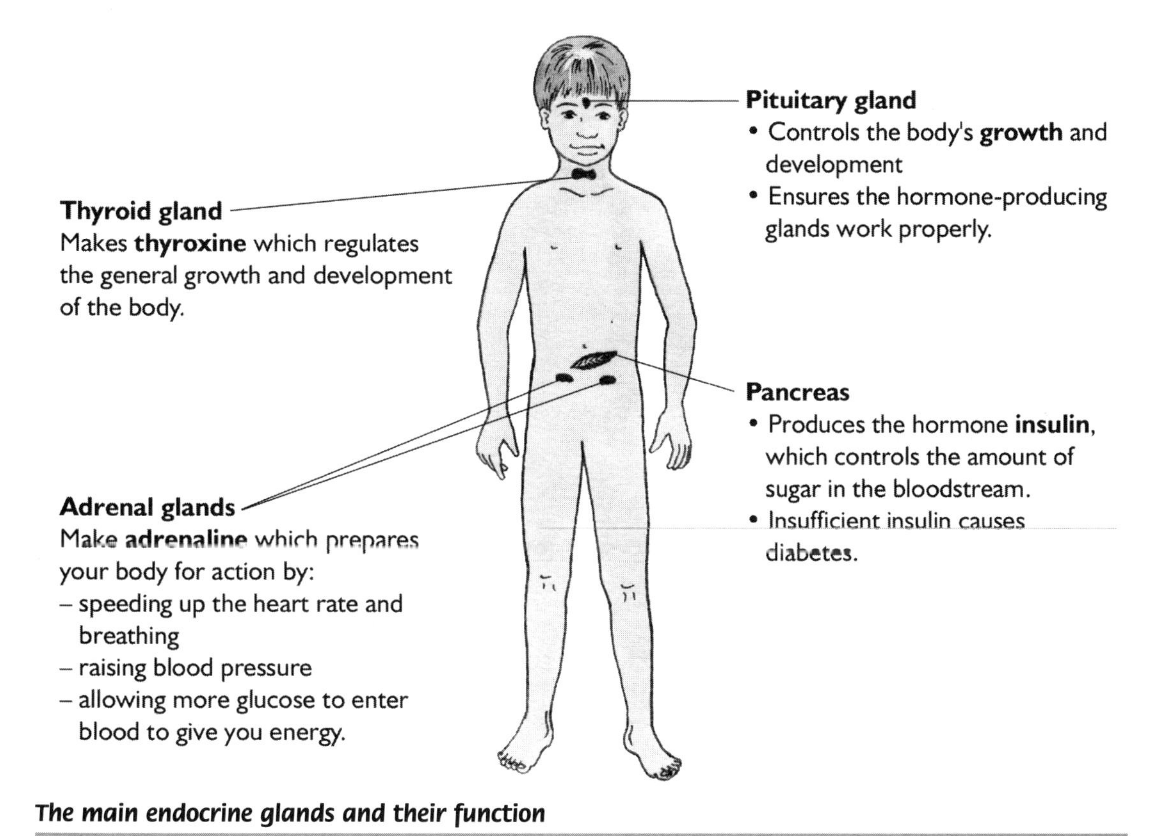

The main endocrine glands and their function

products and is important in fighting infection and in controlling bleeding. Blood consists of 60 per cent plasma (fluid) and 40 per cent blood cells. The three most important types of cells are:

- **Red blood cells**
- **White blood cells**
- **Platelets**.

Although we think of blood as a fluid, it is actually made up of both fluid and cells. These can be seen under a microscope.

Bone marrow is the 'blood cell factory' and is found filling up the cavities of bones. All blood cells originate and are produced from a single 'stem cell'.

- **Red blood cells** are made in the bone marrow of the body's long bones, e.g. the femur. They contain the pigment **haemoglobin**, which gives them their colour and carries oxygen from your lungs to all parts of your body. If you don't have enough red blood cells you have **anaemia**. Anaemia can make you look pale and may make you feel tired, dizzy, irritable and short of breath. Red blood cells also pick up wastes on their way around the body, carrying them to the lungs to be breathed out as carbon dioxide.
- **White blood cells** are made in the lymph nodes (glands), spleen, bone marrow and thymus. They are the body's infection fighters. Their job is to rid your body of disease-causing bacteria, viruses, fungi and to destroy the body's dead or defective cells. If we do not have enough white blood cells we are at risk of catching all types of infections.
- **Platelets** are small cells that prevent bleeding and makes blood clot following an injury. When a blood vessel is damaged or cut, platelets rush to the area and clump together to plug the bleeding site. If we do not have enough platelets, easy bruising, nose bleeds, prolonged bleeding from cuts, or internal bleeding from the bowel or bladder may occur.

When the body is healthy, the numbers of red cells, white cells and platelets in the blood are kept in balance.

How blood circulates around the body

The tubes that carry blood are called blood vessels. There are three types of blood vessel:

- **Arteries**: Arteries have thick muscular walls that contain elastic fibres. The blood pumps into the artery very fast, at high pressure, so the elastic fibres stretch. Then they contract, and that squeezes the blood towards the capillaries.
- **Veins**: Veins are wider than arteries and have thinner, non-muscular walls. The blood flows through them more slowly, and they contain valves which stop the blood from flowing backwards.
- **Capillaries**: Capillaries are the smallest blood vessels; their walls are so thin that liquid from blood can pass through them. This liquid takes food and oxygen to the cells of the body. It also takes away carbon dioxide and other wastes.

The **heart** and blood vessels together make up the **circulatory system**, which has two parts:

1 **The right side of the heart pumps blood to the lungs and back again**. In the lungs it loses carbon dioxide and picks up oxygen. This oxygenated blood is bright red in colour. It is circulated under considerable pressure and the main arteries pulsate due to the pumping of the heart. Small arteries are called **arterioles** and these then pass this bright red oxygenated blood into the delicate **capillaries** where the pressure is quite low and where it can release its oxygen.

2 **The left side of the heart pumps blood to the rest of the body and back**. On its way around the body the blood loses oxygen to the body cells and picks up carbon dioxide. The blood collects in small veins, once it has lost its oxygen. **Veins** have thinner walls than arteries and valves that ensure that one-way flow. Exercise helps blood return in veins. On release of oxygen the blood has gained back in exchange much carbon dioxide gas that it carries in dissolved form. The dark red de-oxygenated blood is then pumped back to the lungs by the right side of the heart under much lower pressure. Further gas exchange takes place at the lungs.

ACTIVITY

Select the correct multiple choice response:

1 Which part of the blood carries oxygen to the body cells?
- **a** Plasma
- **b** Platelets
- **c** Red blood cells.

2 What is the function of white blood cells?
- **a** Clotting
- **b** Fighting and preventing infection
- **c** Carrying waste.

3 How is carbon dioxide returned to the lungs? It is transported by the:
- **a** Red blood cells
- **b** White blood cells
- **c** Platelets.

4 The sequence of vessels through which blood leaves and returns to the heart is:
- **a** Veins – venules – capillaries – arterioles – arteries
- **b** Arteries – arterioles – capillaries – venules – veins
- **c** Veins – arterioles – capillaries – venules – arteries.

5 Red blood cells are made in:
- **a** The liver
- **b** The bone marrow of long bones
- **c** The heart.

6 The beating of the heart causes pressure pulsation in:
- **a** The arteries
- **b** The veins
- **c** The capillaries.

Note: For answers see page 72.

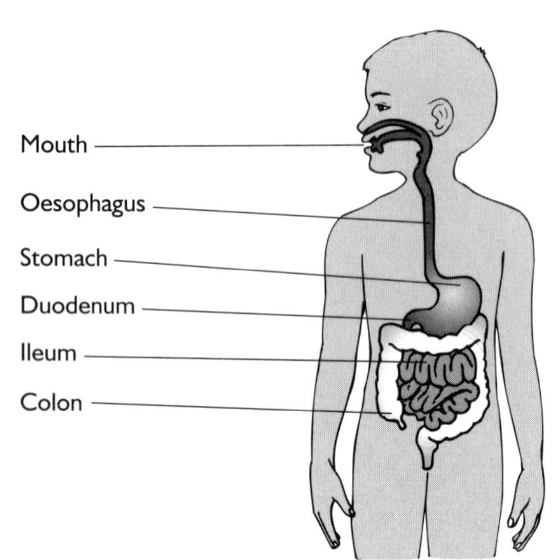

The digestive system

- maintain the proper functioning of body systems
- provide warmth and energy.

Food contains substances that cannot be absorbed into our blood until they have been digested. This means that they are converted into small soluble chemicals. In the case of minerals and vitamins this is not necessary, as they are already small molecules.

Component	Use in the body	Typical food source
Carbohydrates	provide energy	bread, potatoes
Fats	store energy, insulate	butter, oil
Fibre	provide roughage	vegetables, bran
Minerals	maintain cells	spinach, milk, salt
Proteins	growth and repair	meat, fish, cheese
Vitamins	maintain cell processes	dairy foods, fruit, vegetables
Water	cell and body fluids	fruit juice, milk, vegetables

The digestion process involves **four** linked stages

1. **Ingestion**: Food is taken into the body and physically broken down.
2. **Digestion**: The particles of food are surrounded by digestive juices. This is the true **digestion** stage. The fibre or roughage in our diet is not digested. Fibre is important because it allows the muscles in our intestines to move the material by muscle waves called **peristalsis**.
3. **Absorption**: The enzymes (biological protein catalysts) speed up the chemical changes in the food. They speed up the breakdown of large molecules so they can be absorbed as smaller soluble units through the intestinal wall and carried by the bloodstream to be used in the cells of the body.

4 **Egestion**: Water is taken back (re-absorbed) and then all undigested solid matter is pushed out as faeces (solid waste).

Most digested food passes into the blood plasma via the small finger-like projections rich in blood capillaries that greatly increase the surface of the **small intestine**. The projections are called **villi**. The absorbed food passes via the bloodstream to the **liver**, where it is either stored or transported further to the rest of the body.

During this process of digestion the following takes place:

- Carbohydrate is broken down to glucose.
- Protein is broken down to amino acids.
- Fats and oils are emulsified by bile salts and then broken down to fatty acids and glycerol.

A balanced diet

There is a relationship between our food intake and the energy we use up. The amount of food needed depends on age, body mass and energy requirements. The energy value of foods is measured in calories or **kilojoules (kJ)**.

A small one-year-old baby needs 3,850 kJ daily to maintain body mass and continue to grow, whereas an adult Olympic swimmer in training needs 15,600 kJ daily. When the amount of food eaten equals the amount of food needed for energy, growth and repair, the diet is described as **balanced**. An unbalanced diet with over-eating and lack of exercise can lead to **obesity**.

ACTIVITY

Look at the data in the table on different types of milk and answer the following questions.

	Human breast milk	**Cows' milk (Whole)**	**Cows' milk (Skimmed)**
Energy (kJ/100g)	295	276	146
Protein (%)	1.3	3.3	3.4
Fat (%)	4.1	3.8	0.1
Carbohydrate (%)	7.2	4.7	5.0
Minerals (%)	0.2	0.6	0.5
Water (%)	87.1	87.6	90.9

1 Which milk has the greatest energy value and why?

2 Cows' milk has high levels of two food types compared to human breast milk and so should **not** be given to babies under six months as it may cause kidney failure. What are these food types?

3 Why is skimmed milk recommended for low-cholesterol diets where humans are at risk from heart disease?

For answers see page 72.

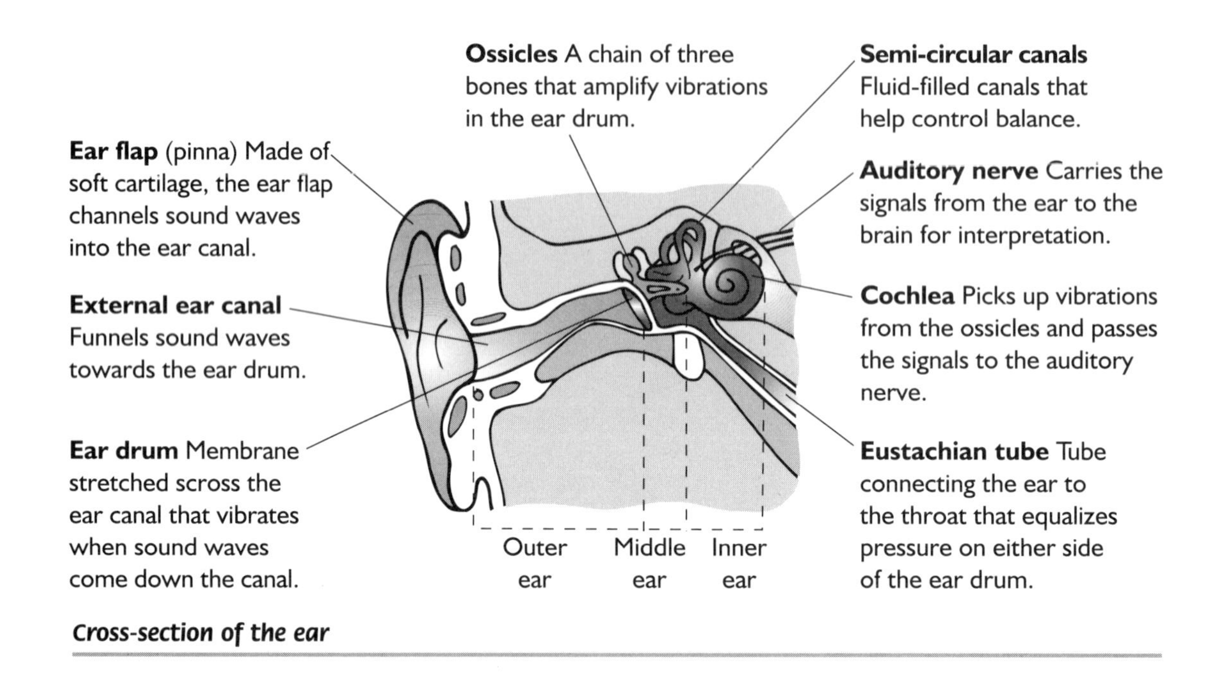

Cross-section of the ear

The outer ear is connected by a short passage, called the canal, to the eardrum and middle ear, which in turn leads to the inner ear. The middle ear is filled with air and the inner ear is filled with fluid. A tube called the **Eustachian tube** leads from the middle ear to the back of the throat.

How does the middle ear function?

The middle ear is a pea-sized, air-filled cavity separated from the outer ear by the paper-thin eardrum. Attached to the eardrum are three tiny ear bones or **ossicles** (see diagram). When sound waves strike the eardrum, it vibrates and sets the bones into a motion that is transmitted to the inner ear, which generates nerve impulses that are sent to the brain.

A healthy middle ear must contain air at the same atmospheric pressure as the outside of the ear, so all these structures can vibrate freely. Air enters the middle ear through the narrow Eustachian tube, which passes from the back of the nose up into the ear. When you yawn or swallow and hear a pop (or click) in your ear, that means your Eustachian tube has just sent a tiny little bubble of air up into your middle ear to equalise the air pressure. (This happens automatically over 1000 times a day.)

How does the urinary system work?

The organs, tubes, muscles, and nerves that work together to create, store, and carry urine are the **urinary system**. The urinary system includes:

- two kidneys
- two ureters
- the bladder
- two sphincter muscles
- the urethra.

How the urinary system works

- **The kidneys**: The kidneys are paired bean-shaped organs lying at the back of the abdomen. They filter and remove waste and water from the blood to produce **urine**. They get rid of about 134 litres of urine per day in an adult and less in a child, depending on the child's age. The amount depends on many factors, the major ones being the amount of fluid and foods a person consumes and how much fluid is lost through sweat and breathing.
- **The ureters**: The urine travels from the kidneys down two narrow tubes called the ureters.
- **The bladder**: The urine is then stored in a muscular balloon-like container called the bladder; in a child, the bladder can hold about 30–45 millilitres of urine for each year of the child's age. So, the bladder of a 4-year-old child may hold about 120 to 180 mls (less than 1 cup); an 8-year-old can hold 240 to 360 mls.
- **The sphincter muscles**: Circular muscles called **sphincters** help keep urine from leaking. The sphincter muscles close tightly like a rubber band around the opening of the bladder into the **urethra**, the tube that allows urine to pass outside the body.
- **The urethra**: When the bladder empties, urine flows out of the body through the urethra, a tube at the bottom of the bladder. The opening of the urethra is at the end of the penis in boys and in front of the vagina in girls (see below).

Your body takes **nutrients** from food and uses them to maintain all bodily functions, including energy and self-repair. After your body has taken what it needs from the food, **waste products** are left behind in the blood and in the bowel. The urinary system works with the lungs, skin, and intestines – all of which also excrete waste products – to keep the chemicals and water in your body balanced.

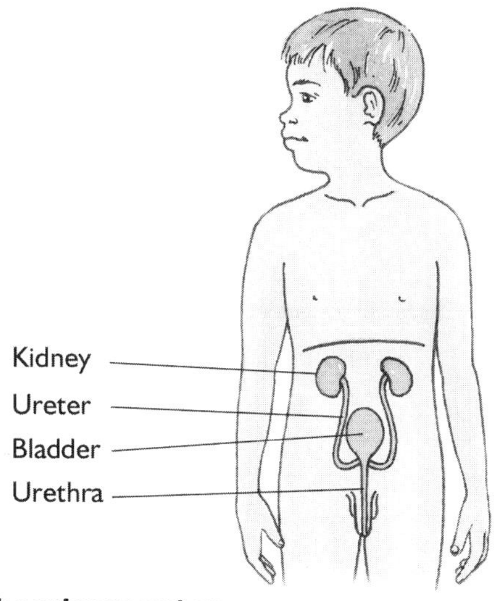

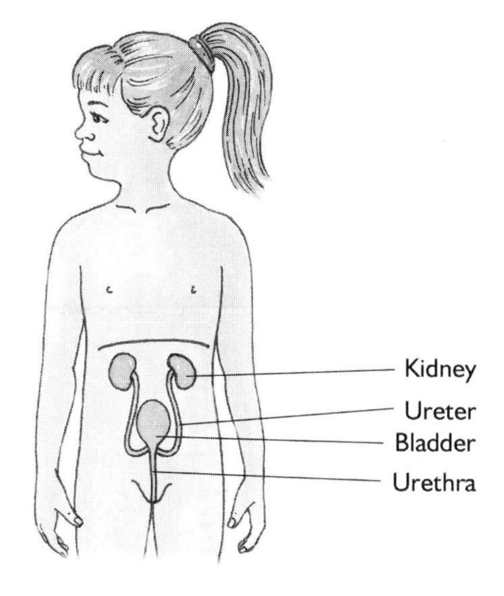

The urinary system

◆ The pupils in your eye get smaller in bright light to protect the retina, and larger in dim light to help you to see.

Voluntary actions

Voluntary actions are actions which need thought, such as speaking to a friend or writing a letter.

ACTIVITY

Which part of the brain:

a helps you balance while cycling?

b gives you the sensation of touch?

c controls the involuntary functions of your body, such as heartbeat and breathing rate?

d controls your speech?

e controls your emotions?

NOTE: For answers see page 72.

Maintaining health in childhood

◆ *Hygiene* ◆ *Nutrition* ◆ *Exercise* ◆ *Rest and sleep* ◆ *Preventing infection* ◆ *Immunisation* ◆ *Providing a safe, hygienic environment*

Hygiene

A good standard of hygiene is important because:

◆ it helps to prevent infection and the spread of disease

◆ being clean increases self-esteem and social acceptance

◆ it helps to prepare children in skills of independence and self-caring.

All children need adult help and supervision to keep their skin, hair and teeth clean. A balance has to be struck where a child is allowed to get dirty when playing, but knows that a bath will be needed at the end of the day.

Care of the skin and hair

As children grow and become involved in more vigorous exercise, especially outside, a daily bath or shower becomes necessary. Most young children love bath-time and adding bubble bath to the water adds to the fun of getting clean.

Remember: Children should never be left alone in the bath or shower, because of the risk of drowning and scalding.

Establishing hygiene routines

All children benefit from regular routines in daily care. You need to encourage children to become independent by helping them to learn how to take care of themselves. You can help children to become independent in these ways:

◆ Teach children how to wash and dry their hands before eating or drinking.

General guidelines for looking after children's skin and hair

- ☐ Wash face and hands in the morning (**NOTE:** Muslims always wash under running water).
- ☐ Always wash hands after using the toilet and before meals; dry hands thoroughly – young children will need supervision.
- ☐ After using the toilet, girls should be taught to wipe their bottom from front to back to prevent germs from the anus entering the vagina and urethra.
- ☐ Wash hands after playing outside or after handling animals.
- ☐ Nails should be scrubbed with a soft nailbrush and trimmed regularly by cutting straight across; never cut into the sides of the nails as this can cause sores and infections.
- ☐ Find out about any special skin conditions, such as eczema or dry skin, and be guided by the parents' advice concerning the use of soap and creams.
- ☐ Hair usually only needs washing twice a week; children with long or curly hair benefit from the use of a conditioning shampoo which helps to reduce tangles. Hair should always be rinsed thoroughly in clean water and not brushed until it is dry – brushing wet hair damages the hair shafts. A wide-toothed comb is useful for combing wet hair.
- ☐ Afro-Caribbean hair tends to dryness and may need special oil or moisturisers; if the hair is braided (with or without beads), it may be washed with the braids left intact, unless otherwise advised.
- ☐ Rastafarian children with hair styled in dreadlocks may not use either combs or shampoo, preferring to brush the dreadlocks gently and secure them with braid.
- ☐ Children should have their own flannel, comb and brush which should be cleaned regularly.
- ☐ Skin should always be dried thoroughly, taking special care of such areas as between the toes and under the armpits; black skin tends to dryness and may need massaging with special oils or moisturisers.
- ☐ Children do not need deodorants or anti-perspirants, although these are now marketed as essential products.

- ◆ Make sure that children *always* wash and dry their hands after going to the toilet and after playing outdoors.
- ◆ Provide children with their own combs and brushes and encourage them to use them every day.
- ◆ Provide a soft toothbrush and teach children how and when to brush their teeth.
- ◆ Ensure that you are **good role models** for children; for example, when you cough or sneeze, you always cover your mouth.
- ◆ Devise activities which develop an awareness in children of the importance of hygiene routines; for example, you could invite a dental hygienist or dental nurse to the nursery to talk to children about daily teeth care.

Toilet training

There is no point in attempting to start toilet training until the toddler shows that they are ready, and this rarely occurs before the age of 18 months. Before attempting to toilet train a child, make sure they have shown that they are *ready* to be trained, and remember that there is, as with all other developmental milestones, a wide variation in the age range at which children achieve bowel and bladder control.

The signs that a child is ready to start toilet training are when they:

- show increased interest when passing urine or a motion; or start to play with toys and teddies on the potty
- tell you just after passing urine or a bowel motion or look very uncomfortable
- begin to be more regular with bowel motions, or the wet nappies may become rarer.

Toilet training can be over in a few days or may take some months. Becoming dry at night takes longer, but most children manage this before the age of five.

Guidelines for toilet training

- Be relaxed about toilet training and be prepared for accidents.
- Have the potty in the home so that the child becomes familiar with it and can include it in their play.
- Some children feel insecure when sitting on a potty with no nappy on – try it first with nappy or pants if this is the case.
- It is easier to attempt toilet training in fine weather when the child can run around without nappies or pants on.
- It helps if the child sees other children using the toilet or potty.
- If you start training when there is a new baby expected, be prepared for some accidents as many children like to remain babies themselves.
- Don't show any disgust for the child's faeces. Children have no natural shame about their bodily functions (unless adults make them ashamed). Children will regard using the potty as an achievement and will be proud of their results.
- Training pants, similar to ordinary pants but with a waterproof covering, are useful in the early stages of training – and having more than one potty in the house makes life easier.
- Always praise children when they succeed and do not show anger or disapproval if they don't – they may be upset by any accident.
- Offer the potty regularly so that the child becomes used to the idea of a routine, and get used to the signs that a child needs to use it.
- Always liaise with the child's parents about how they would like their child to be toilet trained.
- The child may prefer to try the 'big' toilet seat straight away; a toddler seat fixed onto the normal seat makes this easier.
- Encourage good hygiene right from the start, washing the child's hands after every visit to the potty.

Nutrition

Feeding babies

The way babies and children are fed is much more than simply providing enough food to meet nutritional requirements; for the new-born baby, sucking milk is a great source of pleasure and is also rewarding and enjoyable for the mother. The ideal food for babies to start life with is breast milk and breastfeeding should always be encouraged as the first choice in infant feeding. However mothers should not be made to feel guilty or inadequate if they choose not to breastfeed their babies.

Weaning

Weaning is the gradual introduction of solid food to the baby's diet of milk alone (see Table 3.1). The reasons for weaning are:

- to meet the baby's nutritional needs – from about six months of age, milk alone will not satisfy the baby's increased nutritional requirements, especially for iron
- to develop the chewing mechanism; the muscular movement of the mouth and jaw also aids the development of speech
- to satisfy increasing appetite
- to introduce new tastes and textures; this enables the baby to join in family meals, and so promotes cognitive and social development
- to develop new skills – use of feeding beaker, cup and cutlery.

Planning a healthy diet for children

A healthy balance of foods provides the energy and nourishment everyone needs to survive and to enjoy life. Eating too little food soon leads to illness, but eating too much or the wrong balance of foods can lead to problems in the long term. So it's important to get the balance right – both in the amount and in the type of foods eaten. A healthy and balanced diet in childhood can reduce the risk of anaemia and dental decay.

Table 3.2 on page 55 shows the types and proportions of foods needed for a well-balanced and healthy diet.

How much food should children be given?

Children's appetites vary enormously, so common sense is a good guide on how big a portion should be. Always be guided by the individual child and remember:

- don't force them to eat when they no longer wish to, but
- don't refuse to give more if they really are hungry.

Some children always feel hungry at one particular mealtime. Others require little food but often. You should always offer a child food that is nourishing as well as satisfying their hunger.

Meals and snacks

Some children really *do* need to eat between meals. Their stomachs are relatively small and so they fill up and empty faster than adult stomachs. Sugary foods should *not* be given as a snack, because sugar is an appetite depressant and may spoil the child's appetite for the main meal to follow. Healthy snack foods include:

The main vitamins and minerals needed			
Substance	**Where you find it**	**Why you need it**	**Lack of it can cause**
Vitamin C	Oranges, lemons, grapefruit, tangerines, green vegetables, potatoes	For healthy skin and gums To heal wounds quickly	**Scurvy**: gums and nose bleed and the body bleeds inside
Vitamin D	Milk, butter, eggs, fish, liver (also made by the skin in sunshine)	For strong bones and teeth	**Rickets**: the bones become soft and bend
Calcium	Milk, eggs, nuts, fish with edible bones	For strong bones and teeth	**Rickets**
Iron	Liver, lean red meat, wholemeal bread, dried fruit, spinach	For making red blood cells	**Anaemia**: the child is pale and lacks energy

Providing drinks for children

You need to offer children drinks several times during the day. The best drinks for young children are water and milk:

- Water is a very underrated drink for the whole family as it quenches thirst without spoiling the appetite; if bottled water is used it should be still, not carbonated (fizzy), which is acidic. More water should be given in hot weather in order to prevent dehydration.
- Milk is an excellent nourishing drink. Reduced-fat milks should not normally be given to children under the age of five because of their lower energy and fat-soluble content; however, semi-skimmed milk may be offered from two years of age, provided that the child's overall diet is adequate.

Other drinks

All drinks that contain sugar can be harmful to teeth and can also take the edge off children's appetites. Examples are:

- flavoured milks
- fruit squashes
- flavoured fizzy drinks
- fruit juices (containing natural sugar)

Unsweetened diluted fruit juice is the best drink – other than water or milk – for children, however ideally it should only be offered at mealtimes. The low-sugar or diet fruit drinks contain artificial sweeteners and are best avoided.

Tea and coffee should not be given to children under five, as they prevent the absorption of iron from foods. They also fill children easily without providing nourishment.

The importance of a good breakfast

Breakfast is an important meal. Breakfast sets the pattern for eating for the rest of the day. If children miss that first important meal to save time, then they are more likely to crave junk food and to overeat during the rest of the day.

Recent research has proved that children who eat a nutritious breakfast are:

- ✓ better behaved
- ✓ pay closer attention
- ✓ participate more in class discussions
- ✓ can manage more complex academic problems
- ✓ generally do better at schoolwork than children who miss out on a good breakfast.

What is a good breakfast?
A nutritious breakfast should be a balance of complex carbohydrates and proteins. A breakfast composed primarily of only one or the other will not provide the correct balance. The reasons are that carbohydrates have a sedative effect upon the brain, and proteins have a stimulating effect. But when they are combined, they help to release the amino acids from the proteins into the brain and this helps to further the learning processes. Some examples of a good breakfast may be:

- Whole wheat cereal, yoghurt and sliced apple
- Scrambled eggs, toast and orange juice
- Plain omelette, brown toast and fruit with yoghurt
- French toast topped with fruit and a glass of orange juice.

Establishing healthy eating habits

Some children can be choosy about the food they eat, and this can be a source of anxiety for parents and for those who work with children. However, as long as children eat some food from each of the five food groups – even if they are the same old favourites – there is no cause for worry.

Guidelines for making mealtimes healthy and fun

- ☐ **Set an example**. Children imitate both what you eat and how you eat it. Sit down to eat alongside the children. Try not to rush mealtimes: be relaxed, patient and friendly.
- ☐ **Be prepared for messy mealtimes**! Present the food in a form that is fairly easy for children to manage by themselves (e.g. not difficult to chew).
- ☐ **Be imaginative with presentation**, e.g. cut slices of pizza into interesting shapes. Use ideas from children's food manufacturers. (See also colour section after page 60.)
- ☐ **Encourage children to feed themselves**, either with a spoon or by offering suitable finger foods.
- ☐ **Respect individual preferences**. Some families prefer to eat with their fingers, while others use chopsticks or cutlery. Whatever tool is preferred, be patient as children need time to get used to them. If a child prefers drink to food, cut down on the amount of drinks you give just before mealtimes.

▶

Exercise

Children need opportunities for physical activity or exercise. Exercise is important because it keeps children's bodies – and minds – healthy. Regular exercise reduces the risk of children developing heart disease in later life. Physical activity is essential for children because it:

- ✓ **Makes the heart strong**. The heart needs **aerobic exercise** to keep bringing fresh oxygen to *all* the muscles in the body. Children need to do some kind of aerobic exercise two or three times a week, for 20 to 30 minutes at a time. Examples of aerobic activities: swimming, basketball, running, jogging (or walking quickly), inline skating, soccer, cycling, dancing, skipping, and playing hopscotch.
- ✓ **Develops the muscles**. Exercise makes the muscles stronger and sometimes larger. As the muscles become stronger, children can do more active things for longer periods of time. Children can strengthen their arm muscles by using climbing equipment and by playing tug-of-war games. For strong leg muscles, they can run, ride a bike or try inline skating.

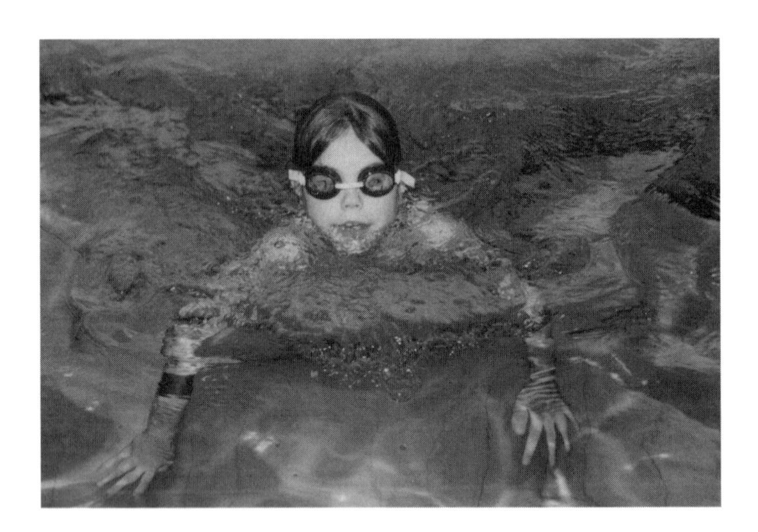

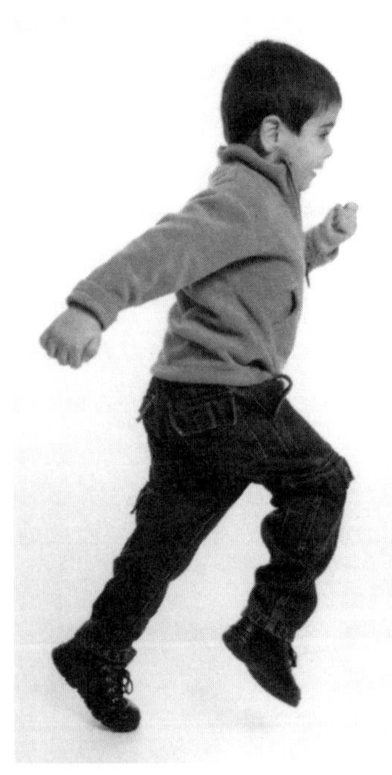

- ✓ **Makes children more flexible**. Most children are very flexible, which means that they can bend and stretch their bodies without too much trouble. Dancing, yoga, gymnastics and martial arts (such as karate and tae-kwon-do) are very good ways to become more flexible.
- ✓ **Keeps children at a healthy weight**. Every time you eat food, your body does the same thing and uses some of the nutrients in the food as fuel. It burns these nutrients to give us energy or **calories**. However, if the body is unable to *use* all the calories that are coming from food, it stores them away as fat. Exercise helps to keep a child at the right weight for their height, by burning up *extra* calories.

✓ **Makes children feel good**. Exercising is a very good way to feel happy, because when you exercise your body can release **endorphins**, which are chemicals that create a happy feeling in your brain. Also, when you are breathing deeply during exercise and bringing more air into your lungs, your brain is receiving extra oxygen.

✓ **Helps children to develop self-esteem and independence**. Exercise can make children feel better about themselves; when they have mastered a certain skill, such as climbing a rope ladder or swimming, they feel a sense of achievement and independence.

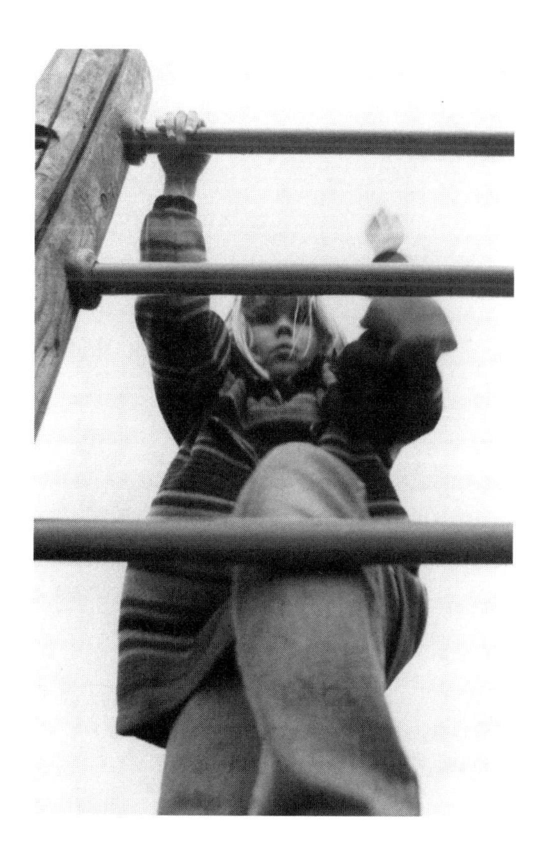

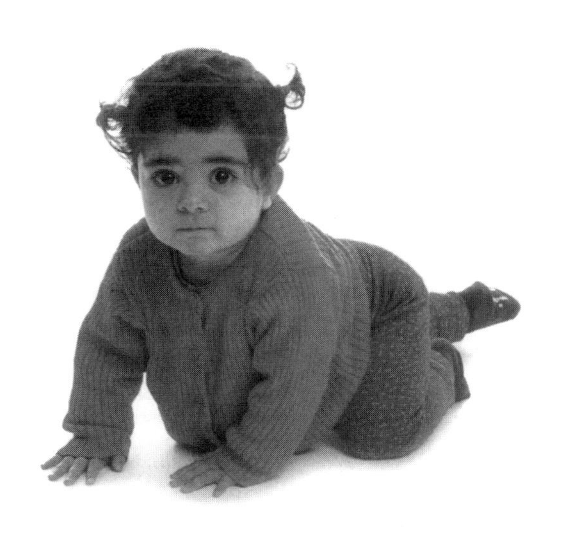

✓ **Helps to promote sleep**. Children need to relax after physical activity; this does not necessarily mean that they will need to sleep more, but they will need to *rest* after exercise.

✓ **Promotes social skills and mutual understanding**. Children learn to share when using play equipment and to take turns. They also learn how to play and work together in team games and in co-operative play, e.g. pulling each other along in a cart.

Viruses

Many viruses invade the body by crossing the moist mucus membranes that line the breathing passages, eyes, intestines, or reproductive tracts. They can spread in the following ways:

- in an infected person's body fluids
- or in the airborne droplets of coughs and sneezes.

Once inside the body, viruses can spread from one area to another through the blood vessels and arteries, the fluid-filled channels between tissues, and even along the length of nerve cells. Once they invade and cause illness, some forms of viruses can be totally defeated by the **immune system**. Others can lie dormant in our cells and cause more than one episode of illness, even years after infection, for example the chickenpox virus and herpes simplex virus. Once a child has been infected with a viral illness, they are usually immune for life. In the case of colds, however, there are so many different cold viruses that they cannot build up an immunity to all of them.

Fungi

There are only a few fungi which cause harm to humans. Fungi are spread by:

- airborne spores
- contact with an infected person
- walking barefoot on infected floor areas.

Because fungi prefer warm, damp areas, they love to grow on moist parts of our bodies; athlete's foot, ringworm and thrush are three common fungal infections. Since our breathing passages are moist, some forms of fungi can invade them as well.

Persons whose immune systems are weakened by cancer, AIDS, or certain medicines have an increased risk for serious fungal infections. In these persons, a fungus can spread throughout the body, even to the brain, and be deadly.

Parasites

Parasites are organisms which live in or on any other living creature. They obtain their food from the host's blood or tissues and then can multiply. Parasites may remain permanently with their host or may spend only part of their life-cycles in association. The main parasites that commonly affect children are **fleas**, **head lice**, **scabies mites**, and **threadworms**. For further information see the sections on skin disorders and digestive conditions in Part 2, Chapter 6.

How infection is spread

Infection enters the body in several ways:

- **Droplet infection**. This occurs by breathing in air containing tiny droplets of infected mucus from an infected person's sneeze or cough. Colds, flu, pneumonia and whooping cough are spread by coughs and sneezes.
- **By touching infected people**. Germs can be spread by touching someone who is infected or the things they have used, e.g. towels, combs and cups. Chickenpox and measles can be caught by touching infected people, and athlete's foot can be caught by walking on wet floors or mats used by infected people.
- **Through infected food or drink**. Food and drink can be infected with germs by coughs and sneezes, dirty hands, flies, mice and pet animals. Infected food and drink cause food poisoning and dysentery.

Healthy meals for children

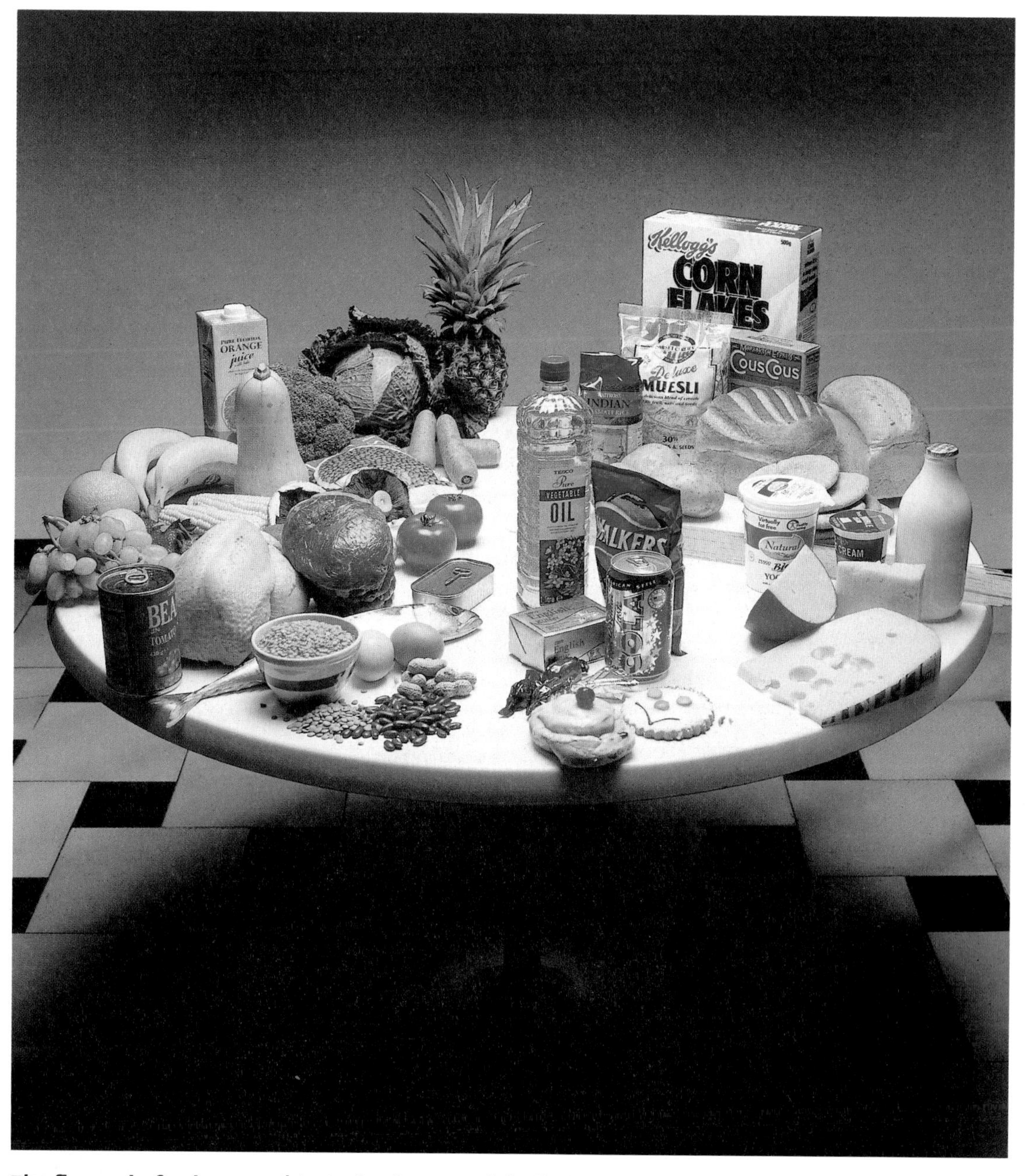

The five main food groups (clockwise from top left: fruit and vegetables; bread, other cereals and potatoes; milk and dairy foods; fatty and sugary foods; meat, fish and alternatives)

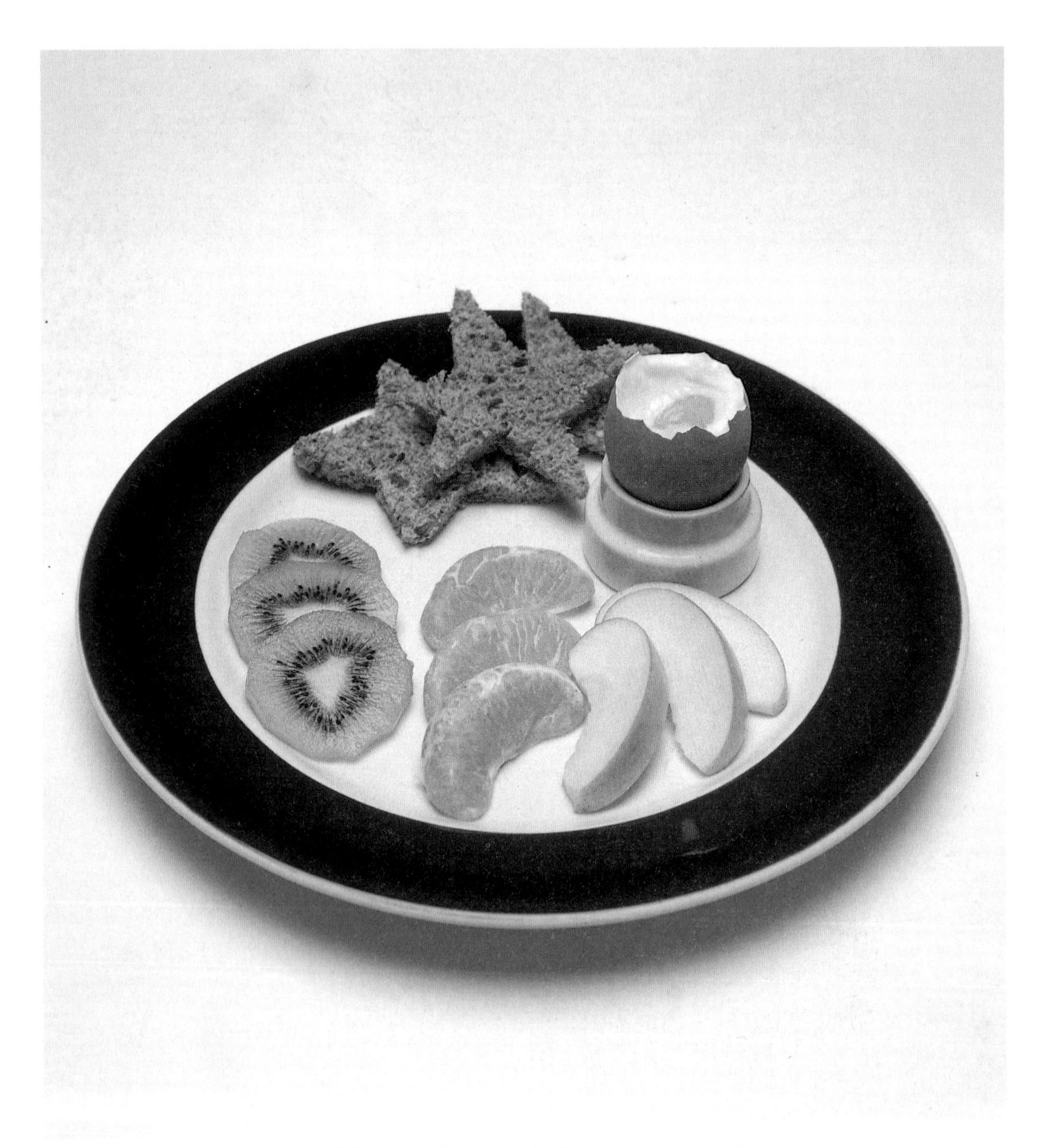

A balanced meal for young children and babies who have been weaned – a boiled egg and some finger foods

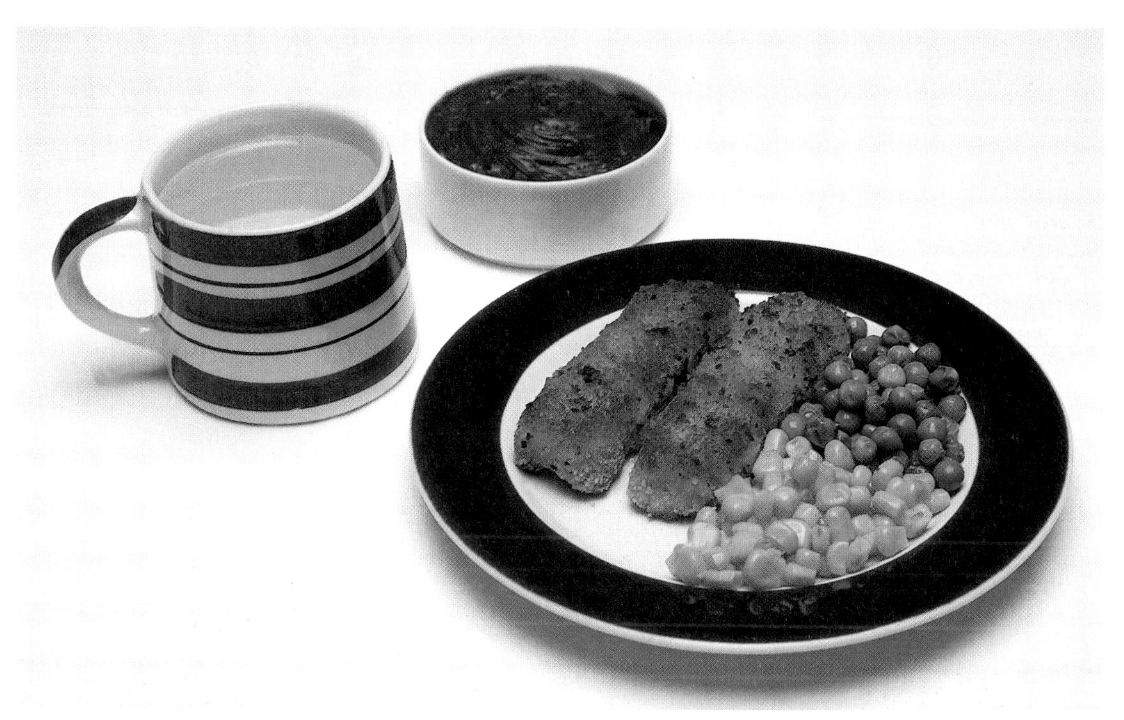

A healthy lunch – fish fingers, sweetcorn, peas, chocolate mousse, mug of water

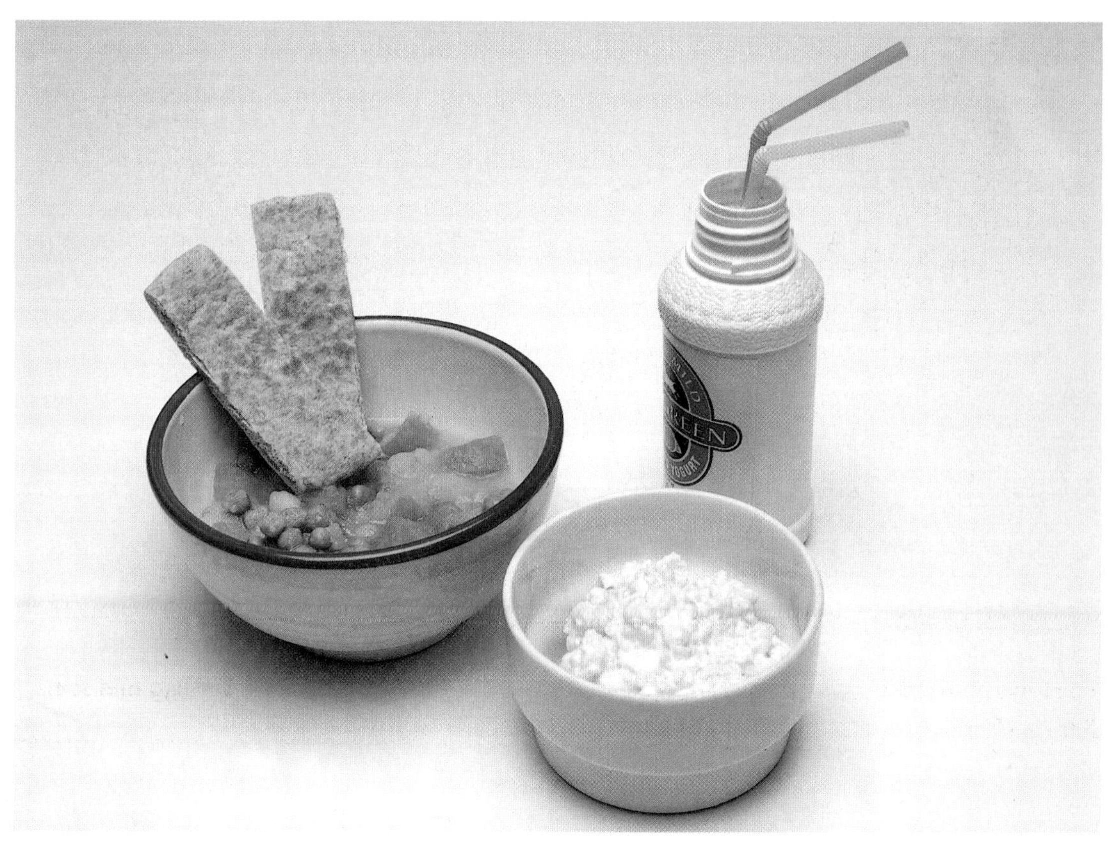

A healthy supper – thick vegetable soup, wholemeal pitta bread, rice pudding, yoghurt drink

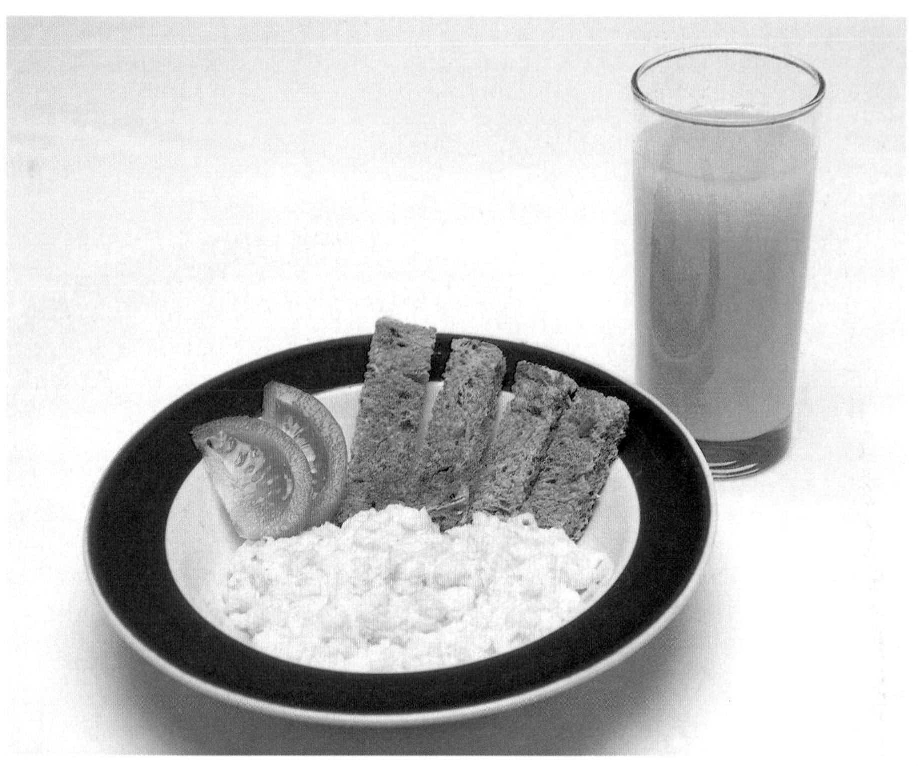

A healthy breakfast – scrambled eggs, wholemeal toast fingers, orange juice

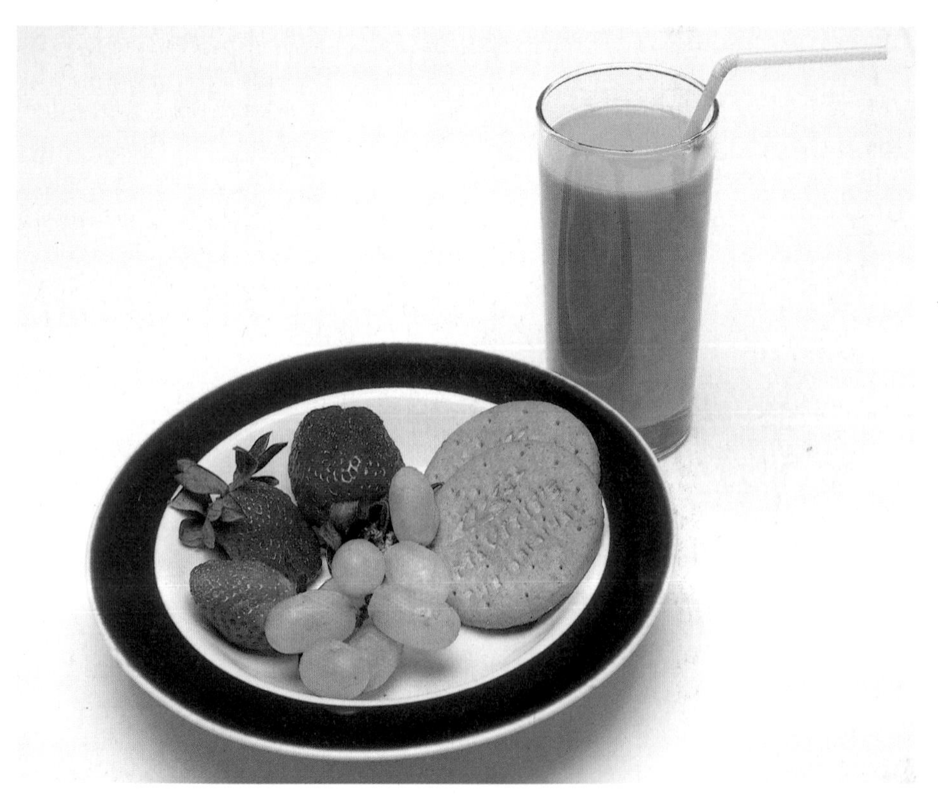

A healthy snack – digestive biscuits, grapes, strawberries, strawberry milkshake

How infection is prevented

Natural defences against infection

We are all born with **natural immunity** – which is the ability of the body to resist infection.

The body has a complex immune system which works in partnership with other protective body systems.

- The skin forms a physical barrier against germs entering your body. Skin is tough and generally impermeable to bacteria and viruses. The epidermis contains special cells called Langerhans cells that are an important early-warning feature of the immune system. The skin also secretes **anti-bacterial** substances – most bacteria and spores that land on the skin die quickly.
- Your nose, mouth and eyes are also obvious entry points for germs. Tears and mucus contain an **enzyme** (lysozyme) that breaks down the cell wall of many bacteria. **Saliva** is also anti-bacterial. Since the nasal passage and lungs are coated in mucus, many germs not killed immediately are trapped in the mucus and soon swallowed.
- The respiratory system uses **cilia**, mucus and coughing to rid the body of inhaled microbes and pollutants.

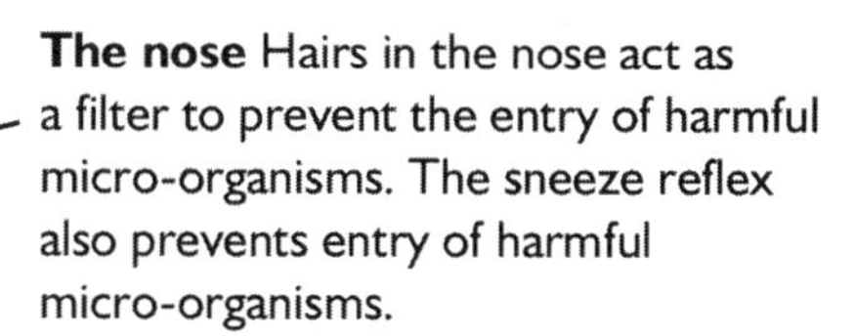
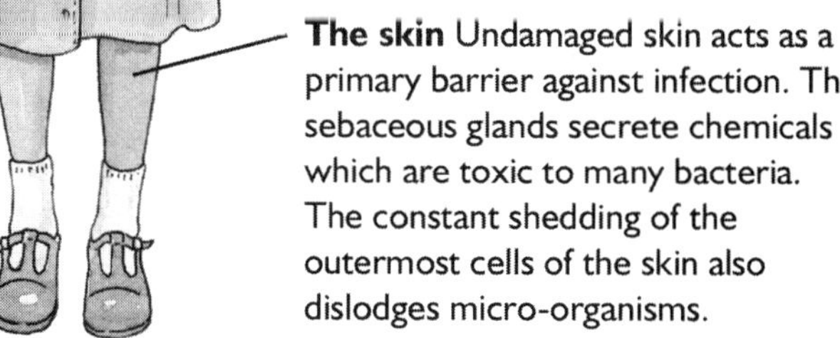

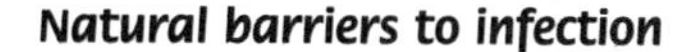

Natural barriers to infection

- Acid in the **stomach** and enzymes in the **intestines** destroy many harmful micro-organisms.

If foreign materials enter the body despite these protective mechanisms, then the immune and defence systems begin to operate.

The **immune system** includes:

- lymph nodes
- blood proteins
- specialised blood cells such as **lymphocytes**, as well as the organs that produce these cells and the blood vessels that transport them.

These are all designed to react rapidly against foreign organisms and their substances.

The main job of the immune system is to keep your body protected from invasion both by other organisms and by your own cells, which may develop incorrectly and cause harm to the fine balance of the body's systems, as in the case of cancer.

How does the immune system work?

The natural barriers of the immune system are the skin and the **mucosal membranes** which line the digestive, the respiratory and the **genito-urinary** systems, which can be accessed from outside the body. If this physical and chemical barrier is broken down by **trauma** or as a result of infection on the surface, the invading micro-organisms can enter the body, the blood stream and the lymphatic system and potentially find a niche elsewhere in the body tissue to multiply and form a colony.

The immune system works by using a collection of specialised cells:

1. **White blood cells**

   All white blood cells are known as **leucocytes**. White blood cells are not like normal cells in the body – they actually act like independent, living single-cell organisms able to move and capture things on their own. The two most important white blood cells in our immune system are phagocytes and lymphocytes:

   - **Phagocytes**. These cells fight infection by surrounding and engulfing the harmful micro-organisms – or **germs** – and then attacking them with a range of chemicals and enzymes. They are not effective against viruses.
   - **Lymphocytes**. Once the phagocytes have attacked the invaders, the resultant parts would then be processed by other white blood cells, including the lymphocytes. If there have been similar invaders before, the lymphocytes may have a 'memory' of this and rapidly produce **antibodies** to set an early attack before the invading germs get a chance to multiply.

2. **Antibodies**

   Once the lymphocytes have made a particular kind of antibody they can make it faster next time; also it may stay in your blood for a while. This makes you immune to the disease. You may never catch it again, or if you do, you will only have it mildly. You can also get **vaccinated** against certain diseases. Specially treated germs are injected into you, to give you a mild attack of the disease. Your body responds by making antibodies, so you become immune for the future.

The lymphatic system

The lymphatic system plays an important part in our defence against infection. **Lymph** is a clearish liquid that contains some white blood cells and some chemicals that are also found in blood. Lymph helps fight infections and drains fluid from body tissues back into the bloodstream. The lymph permeates the body just as blood does, but it circulates through muscle movements rather than being pumped around the body like blood. Any random bacteria that enter the body also find their way into the lymphatic system. One job of the lymph system is to drain and filter these fluids to detect and remove the bacteria. Small lymph vessels collect the liquid and move it towards larger vessels so that the fluid finally arrives at the lymph nodes for processing.

Lymph nodes contain filtering tissue and a large number of lymph cells. When fighting certain bacterial infections, the lymph nodes swell with bacteria and the cells fighting the bacteria, to the point where you can actually feel them. Swollen lymph nodes – often called **swollen glands** – are therefore a good indication that you have an infection of some sort. These swollen glands may be felt in the neck, in the armpits and in the groin area.

How antibiotics work

Normally our bodies are fit enough to fight an infection with all the parts of our immune system. **Antibiotics** are chemicals developed to help us in the fight. They reduce the risk of tissue damage while the immune system fights off the infection, and reduce the risk of death if it is unsuccessful. There is an argument that antibiotics are used too much; for minor infections with low risks we should wait for the body's own defences. One problem of giving a course of antibiotics for an infection is that as well as killing off the *harmful* bacteria causing the infection, some of your '**commensal flora**' will die too, leaving an opportunity for others to grow. A good example is 'thrush' or candida infection. This yeast-like fungus normally lives on the skin and in the gut and vagina in small, well-controlled numbers but after a dose of antibiotics it gets a chance to multiply and cause further harm.

There is also a danger that people will develop resistance to antibiotics.

The immune system in children

A baby is born with some natural immunity and can be further protected by:

- infection-fighting cells
- antibodies and other substances found in breast milk.

A child's own experiences of infection boost his or her immunity. For some infections, immunity is life-long while for others it is short-lived. Some illnesses, such as the common cold, are caused by one of several strains of virus, which is why having one cold doesn't automatically prevent another one later. **Immunisation** makes a child immune without having the illness itself.

Sometimes the immune system doesn't work properly, as with **AIDS** and some rare conditions; sometimes it over-works and causes **allergy**. It can also be affected by emotional distress and physical exhaustion.

ACTIVITY

1 What are the natural defences to infection?
2 Which part of the blood protects you against infection?
3 What is the role of the lymphatic system in preventing infection?
4 Describe two ways in which your body can become immune to a disease.

Understanding infection: some common terms

Antibiotics Drugs used to prevent and treat infection.

Communicable disease A disease which is passed from one person to another by direct or indirect contact.

Contagious An infectious disease which is transmitted by contact, i.e. not transmitted through atmosphere.

Infectious disease A communicable disease.

Endemic A disease which occurs frequently in a particular locality.

Epidemic An infectious disease attacking a number of people in the same locality at one time.

Fomites Inanimate articles – such as clothing, books, toys or a telephone receiver – which are not harmful in themselves but may harbour infection which can then be passed on to another person.

Incubation period The time gap between the entry of the infective organism and the first appearance of symptoms.

Isolation The act of setting apart; an isolation room or ward is one kept for infectious diseases and nurses follow strict rules to prevent the disease from spreading.

Pathogen Any micro-organism capable of causing disease.

Quarantine The amount of time for which children are advised to remain at home or otherwise isolated. This has little relevance in cases such as chickenpox, when the disease is highly infectious even before symptoms appear.

Types of immunity

There are two types of immunity: **active** and **passive**.

1 **Active immunity**. In this type of immunity, the body is *active* and works to produce its own antibodies to defend against a certain antigen. Active immunity may result from having a certain disease once and then getting it again. For some diseases a person usually only gets them once, such as the chickenpox. If a particular virus that has been in the body before enters, the memory cells within the body tissue will produce antibodies or killer T cells.

2 **Passive immunity**. The body is *passive*; it relies on being given the antibodies required to defend against the antigen. You may receive passive immunity through a **vaccine**. The vaccine consists of dead or weakened viruses or bacteria. These organisms can act as antigens and cannot cause diseases because they are weakened. When the vaccine enters the body, the immune system reacts to it the same way as it would to a **pathogen**. This way a person can actually develop immunity without even getting the disease.

Immunisation

Immunisation is the use of vaccines to protect people from disease. Because babies and children are particularly vulnerable to infection, they are offered immunisation, but their parents must give their written consent. In the UK parents can choose whether to have their children immunised. The advantages of immunisation include:

- Children who are not immunised run a risk of catching diseases and having complications.

- Immunisation is the safest way to protect children from particular diseases which may have long-lasting effects.
- Having children immunised at an early age means they are well protected by the time they start playgroup or school where they are in contact with lots of children.
- Immunisation also protects those children who are unable to receive immunisation, by providing what is called **herd immunity**. This describes the *partial* uptake of immunisation, where enough people are immunised to prevent the spread of the disease.

The tables below give the current recommended immunisation schedules in the UK:

Age	Children's vaccination	Type
2 months	Polio Hib Diphtheria Tetanus Whooping cough	By mouth One injection
3 months	Polio Hib Diphtheria Tetanus Whooping cough	By mouth One injection
4 months	Polio Hib Diphtheria Tetanus Whooping cough	By mouth One injection
12–15 months	Measles Mumps Rubella	One injection
3–5 years	Measles Mumps Rubella Diphtheria Tetanus Polio	One injection One injection By mouth
10–14 years	BCG (tuberculosis)	Skin test followed by one injection, if required
School leavers 13–18 years	Diphtheria Tetanus Polio	One injection By mouth

▶

Meningitis C vaccine: This new immunisation is given to children aged 2, 3 and 4 months and around 13 months with their routine immunisations. Extra appointments will be organised where necessary. Depending on their age, all other children will be invited through their GP, school or college to have the vaccine in a special catch up programme. (See the table below.)

	When will the vaccine be available?	Where will the vaccine be given?
From January 2000	Given to babies over 4 months and under 12 months.	At the surgery or health clinic – special appointments will be arranged. Please wait to be called.
	Given to children aged 1 to 4 years.	At the surgery or health clinic – special appointments will be arranged. Please wait to be called.
	Given to children aged 5 to 14 years.	At school. Please wait to be called.

Abbreviations

Hib Vaccination against the bacteria haemophilus influenzae, type B, which may cause meningitis (cerebrospinal meningitis) and infection of the epiglottis (back of the throat).

MMR Vaccination against measles, mumps and rubella (German measles).

The vaccinations at the ages of 2 months and 3–5 years are usually combined with routine children's medical examinations.

The Department of Health issues the following guidelines:

- **Children should not be vaccinated if they have a fever**. When children have a fever, the vaccination should be postponed. If the child just has an ordinary cold, but their temperature is normal, it is safe for them to be vaccinated.
- **Side-effects** to the vaccines do occur, but **allergy** to the vaccines is *very* rare:
  - The vaccines for diphtheria-tetanus-whooping cough, Hib and diphtheria-tetanus may cause a red area and swelling to occur on the vaccination spot. However, it will disappear within a few days. A fever may also be noticed on the day of the jabs and for a week to 10 days later.
  - The MMR vaccine may cause a brief reaction that may begin at any time from a few days to three weeks after the vaccination. The child may have symptoms like the diseases which are being vaccinated against, but only in a mild form. That is, a cold, a skin reaction, a fever and perhaps swollen salivary glands. The child will not be contagious.

The meningitis C vaccine may have the following effects:

- **Babies**. Some swelling and redness where the injection is given.
- **Toddlers over 12 months**. Some swelling and redness where the injection is given. About 1 in 4 toddlers may have disturbed sleep. About 1 in 20 toddlers may have a mild fever.
- **Pre-school children**. About 1 in 20 may have some swelling at the injection site. About 1 in 50 may have a mild fever within a few days of the vaccination.
- **Children and young people**. About 1 in 4 may have some swelling and redness at the injection site. About 1 in 50 may have a mild fever. About 1 in 100 may have a very sore arm from the injection, which may last a day or so.
- **On very rare occasions, vaccinations may cause serious complications**.

Care of children after immunisations

Children should be closely observed after any immunisation. Look out for any of the signs and symptoms listed above:

- If fever occurs, keep them cool, offer plenty to drink and give them children's paracetamol.
- If the temperature remains high, or if there are any other symptoms, such as convulsions, call a doctor immediately.

Alternatives to immunisation

There is no proven, effective alternative to conventional immunisation. **Homeopathic medicine** has been tried as an alternative to the whooping cough vaccine but it was not effective.

The Council of the Faculty of Homeopathy (the registered organisation for doctors qualified in homeopathy) advises parents to have their children immunised with conventional vaccines.

ACTIVITY

Prepare a large colourful poster, to be put on the parent's notice board in your nursery placement, which explains the current **immunisation schedule** for babies and children. Include phone numbers of local GPs and health visitors who can advise parents on all aspects of immunisation.

Providing a safe, hygienic environment

Children are more likely than adults to develop an infection because:

- they have immature immune systems
- they are not usually aware of the need for hygiene; they need to be taught and reminded to wash their hands
- they tend to play closely with other children for long periods of time.

Good hygiene routines will help to prevent infection. Children will take their cue from you, so you need to ensure that you are a good role model by setting a high standard of personal hygiene.

Personal hygiene

Personal hygiene involves regular and thorough cleaning of your skin, hair, teeth and clothes. The following are particularly important:

- The most important defence against the spread of infection is **hand washing**; wash your hands frequently – especially before eating, or before touching your mouth or nose.
- Parents and carers must make sure to wash their hands after they blow their nose or wipe the mouth of a sick child.
- Use paper towels to dry your hands if possible; if cloth towels are used, make sure they are washed daily in hot water.
- Keep your nails clean and short.
- Avoid contact with the secretions (especially on paper tissues) of somebody with a runny nose, sore throat or cough.
- Cover any cuts or sores on the hands daily with a clean, waterproof plaster.
- Don't share utensils or cups with somebody who has a cold, sore throat or upper respiratory infection.
- Wear disposable gloves when changing nappies or when dealing with blood, urine, faeces or vomit.
- Hair should be kept clean, regularly brushed and tied back.

Promoting children's hygiene

Nobody should expect children to be forever worrying about personal cleanliness, but by encouraging hygiene routines, you will help to prevent the spread of infection. Hand washing is especially important for children who eat with their hands as illness can be spread in saliva, which can contain bacteria. Make sure that children always wash their hands thoroughly, using soap and water:

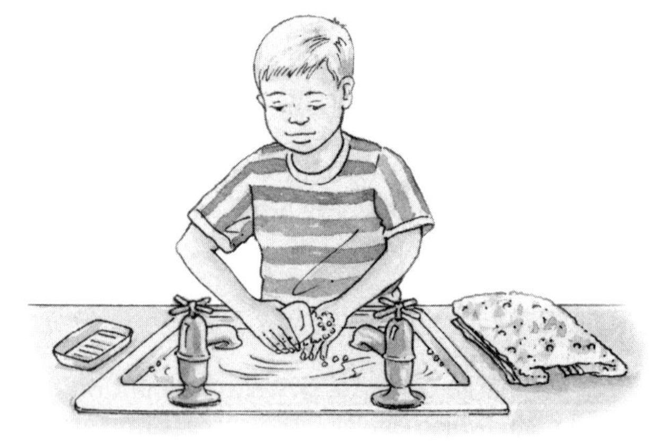

Washing hands will help prevent the spread of bacteria

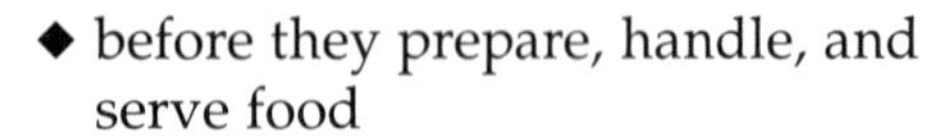

- before they prepare, handle, and serve food
- after using the toilet
- before and after eating meals or snacks
- after handling pets or other animals
- after the child blows their nose
- after being exposed to blood or blood-containing body fluids and tissue discharges.

Also make sure that paper tissues are available for children to use.

ACTIVITY

Encouraging children to wash their hands

Plan an activity to use with small groups of nursery-age children which will teach them about the importance of washing their hands. Children should wash their hands by cleaning them with soap for at least 10 seconds using warm running water. To encourage the right length of time, you could, for example, get them to sing 'Twinkle Twinkle Little Star', or a similar song, slowly all the way through.

You should include:

- A rationale – a reason for doing your particular activity.
- How you plan to carry out the activity, i.e. when, how many children, etc.
- How the activity went – did you achieve your aims?
- A brief summary of the activity and any ideas for improving it in the future.

Bear in mind that you need to make it fun for the children and that you will need to make sure that you have everything you need before beginning – soap, warm water and paper towels or clean cloth towels.

Providing a hygienic indoor environment

All child care establishments should have set routines for tidying up and for cleaning the floors, walls and furniture.

Routines for maintaining a hygienic indoor environment

- ☐ Keep a window open to ventilate rooms, but avoid draughts.
- ☐ All surfaces should be damp dusted daily.
- ☐ Teach children how to wash their hands properly, and supervise them.
- ☐ Clean up any spills and accidents straightaway.
- ☐ Check the toilet area for cleanliness on a regular basis.
- ☐ Use paper towels and tissues and dispose of them in covered bins.
- ☐ Use antiseptic solutions, such as Savlon, to disinfect toys and play equipment regularly; toys used by babies under 1 year should be disinfected daily.
- ☐ Make sure the class pet enclosure is cleaned out regularly and that children wash their hands after playing near it.
- ☐ Encourage children to cover their nose and mouth when coughing or sneezing.
- ☐ Discourage parents from bringing their child into the nursery or school if they have a high temperature or other signs of infection.
- ☐ Empty water containers daily and store in the sinks to dry.
- ☐ Encourage children to play outside whatever the season.
- ☐ Keep sand trays clean by sieving and washing the sand regularly.
- ☐ A no smoking policy must be observed by staff and visitors.

Providing a hygienic outdoor environment

Children benefit from playing in the fresh air, as long as they are dressed for the weather. All child care settings should be regularly checked to make sure they are safe and hygienic environments.

How to make the environment safer and more hygenic

- Check the outdoor play area daily for litter, dog excrement and hazards such as broken glass or rusty cans.
- Keep gates locked and check that hinges are secure.
- Follow the sun safety code; provide floppy hats and use sun cream (SPF15) to prevent sunburn.
- Supervise children at all times.
- Check all play equipment for splinters, jagged edges or protruding nails, etc.
- Keep sand covered and check regularly for insects or litter.

Preventing infection by food and drink

Food hygiene

Young children are particularly vulnerable to the bacteria which can cause food poisoning or gastro-enteritis. Bacteria multiply rapidly in warm, moist conditions and can enter food without causing the food to look, smell or even taste bad. So it is very important to store, prepare and cook food safely, and to keep the kitchen clean.

Food safety

1 Storing food safely

- Keep food cold. The fridge should be kept as cold as it will go without actually freezing the food (1–5 °C or 34–41 °F).
- Always read instructions on the label before storing food.
- Once a tin is opened, store the contents in a covered dish in the fridge.
- Cover or wrap food with food wrap or microwave clingfilm.
- Store raw foods at the bottom of the fridge so that juices cannot drip onto cooked food.
- Never refreeze food which has begun to thaw.
- Do not use foods that are past their sell-by or best-before date.
- Thaw frozen meat completely before cooking.

2 Preparing and cooking food safely

- Always wash hands in warm water and soap and dry on a clean towel, before handling food and after handling raw foods, especially meat.
- Wear clean protective clothing which is solely for use in the kitchen.
- Keep food covered at all times.
- Never cough or sneeze over food.

▶

- ☐ Always cover any septic cuts or boils with a waterproof dressing.
- ☐ Never smoke in any room that is used for food.
- ☐ Keep work surfaces and chopping boards clean and disinfected; use separate boards for raw meat, fish, vegetables, etc.
- ☐ Wash all fruits and vegetables before eating. Peel and top carrots and peel fruits such as apples.
- ☐ Make sure that meat dishes are thoroughly cooked.
- ☐ Avoid raw eggs. They sometimes contain Salmonella bacteria, which may cause food poisoning. (Also avoid giving children uncooked cake mixture, home-made ice creams, mayonnaise, or desserts that contain uncooked raw egg.) When cooking eggs, the egg yolk and white should be firm.
- ☐ When re-heating food, make sure that it is piping hot *all the way through*, and allow to cool slightly before giving it to children. When using a microwave, always stir and check the temperature of the food before feeding children, to avoid burning from hot spots.
- ☐ Avoid having leftovers – they are a common cause of food poisoning.

3 Keeping the kitchen safe

- ☐ Teach children to wash their hands after touching pets and going to the toilet, and before eating.
- ☐ Clean tin-openers, graters and mixers thoroughly after use.
- ☐ Keep flies and other insects away – use a fine mesh over open windows.
- ☐ Stay away from the kitchen if you are suffering from diarrhoea or sickness.
- ☐ Keep the kitchen clean – the floor, work surfaces, sink, utensils, cloths and waste bins should be cleaned regularly.
- ☐ Tea towels should be boiled every day and dishcloths boiled or disinfected.
- ☐ Keep pets away from the kitchen.
- ☐ Keep all waste bins covered, and empty them regularly.
- ☐ Keep sharp knives stored safely where children cannot reach them.

Disposing of waste

All child care settings should have a written policy which explains how waste should be disposed of safely and hygienically:

- Staff should always wear disposable gloves when handling any bodily waste, that is, blood, urine, vomit and faeces. Always wash your hands after dealing with such waste, even if gloves have been worn.
- A dilute bleach (hypochlorite) solution should be used to mop up any spillages.
- Different types of waste should be kept in separate covered bins in designated areas; food waste should be kept well away from toilet waste.
- Soiled nappies, dressings, disposable towels and gloves should be placed in a sealed bag before putting in a plastic-lined, covered bin for incineration.
- Always cover any cuts and open sores with waterproof adhesive plasters.

ACTIVITY

As a full-time early years worker in a day nursery, you have been asked by your manager to help prepare a talk on hygiene and safety for students who are coming to the nursery for work experience. Using the information in this section of the book prepare notes and plan your talk. You will need to:

1 explain briefly how infection spreads in nursery settings
2 outline the measures the nursery uses to maintain a hygienic environment
3 outline the main safety issues.

Don't bombard the students with an overload of information. Keep the talk simple. You might like to prepare a handout to summarise your points.

Revision questions

1 What is plaque?
2 What are the signs that a child is ready to start toilet training?
3 Which five food groups should make up a child's daily diet?
4 List possible food sources of vitamins A, B, C, D, E and K.
5 What deficiency disorders relate to these vitamins?
6 Why are sleep and rest important for health?
7 List the benefits of regular physical exercise.
8 List three ways in which infection can spread and three measures to prevent the spread of infection.
9 List six occasions when children should *always* wash their hands.

Answers

Activity on page 33

1 **c** Red blood cells
2 **b** Fighting and preventing infection
3 **a** Red blood cells
4 **b** Arteries–arterioles–capillaries–venules–veins
5 **b** The bone marrow of long bones
6 **a** The arteries

Activity on page 37

1 Human milk has the highest energy value of 295 kJ/100g because it is high in carbohydrate and fat.
2 The protein and mineral level of cow's milk are three times that of human breast milk. Giving young babies such milk can cause kidney failure.
3 The level of fat in skimmed milk is very low at 0.1% compared with 3.8% in whole milk. High levels of fat in the blood are a cause of heart disease.

Activity on page 38

1 Windpipe–bronchus–bronchiole–alveoli–bloodstream
2 The air leaving the lung is warmer and contains significantly more moisture and carbon dioxide gas

Activity on page 44

a the cerebellum
b sensory cortex
c brain stem
d parietal lobe
e frontal lobes

PART 2

Recognising and dealing with illness

Chapter 4: Recognising general signs of illness in children

◆ *Signs and symptoms* ◆ *General signs of illness in babies* ◆ *Why do babies cry?* ◆ *General signs and symptoms of illness in children: High temperature (fever) – Dehydration – Coughing – Pain – Swollen glands – Loss of appetite – Vomiting – Constipation – Diarrhoea – Emotional and behaviour changes* ◆ *When to call the doctor*

Signs and symptoms

Signs of illness are those that can be directly observed – for example, a change in skin colour, a rash or a swelling.
Symptoms of illness are those experienced by the child – for example, pain or discomfort or generally feeling unwell. These rely on the child being able to describe how they are feeling.

How to recognise a sick child – a checklist

If parents or child care workers can answer 'Yes' to any of these questions, then the child could be sick and the child's parents or doctor should be informed.

- ☐ Is the child complaining of not feeling well?
- ☐ Does the child appear lethargic (more than usual)?
- ☐ Does the child have skin rashes, itchy skin, or scalp?
- ☐ Does the child appear to have a fever? And if so, is their temperature above 38 °C?
- ☐ Does the child vomit?
- ☐ Does the child have an abnormal stool (white or grey bowel movement or diarrhoea)?
- ☐ Does the child have a severe cough?
- ☐ Is the child not urinating?
- ☐ Is the child refusing to eat or drink the amount that is normal for the child (especially when offered favourite foods)?
- ☐ Does the child appear or behave differently than normal?

General signs of illness in babies

Babies are not able to explain how they are feeling to their carers, so it is important to recognise some of the general signs that accompany illness. Some babies may cry in a 'strange' way – or one that is different from their usual cry – indicating hunger or thirst. They may refuse feeds or become unusually listless or lethargic. If the baby has an infection, there will be a raised temperature (or fever).

Some of the common signs of illness in babies are:

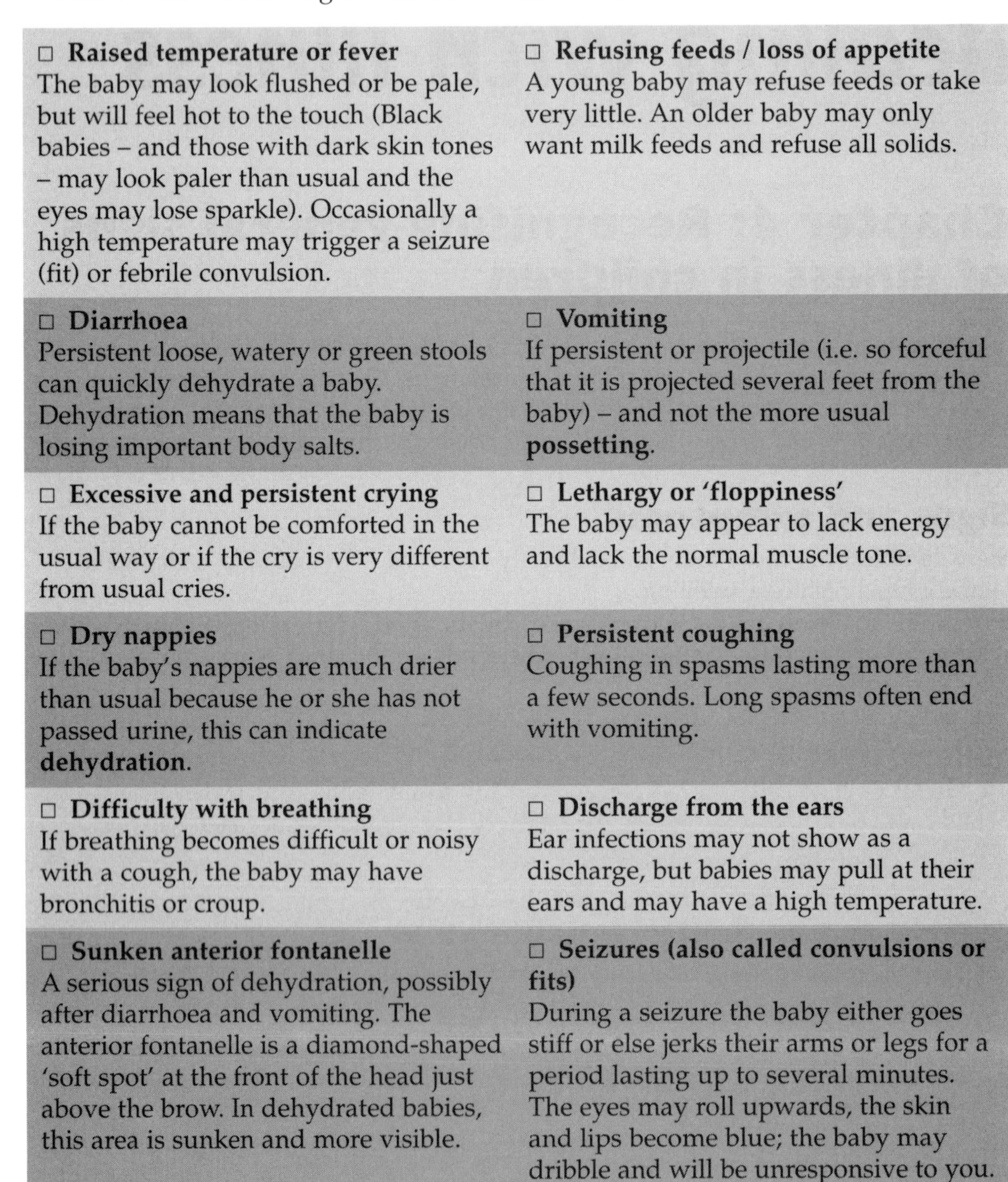

☐ **Raised temperature or fever** The baby may look flushed or be pale, but will feel hot to the touch (Black babies – and those with dark skin tones – may look paler than usual and the eyes may lose sparkle). Occasionally a high temperature may trigger a seizure (fit) or febrile convulsion.	☐ **Refusing feeds / loss of appetite** A young baby may refuse feeds or take very little. An older baby may only want milk feeds and refuse all solids.
☐ **Diarrhoea** Persistent loose, watery or green stools can quickly dehydrate a baby. Dehydration means that the baby is losing important body salts.	☐ **Vomiting** If persistent or projectile (i.e. so forceful that it is projected several feet from the baby) – and not the more usual **possetting**.
☐ **Excessive and persistent crying** If the baby cannot be comforted in the usual way or if the cry is very different from usual cries.	☐ **Lethargy or 'floppiness'** The baby may appear to lack energy and lack the normal muscle tone.
☐ **Dry nappies** If the baby's nappies are much drier than usual because he or she has not passed urine, this can indicate **dehydration**.	☐ **Persistent coughing** Coughing in spasms lasting more than a few seconds. Long spasms often end with vomiting.
☐ **Difficulty with breathing** If breathing becomes difficult or noisy with a cough, the baby may have bronchitis or croup.	☐ **Discharge from the ears** Ear infections may not show as a discharge, but babies may pull at their ears and may have a high temperature.
☐ **Sunken anterior fontanelle** A serious sign of dehydration, possibly after diarrhoea and vomiting. The anterior fontanelle is a diamond-shaped 'soft spot' at the front of the head just above the brow. In dehydrated babies, this area is sunken and more visible.	☐ **Seizures (also called convulsions or fits)** During a seizure the baby either goes stiff or else jerks their arms or legs for a period lasting up to several minutes. The eyes may roll upwards, the skin and lips become blue; the baby may dribble and will be unresponsive to you.

Why do babies cry?

Crying is a way for babies to express their needs – babies never cry for no reason at all. So it is vital that you try to find out just what is causing a crying baby distress. Some reasons are:

- **Hunger**. New-born babies often seem to want to feed all the time. They have small stomachs and they quickly become hungry again. Babies should be fed on demand; as they grow older, the size of the stomach will increase and the space in between feeds will widen.

- **Nappy rash**. A nappy left on for too long can upset any baby as the ammonia in urine can irritate the skin, causing an uncomfortable red rash. If the baby is suffering from nappy rash, change her nappy every couple of hours and leave it off completely when possible, to let the air get to the affected area.

- **Too hot**. Temperature control is not very well developed in young babies. If too hot, the baby will look red in the face, will feel very warm and may be sweaty around the neck folds. In summer babies get hot very quickly and can become dehydrated. Loosen clothes and bedcovers, but watch for signs of chilling.

- **Traumatic birth**. If the baby experienced a traumatic birth, such as a quick or slow delivery, the use of forceps, or if the cord was wrapped around her neck, or if she seems constantly restless and irritable, she may have minor injuries to her delicate skull bones. **Cranial osteopathy** may help relieve this.

- **Pain**. If the baby sounds as if they are in pain, check them over for any obvious signs that may be causing distress. The baby may have a bout of wind, so placing her face down along your forearm and firmly but gently massaging the back will help calm her. You could also try propping the baby over your shoulder and massaging the back in circular movements to bring up the wind.

- **Colic**. If the baby cries soon after being fed or has long bouts of crying, especially in the evening, he or she could be suffering from **colic** (see page 96). A baby with colic will be tense and difficult to hold, but will take comfort from you holding her firmly.

- **Too cold**. Babies dislike being cold, so change nappies and clothes as quickly as possible in a warm room. At night, make sure the room stays at a comfortable temperature of about 18 °C (65 °F). If too cold, the baby may be pale or may have a red face; to check, feel the baby's hands, feet, tummy and the back of the neck. Cuddle the baby to you, wrap a blanket around her and try giving a warm feed.

- **Pain or illness**. A baby might have a cold or snuffles and be generally fretful, or may have an itchy rash, such as eczema.

How to soothe a crying baby

First, check that the baby is not hungry, thirsty, too hot, too cold or showing signs of illness – see page 74. Try the following techniques:

- **Swaddling**. Babies love feeling warm and secure, and wrapping or swaddling them in a blanket can be very reassuring and soothing. You can also place a new-born baby next to your heart, so that he or she can hear its familiar beat.
- **Turn down the noise**. While babies generally enjoy background noise – and can go to sleep to familiar sounds such as the vacuum cleaner – loud or sudden noises can upset them, so keep the noise down to a low level around them and give them a quiet room to sleep in.
- **Breathing**. Match the rhythm of your breathing to theirs, then slow it down while stroking the baby's head more and more slowly.
- **Massage**. Most babies love being massaged. Try placing the baby on a blanket safely on the floor and massage the arms, legs and body in a gentle, circular motion.
- **Motion**. Babies love movement; try gently rocking the baby against your shoulder. The best way to achieve the most effective rate of rocking – 60 rocks a minute – is to walk while rocking the baby from side to side. As a last resort, you could also try a car ride – the sound of the engine and the movement may calm the crying.
- **Something to suck on**. Babies love something to suck, so you could try giving a comforter or teething ring to suck on, or, if old enough to be teething, a rusk to chew.

NOTE: If a baby is crying more often or for longer periods than usual, or if he or she starts crying in a different way, it may mean something is wrong, so always consult a doctor. There is a help-line for parents and carers who are coping with a crying baby:

- **Cry-sis**. Telephone advice on coping with a crying baby. Tel: 020 7404 5011, 24–hours, 7 days a week.

CASE STUDY

The following case study describes something that really happened; names and places have been changed.

'It was just one shake'

Like any proud parent, Sarah Parton has framed photos of her baby daughter, Melanie, all over her living room. But, unlike other parents, Sarah now has nothing left but pictures and memories . . .

Melanie hardly stopped crying in the 16 weeks leading up to her death. One day, Sarah, who was alone at the time and suffering from post-natal depression, snapped. Unable to calm the baby, she picked her up and shook her. Melanie died in hospital the following day.

Sarah, now 23, became pregnant after a brief relationship with the baby's father. He was not aware of the pregnancy and played no part in Melanie's short life. Although Sarah had just gained a certificate in child care studies, she had ▶

more experience with nursery age children and those at primary school than with babies.

Melanie was three weeks premature and was nursed in an incubator for the first few days in hospital. At first, Melanie was a contented baby, only ever crying when she wanted feeding, but all that changed when she was five weeks old. Sarah takes up the story:

'Melanie started screaming at lunch-time and she wouldn't stop. She cried differently from before – as if she was in pain. She refused her feeds, and me cuddling her or changing her didn't make any difference. I went and talked to the health visitor who said it could be colic. I tried everything that was suggested – colic drops, aromatherapy massage, swaddling her securely – but nothing worked. Then, after going every week to the baby clinic, a health visitor suggested I tried switching from cow's milk to soya milk, in case Melanie had an intolerance to cow's milk. It worked for a few days, but then Melanie started screaming all the time again . . . When Melanie was about three months, and I was only getting a couple of hours sleep at night, I went to see my GP and was given anti-depressant tablets – I felt so down and so alone . . . Then Melanie was admitted to hospital for observation – to find out why she cried all the time. The hospital staff said they thought her inability to settle down was caused by my anxiety. When I needed help most, they were telling me *my* illness was causing her crying. One day, when Melanie had been crying constantly all day, I hit rock bottom. I went to the baby clinic and said I couldn't cope any more – I wanted to see if she could be adopted. The health visitor didn't really take me seriously. I went home and sat with Melanie on my lap and I remember saying, "God Melanie, I don't know what to do to make you happy. Please stop it, I can't do anything."

'It was just one shake that I remember, and it wasn't even very hard or violent. I just felt so frustrated. It didn't stop the crying and afterwards I felt really bad about it and immediately gave her a big hug. She seemed to be OK, and then when I went to change her nappy on the changing mat, she stopped breathing. I thought she must be choking – her eyes had rolled back in her head and she was making gasping noises. I just picked up the phone and called an ambulance. At the time I was panicking because my baby was not breathing. I didn't really link it with me shaking her. I tried to give her mouth-to-mouth resuscitation . . . I was in the worst panic you could ever imagine.'

Melanie died the following day after attempts to revive her (by putting her on a life support machine) failed. Sarah was too scared to confess that she had shaken her baby and says she was in a state of complete shock. After an autopsy confirmed that shaking had been the cause of death, Sarah was eventually charged and pleaded guilty to infanticide. Sarah's depression became worse and on the night of Melanie's funeral, she took an overdose of her prescription pills. Sarah spent two weeks in a psychiatric unit and now receives support from a probation officer, a social worker, a psychiatrist and a community psychiatric nurse. She says she doesn't know how to make her life worth living any more. She knows that she has ruined any chance of a much-wanted career with children and also realises that if she *does* have children in the future, she would need to be closely supervised. She wishes the support she is receiving now had been available to her when she most needed it – but it is too late now.

▶

Questions

1 What factors might have contributed to Melanie's constant crying?
2 What were the events leading up to Melanie's death?
3 Describe the part played by the professionals in this case.
4 How might Sarah have been helped to cope with her problems?
5 In groups, prepare a poster that includes the following information:
   - What to do if a baby in your care won't stop crying.
   - Why one must never shake a baby.
   - Where to obtain help if dealing with a baby who constantly cries.

Although this is a tragic story, it is fortunately very rare. Thousands of women suffer post-natal depression, yet do not harm their babies.

General signs and symptoms of illness in children

When children feel generally unwell, you should ask them if they have any pain or discomfort and treat it appropriately. Take their temperature and look for other signs of illness such as a rash or swollen glands. Often, the signs of feeling generally unwell are the first signs that the child is developing an **infectious disease**. Some children can also show general signs of illness if they are anxious or worried about something either at home or at school. Common signs and symptoms of illness in children are:

Loss of appetite May not want to eat or drink; this could be because of a sore, painful throat or a sign of a developing infection.	**Lethargy or listlessness** May be drowsy and prefer to sit quietly with a favourite toy or comfort blanket.
Lacking interest in play May not want to join in play without being able to explain why.	**Irritability and fretfulness** The child may have a change in behaviour, being easily upset and tearful.
Abdominal pain May rub his or her tummy and say that it hurts – could be a sign of gastro-enteritis.	**Pallor** A white child will look paler than usual and may have dark shadows under the eyes; a black child may have a paler area around the lips and the **conjunctiva** may be pale pink instead of the normal dark pink.
Raised temperature (fever) A fever (a temperature above 38 °C) is usually an indication of viral or bacterial infection, but can also result from over-heating.	**Rash** Any rash appearing on the child's body should be investigated – it is usually a sign of an infectious disease.
Diarrhoea and vomiting Attacks of diarrhoea and/or vomiting are usually a sign of gastro-enteritis.	

High temperature (fever)

The normal body temperature is between 36–37 °C. A temperature of above 37.5 °C means that the child has a fever. Common sense, and using the back of your hand to feel the forehead of an ill child, is almost as reliable in detecting a fever as using a thermometer. The child will:

- look hot and flushed: the child may complain of feeling cold and be shivering. This is a natural reflex due to the increased heat loss and a temporary disabling of the usual internal temperature control of the brain.
- complain of thirst
- be either irritable or subdued
- usually go off their food
- may be unusually sleepy.

Children can develop high temperatures very quickly. You need to know how to bring the temperature down to avoid complications, such as dehydration and **febrile convulsions**.

How to take a temperature

All family first-aid kits should contain a thermometer. This may be a:

- Clinical thermometer
- Digital thermometer
- Temperature strip.

Clinical thermometer

This is a glass tube with a bulb at one end containing mercury. The tube is marked with gradations of temperature in degrees Centigrade and Fahrenheit. When the bulb end is placed under the child's armpit, the mercury will expand and so move up the tube until the temperature of the child's body is reached.

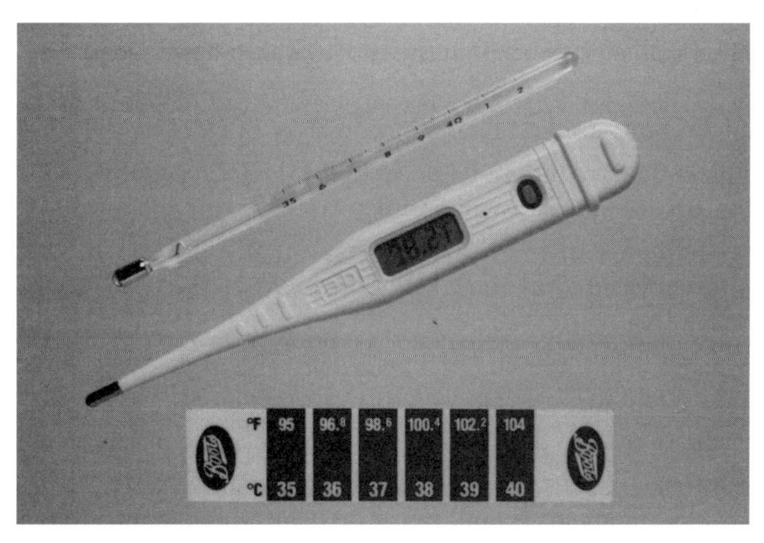

Three types of thermometer:
(Top) clinical, (Middle) digital, (Bottom) temperature strip

Using a mercury thermometer

Hold the thermometer by the top end and shake it down sharply until the mercury falls below 35 °C (95 °F) mark. Always wash the thermometer in cold water after it has been used. Never wash the thermometer in hot water because this can cause the glass to crack.

Armpit method.

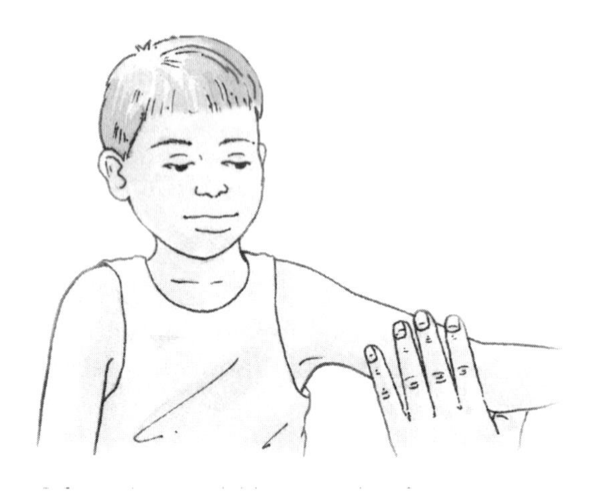

1 Sit the child on your lap, facing away from you. With the thermometer in your right hand, raise the child's left arm to expose the armpit.

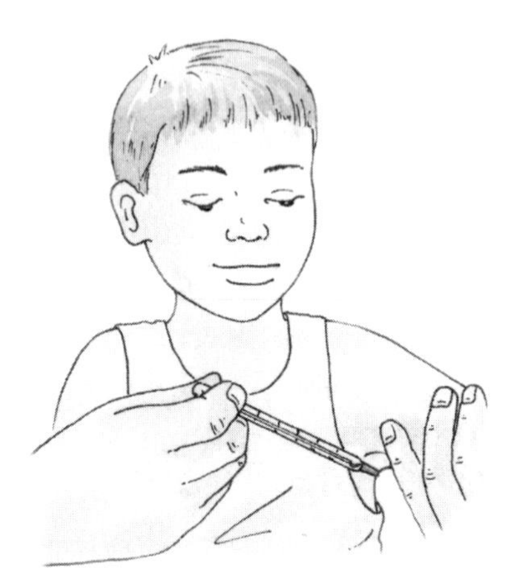

2 Place the thermometer into the armpit and lower the child's arm over it. Hold the arm down for two minutes (or according to manufacturer's instructions), then remove and read. **Note:** The temperature reading when taken will be about 0.6 °C (1 °F) lower than the child's actual body temperature.

Using a clinical thermometer

1. Explain to the child what you are going to do.
2. Collect the thermometer; check that the silvery column of mercury is shaken down to 35 °C.
3. Sit the child on your knee and take their top layer of clothing off.
4. Place the bulb end of the thermometer in the child's armpit, holding their arm close to their side for at least two minutes.
5. Remove the thermometer, and holding it horizontally and in a good light, read off the temperature measured by the level of the mercury. Record the time and the temperature reading.
6. After use, wash the thermometer in tepid water, and shake the column of mercury down again to 35 °C. Dry carefully and replace in case.
7. Decide whether to contact the parents – you may need to obtain their consent to give paracetamol.

NOTE: A clinical thermometer should never be placed in a young child's mouth, because of the danger of biting and breaking the glass.

Digital thermometer
This is battery-operated and consists of a narrow probe with a tip sensitive to temperature. It is easy to read via a display panel and is unbreakable.

1 Place the narrow tip of the thermometer under the child's arm as described above.
2 Read the temperature when it stops rising; some models beep when this point is reached.

Temperature strip
This is a rectangular strip of thin plastic which contains temperature-sensitive crystals that change colour according to the temperature measured. It is not as accurate as the other thermometers, but is a useful check.

1 Hold the plastic strip firmly against the child's forehead for about 30 seconds.
2 Record the temperature revealed by the colour change.

Whatever the cause of the high temperature, it is important to try to reduce it, as there is always the risk of a fever leading to convulsions or fits.

Bringing down a high temperature

- Offer cool drinks; encourage the child to take small, frequent sips of anything he/she will drink (though preferably clear fluids like water or squash rather than milky drinks). Do this even if the child is vomiting, as even then some water will be absorbed in the stomach, though much is vomited up.
- Keep the child as undressed as possible to allow heat to be lost.
- Reduce bedclothes to a cotton sheet if the child is in bed.
- Sponge the child down, using tepid water (see tepid sponging below).
- Give the correct dose of children's paracetamol. (**NOTE:** make sure you have written consent from the parents to use it in case of emergency. If not contact the parents and try to obtain consent.)
- Try to cool the air in the child's room – use an electric fan or open the window.
- Reassure the child who may be very frightened. Remain calm yourself and try to stop a baby from crying as this will tend to push the temperature higher still.
- If the temperature does not come down after appropriate treatment, consult a doctor within 24 hours.

NOTE: Always consult a doctor if a high fever is accompanied by symptoms such as severe headache with stiff neck, abdominal pain or pain when passing urine.

Tepid sponging to reduce a temperature

- Make sure the air in the room is comfortably warm – not hot, cold or draughty.
- Lay the child on a towel on your knee or on the bed and gently remove all but pants or nappy; reassure by talking gently.
- Sponge the child's body, limbs and face with tepid or lukewarm water – *not* cold; as the water evaporates from the skin, it absorbs heat from the blood and so cools the system.

▶

- ☐ As the child cools down, pat the skin dry with a soft towel – don't rub the skin – and dress only in pants or a nappy; cover with a light cotton sheet.
- ☐ Keep checking the child's condition to make sure he or she does not become cold or shivery; put more light covers on if necessary.
- ☐ If the temperature rises again, repeat sponging every 10 minutes.

Febrile convulsions

Febrile convulsions, or fits, affect children under five with very high fevers. They are *not* epilepsy, and do not lead on to epilepsy in later life. It is frightening for parents, but is not as a rule dangerous.

Signs

- ◆ The child will seem to be 'not with it'.
- ◆ Limbs will stiffen and twitch or shake: this can go on for up to five minutes.
- ◆ The eyes may roll back.
- ◆ May be incontinent of urine or faeces.

When the convulsion is over the child may be very drowsy and may be confused and irritable when they wake up.

What to do

It is important to remain calm, and stay with the child until the convulsion is over.

- ◆ Lie the child on their side somewhere where they cannot hurt themself (on a carpeted floor is a good idea). Provide support with a cushion or a rolled-up blanket.
- ◆ Ask a colleague to call a doctor.
- ◆ Don't force anything into the child's mouth – it is not necessary and you could break the teeth. Biting the tongue is rare.
- ◆ Call the doctor when the convulsion is over, if not already called.
- ◆ Contact the child's parents to inform them of what has happened.
- ◆ Continue with tepid sponging and other measures to reduce the child's temperature.

Dehydration

Under normal conditions, we all lose some body water every day in our sweat, tears, urine, and stools. We usually are able to replace this lost water by drinking fluids and eating foods that contain water. Sometimes, however, children lose abnormally large amounts of water through fever, diarrhoea, vomiting, or exercise – this is called **dehydration**. In the most severe cases, they may not be able to replace this water simply by drinking or eating as usual. This is especially true if an illness stops them from taking fluids by mouth or if they have a high fever.

Babies may suffer dehydration if they:

- are vomiting and/or suffering diarrhoea (usually caused by gastro-enteritis)
- have a high fever
- refuse feeds.

Signs of dehydration in babies

- ☐ Sunken fontanelles: these are the areas where the bones of the skull have not yet fused together; they are covered by a tough membrane and a pulse may usually be seen beating under the **anterior fontanelle** in a baby without much hair.
- ☐ Fretfulness.
- ☐ Refusing feeds.
- ☐ Dry nappies because the amount of urine being passed is very small.

Signs of dehydration in children

1 Mild to moderate dehydration

- ☐ Dry mouth
- ☐ No tears when crying
- ☐ Refusing drinks
- ☐ The child is at first thirsty and irritable and then becomes still and quiet
- ☐ Inactivity or lethargy
- ☐ Strong pulse and normal heart rate (for an older child)
- ☐ Restlessness

2 Severe dehydration

- ☐ Very dry mouth
- ☐ Fussy behaviour
- ☐ Sunken eyes
- ☐ Fast and weak pulse
- ☐ Muscle cramps
- ☐ No urination for several hours
- ☐ Dry and wrinkled skin
- ☐ Sleepiness
- ☐ Cool and blotchy hands and feet
- ☐ Disorientation
- ☐ Deep, rapid breathing
- ☐ When you pinch the skin it takes a few seconds to become smooth

What to do

If you think that a baby or child might have signs of dehydration, do not try to treat him or her at home. Call the doctor immediately, or take the child to the nearest accident and emergency department.

The doctor will prescribe oral rehydrating fluid to restore the body salts lost.

Coughing

A cough is a reflex action, caused by the stimulation of nerve endings in the throat. It is usually a symptom of a cold or an upper respiratory infection such as **bronchitis**. There are various types of cough:

- **Dry**: a rasping, painful-sounding cough which does not produce any mucus.
- **Wheezy**: a cough which causes noisy breathing.
- **Productive**: a cough which results in phlegm or mucus being coughed up into the mouth.

- **Barking**: a hard, dry barking cough, common in **croup**.
- **Whooping**: after a spasm of coughing, the child makes a 'whooping' sound when breathing in before the next coughing attack.

Coughs can also be the result of irritants affecting the upper respiratory tract. These include:

- **Cigarette smoke**: some children develop a cough when exposed to smoky atmospheres.
- **Allergens**: certain allergens such as dust mites or animal fur can cause coughs. Coughing which occurs mostly at night is linked with **asthma**.
- **Cold air**: inhaling cold dry air can provoke a cough.

How to soothe a cough

- Keep the air in the room moist by placing wet towels or bowls of warm water over a radiator.
- Spray a menthol preparation near the child's pillow (do not use it for a baby, who should not use pillows).
- Offer plenty of warm, soothing fluids, such as honey and lemon in warm water.
- Avoid overheating the room as a hot, dry atmosphere will irritate the child's air passages.

NOTE: Call an ambulance immediately if a child becomes blue around the mouth or is unable to talk or make any sounds.

Pain

Because pain is the body's warning signal that something is wrong, it should never be ignored. Children can feel pain in any part of the body, but it is not always easy for the parent or carer to know where they are actually hurting. Often the child will say that they 'hurt all over'. A very young child will not have the vocabulary to explain how they are feeling. You may notice that a child is irritable, whiny, pale and not eating. Parents and adults who know the child well will know instinctively when there is something wrong with them. You need to be observant and look for possible clues, for example, children may:

- pull at and rub their ear if they have earache
- hold their tummy if they have tummy ache
- move awkwardly if they have injured their leg.

Babies may feel pain caused by wind, colic, nappy rash, teething and many other reasons, but the only way they can show this is by crying. Sometimes you can tell that a baby is in pain by observing their face; there are three **facial signs** that will tell you if a baby is in pain:

- Squeezing their eyes together to make a bulge of flesh between the eyebrows.
- Squeezing their eyes shut.
- Pulling their mouth very taut.

Earache

Most earache is caused by infection – for example **otitis media** (see page 130). Young children are particularly vulnerable to ear infections because their Eustachian tubes are relatively short.

If the pain is severe and there is also a fever, call the doctor straightaway.

Occasionally, a child pushes a **foreign body** into the ear, such as a bead or a small piece of Lego. Don't try to remove the item unless it is easily reachable, because you may push it in even further. Take the child to a hospital accident and emergency department to have it removed.

Headaches

Most headaches in childhood are not serious, and are usually a symptom of a childhood illness. However, 1 in 5 children suffers from recurrent headaches, which are sometimes linked to anxiety, migraine or eyesight problems. A severe headache is also a symptom of meningitis, encephalitis or concussion. Headaches can be caused by:

- Sinusitis
- Toothache
- A blow to the head
- Meningitis
- A raised temperature
- Earache
- An allergy to foods such as chocolate

Try to find out what is causing the child's headache; one of the first symptoms of **meningitis** is a headache and an intolerance of light, so check for other symptoms such as:

- fever
- vomiting
- neck stiffness
- drowsiness or confusion.

These symptoms are also present in the rarer **encephalitis**, inflammation of the brain (see page 189). **Call the doctor immediately if:**

- you suspect meningitis or encephalitis
- if the child has a headache after a recent fall or blow to the head – it could be a sign of concussion.

How to relieve a headache

1. If the child's temperature is normal, encourage him or her to get some fresh air.
2. If the child has not eaten for a while, offer something light to eat and drink; some headaches are made worse when blood sugar is low.
3. Encourage the child to rest, preferably in a darkened room.
4. If the headache lasts for longer than an hour, give children's paracetamol, with the parent's consent.

Abdominal pain

All children experience abdominal pain at some stage. Any virus infection, not just those that cause diarrhoea, can cause tummy pain. This is because the bowels are surrounded by lymph glands like those in the neck, groins and armpits, and during a general viral illness, they swell too. These swollen glands (the **mesenteric glands**) can become sore and press on the bowel, so that there is discomfort and colicky tummy ache, though this is usually less severe than the colic of diarrhoea.

When in pain, babies tend to pull their knees up to their chest – a classic sign that their tummy hurts. Older children can usually describe the pain.

Causes of abdominal pain, signs and symptoms, and what do do are listed below.

Cause of abdominal pain	Signs and symptoms	What to do
Colic	Babies draw up their knees to their chest and cry constantly; the pain seems only to be relieved by being walked around held upright for hours on end.	The doctor may prescribe medicine to reduce the pain, or a bottle-fed baby may be changed to a lactose-free formula. Colic usually clears up by the 3rd or 4th month.
Intussusception (A rare condition affecting babies between 3 and 18 months, in which a portion of the bowel telescopes in on itself.)	The baby may vomit and have bouts of screaming, drawing up the knees to the chest; will have pallor when not red in the face from crying. The stools are normal in the early stages but may show blood-stained mucus later.	Call the doctor. An ultrasound examination or X-ray will confirm the diagnosis. Some babies need surgery to correct or remove the affected part of the bowel. In less severe cases, a special X-ray technique can straighten the bowel by using pressure.
Appendicitis	Pain in the bottom right-hand corner of the abdomen to start with. Refusal to eat, slight fever and may vomit; pain is more severe when abdomen is pressed.	Contact parents. Call the doctor. The pain is not relieved using the advice below (How to soothe abdominal pain.)
Mesenteric adenitis (Inflammation of the mesenteric glands in the abdomen.)	Pain (usually not severe) in the centre of the abdomen; upper respiratory tract infection, headache, fever (above 38 °C), enlarged neck glands and lymph nodes.	Call the doctor. Usually no treatment necessary; the pain goes away as the lymph nodes become less inflamed. Sometimes mistaken for appendicitis.

▶

Urinary tract infection	Pain in the lower back and/ or on one side of the abdomen.	Contact parents. Call the doctor.
Gastro-enteritis	Pain all over the abdomen with vomiting/diarrhoea and fever.	Call the doctor if the baby is under 1 year. Offer clear fluids and rehydrating solutions for older children: call the doctor if symptoms persist beyond 24 hours.
Recurrent abdominal pain syndrome	This syndrome usually starts after the age of five and is sometimes, but not always, accompanied by vomiting, headaches and occasionally diarrhoea with no other signs of illness.	The condition is thought to be linked to stress and anxiety, both at school and at home, e.g. bullying, emotional problems, etc. Try to soothe the pain. Discuss with parents to find the possible cause. See the doctor, who may refer the child and family for specialist help.

How to soothe abdominal pain

- Contact parents and describe their child's symptoms.
- Ask the child if they have been to the toilet; if not, encourage them to try to open their bowels.
- Try wrapping a warm, but not boiling hot, hot water bottle in a towel and encourage the child to lie with it against their tummy to relieve the pain.
- Offer water to drink but no food while the pain persists.
- If the child has a tummy ache with a sore throat or cough, use children's paracetamol to ease the pain (if the parents have given consent).

Call an ambulance if:

- the pain becomes constant or fixed in one place for six hours or more
- the child's vomit is green or yellow (bile)
- if the pain is in the groin or scrotum – it could be a **hernia**.

Muscular aches and pains

Children don't suffer muscular aches and pains to the same degree as adults do. Painful injury to arms and legs include fractures, sprains and strains, which become more common when children start school and take more vigorous exercise. For children suffering growing pains you can give them paracetamol, with written consent from their parents. Guidelines for dealing with **fractures**, **strains** and **sprains** are given in Chapter 7.

Cramp

Cramps are caused by the sudden and involuntary contraction of a muscle or group of muscles that then fail to relax. No one knows exactly why cramps occur, but they usually follow strenuous or repetitive exercises and are linked to a reduction in body salts in the body after excessive sweating or diarrhoea. Cramps can cause intense pain, usually in the calf muscles, but they are not dangerous. See page 183 for how to relieve a cramp.

Swollen glands

The glands that swell during an illness are not glands in the true sense, because they do not secrete hormones. They are enlarged **lymph nodes**. They are particularly common in children because the lymphatic system plays a greater role in fighting infection during childhood. Swollen glands are usually caused by a minor viral or bacterial infection. The swelling is a result of the accumulation of white blood cells which are produced by the immune system to fight infection.

They commonly occur in the neck, armpit and groin; those that swell tend to be the ones nearest to the site of infection. The diagram below shows the sites where swollen glands may occur.

Swollen glands in the neck

Swollen glands in the neck are common in children with a throat infection, an ear infection or **German measles** (rubella).

Signs and symptoms

- The child will complain that their neck hurts.
- The glands may be felt as tender, slightly warm smooth lumps about the size of a large pea.
- Glands felt below the ear and jaw are usually affected by **tonsillitis**.
- Glands felt behind the ear are usually caused by an ear infection and are usually present only on the affected side of the neck.
- Glands in the back of the neck are usually caused by **German measles (rubella)**.

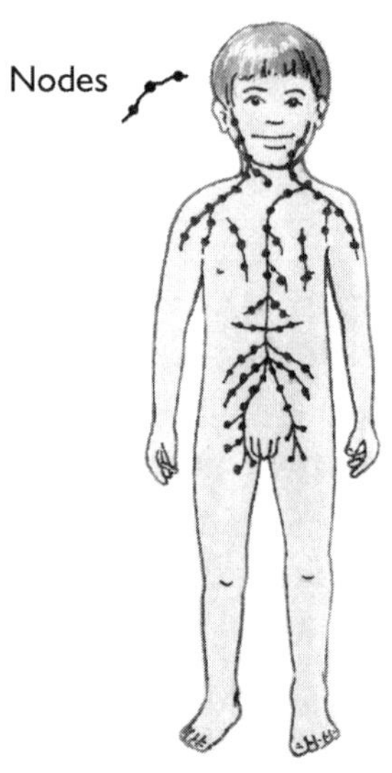

The sites of lymph nodes

What to do

- ☐ If the swollen glands are obviously linked with an infection which is getting better, there is no need to call a doctor.
- ☐ See the doctor if:
  - the glands are swollen with no other signs of illness
  - the swollen glands do not improve within two weeks.

The doctor may check for swollen glands in other areas, such as in the armpits, the groin and the abdomen. If these are also enlarged there may be a more widespread infection.

Loss of appetite

As long as a child is generally well and gaining weight, a temporary loss of appetite is not a problem. Children may not want to eat, for example, if they are very tired or if they have travel sickness. However, appetite loss nearly always accompanies illness, especially when there is a fever.

What to do

Try to find out what is causing the problem; look for other signs of illness, such as:

- **fever**: check the child's temperature
- **sore throat**: check the child's throat to see if the tonsils are inflamed; do this by gently holding the child's tongue down with the handle of a clean spoon and asking them to say 'aaah'. (Tonsillitis will make swallowing very painful.)
- **earache**: otitis media can be painful enough to put a child off eating
- **swollen glands**
- **urinary tract infection**: check if the child is passing urine frequently or having pain when urinating
- **appendicitis**: examine the lower right of the abdomen.

What to do if the child's temperature is normal and there is no evidence of illness, although the child is still refusing to eat:

- Encourage plenty of fluids; make sure the child gets plenty of nutrients by disguising them in drinks, for example a milkshake enriched with banana and wheatgerm.
- **Consult a doctor if**:
  - the loss of appetite persists, even without any other symptoms, for more than 24 hours. The doctor will examine the child to see if there is any physical reason for the loss of appetite.

See pages 239–240 for ideas to encourage a sick child to eat.

Vomiting

Vomiting is the violent expulsion of the contents of the stomach through the mouth. A single episode of vomiting without other symptoms is something that happens frequently in childhood. It could be a result of overeating or too much excitement. Vomiting has many causes, but in the majority of cases there is little warning and after a single bout the child recovers and quickly gets back to normal.

Accompanying symptoms	Possible causes and what to do
In babies:	
The baby brings up a little milk during or after a feed, but seems contented, generally feeds well and is gaining weight.	This is **possetting** and is harmless.
The baby is under 2 months and vomits forcibly after every feed.	**Pyloric stenosis** (see page 106). Call the doctor.

▶

The baby has a runny or blocked nose, snuffly breathing or a cough.	**Common cold** (see page 198). **Cough** Take no action unless the vomiting persists.
The baby is in severe pain and is passing stools that contain mucus and blood.	**Intussusception** (a bowel blockage) see page 86. Call the doctor immediately.
The baby seems unwell and is passing frequent watery stools.	**Gastro-enteritis** (see page 100). Call the doctor immediately.
□ **In children over 1 year**:	
The child's vomit is greenish-yellow.	**Intestinal obstruction**. **Call an ambulance**; do not give the child anything to eat or drink.
The child has continuous abdominal pain around the navel and to the right side of the abdomen.	**Appendicitis** (see page 119). **Call an ambulance**; do not give anything to eat or drink.
The child seems unwell, looks flushed and feels hot.	**Infection** Reduce the fever (see page 81). See the doctor within 24 hours.
The child has diarrhoea.	**Gastro-enteritis**. See the doctor within 24 hours. Follow guidelines to prevent **dehydration** – see page 101.
The child complains of a severe headache on one side of the forehead.	**Migraine**. See the doctor if accompanied by severe abdominal pain (it could be appendicitis).
The child has pale faeces and dark urine	**Hepatitis** (see page 125). See the doctor within 24 hours.
The child has recently suffered a blow to the head.	**Head injury**. **Call an ambulance**; do not give anything to eat or drink.
The child has a fever, a stiff neck or flat purplish spots that do not disappear when pressed.	**Meningitis** (see page 103). **Call an ambulance**.
When travelling, the child seems pale and quiet and complains of nausea.	**Travel sickness**. Give the child a travel-sickness remedy before starting a journey; take plenty of drinks to prevent dehydration.
The child vomits after a bout of coughing.	**Whooping cough** (see page 173). See the doctor within 24 hours.

Helping a child who is vomiting

- Reassure the child, who may be very frightened.
- Stay with the child and support their head by putting your hand on their forehead.
- Keep the child cool by wiping the face with a cool, damp cloth.
- Offer mouthwash or sips of water after vomiting.
- Give frequent small drinks of cold water with a pinch of salt and a teaspoon of glucose added – or you can buy special rehydrating powders.
- Encourage the child to rest in bed with a bowl by their side. Don't leave them until they have fallen asleep, and stay within call in case they vomit again.

Constipation

Sometimes constipation occurs briefly in a child recovering from a high fever. During the heat of a fever, a child's body loses some of its water to evaporation. The child also sweats more and may vomit. If the sick child doesn't feel like drinking, their body may try to recover as much water as possible by absorbing it from inside the intestines. The intestines then temporarily form bowel movements that are dry and hard. Once the child returns to their normal pattern of diet and exercise, bowel movements usually also return to normal.

Diarrhoea

Most children have diarrhoea at some time, usually after an infection involving the digestive tract. If the fluid lost through passing frequent loose, watery stools is not replaced, there is a danger the child will become **dehydrated**. Babies become dehydrated very quickly and can become seriously ill as the result of diarrhoea.

Diarrhoea can also be caused by:

- emotional factors – over-tiredness, excitement and anxiety
- allergy
- reaction to certain drugs and medicines.

Emotional and behaviour changes

Children react in certain characteristic ways when they are unwell. Some of the more common emotional and behaviour changes include:

- Being quieter than usual.
- Becoming more clingy to their parents or primary carer.
- Attention-seeking behaviour.
- Changed sleeping patterns; some children sleep more than usual, others less.
- Lack of energy.
- Crying: babies cry for a variety of reasons (see page 75). Older children who cry more than usual may be physically unwell or you may need to explore the reasons for their unhappiness.
- Regression: children who are unwell often regress in their development and behaviour. They revert to an earlier stage of development. They may:
  - want to be carried everywhere instead of walking independently

– go back to nappies after having been toilet-trained
– start to wet the bed
– play with familiar, previously outgrown toys.

When to call the doctor

If you think the child's life is in danger, dial 999 if you are in the UK, ask for an ambulance urgently and explain the situation.

For babies under 1 year

Contact the family doctor (GP) if the baby has *any* of the following symptoms. If the doctor cannot reach you quickly, take the child to the accident and emergency department of the nearest hospital.

□ A temperature of 38.5 °C which is not lowered by measures to reduce fever, or a temperature over 37.5 °C for more than one day.	□ Convulsions, or is limp and floppy. □ Cannot be woken, is unusually drowsy or may be losing consciousness.
□ Severe or persistent vomiting and/or diarrhoea, or projectile vomiting.	□ Seems dehydrated – a sunken anterior fontanelle can indicate dehydration (see page 83).
□ Symptoms of **meningitis**.	□ **Croup** symptoms.
□ A pallor, listless, and does not respond to usual stimulation.	□ Cries or screams inconsolably and may have severe pain.
□ A bulging **fontanelle** (soft spot on top of head) when not crying.	□ Appears to have severe abdominal pain, with symptoms of **shock**.
□ Refuses two successive feeds.	□ Develops **purple-red rash** anywhere on body. Could be **meningitis**
□ Passes bowel motions (stools) containing blood.	□ Has jaundice.
□ A suspected ear infection.	□ Has been injured, e.g. by a burn which blisters and covers more than 10% of the body surface.
□ Has inhaled something, such as a peanut, into the air passages and may be choking.	□ Has swallowed a poisonous substance, or an object, e.g. a safety pin or button.
□ Has bright pink cheeks and swollen hands and feet (could be due to **hypothermia**).	□ Has difficulty in **breathing;** rapid, difficult or noisy breathing.

NOTE: Babies with black skins will show darker coloured rashes than those on fair-skinned babies.

▶

In children over 1 year

Contact the family doctor (GP) if the child has *any* of the following symptoms. If the doctor cannot reach you quickly, take the child to the accident and emergency department of the nearest hospital.

□ A temperature of over 39 °C	□ Drowsy and difficult to wake up.
□ Pain or stiffness in their neck or a severe headache.	□ Convulsion or a seizure for the first time.
□ Unusually confused, very ill, or seems to be getting worse.	□ Signs of meningitis, such as headache, photophobia or a stiff neck.
□ Breathing so hard or fast that he or she cannot speak, cry, or swallow.	□ Severe stomach ache that causes them to double up and scream, but does not experience vomiting or diarrhoea.
□ Stools that are black or bloody.	□ Has not urinated in an 8-hour period and the mouth and tongue appear to be dry.
□ Drowsy or confused after a blow to the head.	□ Hypothermia.
□ Vomiting for more than 24 hours *or* if associated with pain.	□ Pain in any part of the body.

Revision questions

1 What is the normal body temperature for a child?
2 What are febrile convulsions? How can you reduce a high temperature?
3 What is dehydration and how can it be recognised?
4 Note down four signs and symptoms of a childhood infection.
5 Give six reasons why a baby might cry.

Chapter 5: The main conditions affecting babies under 1 year

◆ Bronchiolitis ◆ Coeliac disease ◆ Colic ◆ Cow's milk protein intolerance ◆ Cradle cap ◆ Croup ◆ Failure to thrive ◆ Gastro-enteritis ◆ Heat rash ◆ Hypothermia ◆ Lactose intolerance ◆ Meningitis ◆ Milk spots ◆ Nappy rash ◆ Pyloric stenosis ◆ Squint ◆ Sticky eyes ◆ Sudden infant death syndrome (SIDS) ◆ Thrush ◆ Umbilical hernia

Bronchiolitis

What is it? Bronchiolitis is an acute lung infection of the smaller airways – the bronchioles – which affects babies under one year of age. It is a seasonal infection, occurring in the winter months. Each year the virus changes slightly, so a new form spreads among babies who have not come across the virus before. It is one of the commonest childhood diseases – about 1 in 10 babies under the age of one suffer from it and many end up needing treatment in hospital.

Cause: Bronchiolitis is caused by a virus, usually one called RSV or respiratory syncitial virus, which infects the tiny air passages in the baby's lungs called the bronchioles. When they are infected by the virus, there is a dramatic reaction by the white cells of the immune system, which can cause the walls of the tubes to become thicker. This makes the air passages become smaller, making it harder for the baby to move air in and out of the lungs.

Signs and symptoms:

- It usually starts with a cold, cough and fever.
- The baby starts to breathe faster – up to 60 breaths a minute.
- There may be wheezing and difficulty in breathing.
- The baby cannot feed properly and may vomit.
- Abnormal drowsiness.
- Bluish tinge to lips and tongue (**cyanosis**).

What to do immediately:

- Call an ambulance immediately if the baby has difficulty in breathing; the baby may need to be given oxygen in a plastic head box, and may require further hospital care.
- Send for the doctor if there is wheezing and/or a dry, rasping cough.
- Ease the cough by placing the baby across your lap and patting gently on the back; this will help to loosen the build-up of thick mucus.

General care:

- In mild attacks, the doctor usually prescribes a bronchodilator drug, in syrup form.
- Hold the baby snuggled against you in an upright position to ease breathing – propped against your shoulder is ideal.
- Offer plenty of fluids and small regular feeds; some babies refuse solid foods and prefer to feed from the breast or bottle.
- Babies with mild bronchiolitis usually recover within one week, although the cough may persist for several weeks.

Possible complications:

- Most babies make a complete recovery. Bronchiolitis does not cause any permanent damage to the lungs. ➲

➲ Bronchiolitis continued

- Babies who have had bronchiolitis tend to wheeze whenever they have a cold. Bronchiolitis is very difficult to avoid because the virus is so widespread throughout the environment. However, it is worth keeping babies away from others who currently have the infection.

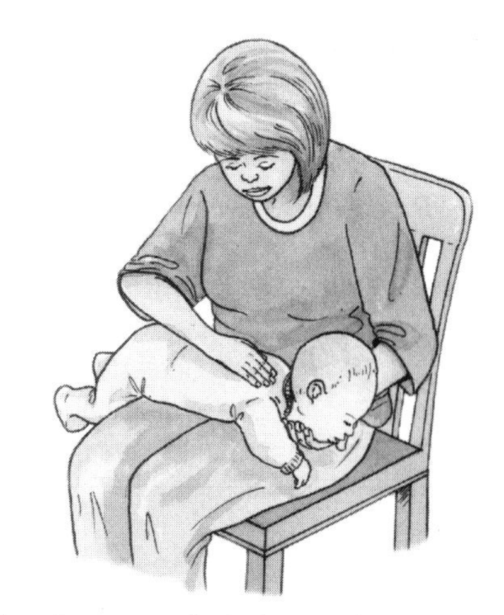

How to ease a baby's cough

Coeliac disease

What is it? A rare disease which affects the small intestine and prevents the absorption of nutrients.

Cause: Coeliac disease is caused by an extreme sensitivity of the small intestine to a protein (gluten) present in the cereals of wheat, rye, barley and oats. Gluten damages the small finger-like projections (the villi) that line the small intestine and play a significant role in digestion. When damaged and inflamed, the villi are unable to absorb food properly, and this often causes diarrhoea and malnutrition.

Signs and symptoms: In babies, symptoms of the condition usually start soon after the baby is weaned onto solid foods. These are:

- Chronic diarrhoea; there will be very pale, floating faeces that have an unpleasant smell – this is due to the poor absorption of fat.
- Abdominal distension (the baby appears to have a 'pot belly').
- Poor feeding and poor weight gain or weight loss, resulting in failure to thrive.
- Muscle wasting.
- Irritability and lack of appetite.

Later on, the child will show signs of:

- Anaemia – shown by breathlessness, pallor and a general lack of energy.

What to do:

- Any child who shows the signs and symptoms of coeliac disease should see a doctor for assessment.
- Once coeliac disease is suspected, the diagnosis is made by taking a blood test to detect antibodies to gluten and a stool sample to measure the amount of fat excreted in the faeces. If these are positive then a **biopsy** is performed on the small intestine to examine the cells that line it and to confirm the diagnosis.

General care:

- A **gluten-free diet** for life. Once diagnosed, it is necessary to completely eliminate gluten and related proteins from the diet.
- Once this is done, recovery is speedy and the symptoms quickly disappear.
- The help of a dietician is an essential component of understanding which foods are gluten-free (fruit, vegetables, fresh meat, fish, cheese, eggs, and milk) and those that contain wheat, barley, and rye, which should be avoided and replaced with rice and corn flour, for example.
- Recipe books and gluten-free foods, some of which are available on prescription, are now much more readily available. Support organisations, such as the **Coeliac** ➲

➲ Coeliac disease continued

Society, produce a regularly updated list of gluten-free foods, which helps its members enjoy a healthy and nutritious diet.

Possible complications:

- Symptoms of the disease may recur if gluten is re-introduced into the diet.
- Provided they stick to their gluten-free diet, then the risk of developing bowel cancer is believed to be no more than that of someone who doesn't have coeliac disease.

It has been suggested that breastfeeding and delaying the introduction of gluten-containing foods until a baby is older than four months of age may prevent children from developing coeliac disease.

Colic

What is it? Colic is not a disease but a pattern of persistent, prolonged crying; it is thought to be abdominal pain that causes the baby to cry inconsolably. It usually occurs between 2 weeks and 3 months of age and causes considerable distress for parents and carers.

Cause: The cause is unknown, but babies with colic seem to produce a lot of wind; this causes painful contractions or spasms in the intestines. Experts attribute colic to various factors, including an infant's immature digestive system, allergies, hormones in breast milk and overfeeding.

Signs and symptoms:

- The baby is otherwise healthy but suffers from bouts of apparent abdominal pain.
- Constant crying; the baby appears inconsolable with loud crying lasting three hours or more for three or more days a week, over a period of more than three weeks.
- Prolonged crying between 6 p.m. and midnight in a baby that has been fed, especially breastfed babies.
- While crying, babies draw their legs to the abdomen, clench their hands and curl their toes. ➲

What to do:

- If the bouts of colic are accompanied by fever, diarrhoea, vomiting or constipation, then call the doctor.
- Try to remain calm; communication of your own anxiety or frustration may result in more crying. (See also hints for calming a crying baby on page 76).
- Comfort and reassure the baby; you could try:
  - Lying the baby on your lap and gently rubbing the back; hold the baby, stomach down, along your forearm, with the head facing outward on your palm and legs on either side of your elbow (see photo below). This technique may be more effective if you rock in a rocking chair or walk quietly until the baby falls asleep.
  - Cuddling the baby close and gently rubbing the back.
  - Massaging the abdomen gently in a clockwise direction, using the tips of your middle fingers.
  - Try bathing the baby around the worst time – the warm water can be soothing and may distract the baby for a while.

General care:

- Drugs may be prescribed in severe cases of colic, but these do not always solve the problem; alternative therapies include **homeopathy** (Chamomilla is often used), **cranial osteopathy** and **Traditional Chinese Medicine**.
- Some doctors and health visitors advise breastfeeding mothers to watch their own diet and to cut out foods that could irritate the baby's stomach – e.g. cow's milk, oranges, strawberries, chocolate and coffee. ➲

➲ Colic continued

- The teats for bottle-fed babies should be checked as too small a hole will limit the flow of milk and allow more air to be swallowed with each feed.
- Colic has no lasting effects on the baby and usually resolves by the age of 3 or 4 months.
- Always be sure to exclude other possible causes of crying; if in doubt, consult the doctor.

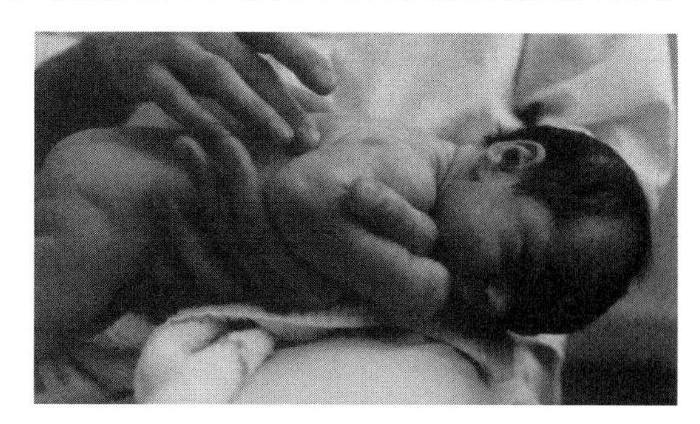

Comforting a baby with colic

Possible complications:
- If milk is introduced too early into the baby's diet following a bout of gastro-enteritis, lactose intolerance may occur and this could cause colic.

Cow's milk protein intolerance

What is it? Cow's milk protein intolerance is an inability to digest the protein in cow's milk. It is *not* an allergy.

Cause: The cause is not known. The problem usually appears between one week and several months after a baby starts on cow's milk.

Signs and symptoms:
- Diarrhoea and/or vomiting, which occurs soon after the introduction of cow's milk into the diet.

What to do:
- Call a doctor if symptoms persist for 24 hours.
- Offer a substitute milk, recommended by a doctor, and exclude all cow's milk and cow's milk products from the baby's diet for about two weeks.

General care:
- After two weeks a trial amount of cow's milk is offered under medical supervision; if the symptoms recur, the diagnosis is confirmed.
- Babies under 1 year may require a milk substitute, in which the cow's milk proteins are broken down into smaller, more easily digested components.
- Breastfeeding mothers are advised to exclude or to reduce dairy products from their diet.
- The cow's milk trial will be repeated every three months, until the baby no longer has an adverse reaction to the protein. The amount of milk given can then be increased over time.

Possible complications:
- By the age of three years, the intolerance to protein in cow's milk usually disappears.
- If not diagnosed early, there is a possibility of failure to thrive (see page 99).

Cradle cap (Seborrhoeic dermatitis)

What is it? Cradle cap is a chronic, recurring condition caused by inflammation of skin glands. It is similar to dandruff in adults.

Cause: There is no known cause.

Signs and symptoms:
- Thick, crusty, yellow scales over the baby's scalp. (Similar scales may also be found on the eyelids, ear, around the nose, and in the groin.) ➲

➲ Cradle cap (Seborrhoeic dermatitis) continued

- Cradle cap may be seen in new-borns and small children up to the age of three years.
- It is not contagious, it is not caused by poor hygiene, it is not an allergy, and it is not dangerous.
- It may or may not itch. If itching is present, excessive scratching of the area may cause additional inflammation and breaks in skin may cause mild infections or bleeding.

What to do:
- Massage the scalp and crust areas with olive oil.
- Allow the oil to soak in overnight.
- The next morning, gently comb the hair to remove the crusts.
- Use a mild shampoo to wash the oil away.

General care:
- If the treatment does not work, ask the pharmacist for a specialist shampoo or lotion.
- Avoid the use of soap on affected areas.

Possible complications:
- **Impetigo** (see page 212) may result if the skin becomes infected.

Croup

What is it? Croup is inflammation and narrowing of the main airway to the lungs. It mainly affects babies and children between 6 months and 3 years of age.

Cause: Usually caused by a virus, but occasionally an allergy.

Signs and symptoms:
- Usually starts with common cold signs – runny nose and sneezing.
- Noisy, rasping breathing.
- Hoarse voice.
- Persistent cough which sounds like a dog barking.
- Usually occurs in the early morning and lasts for a few hours

In severe cases, there may also be:
- difficulty in breathing – indrawing between or below the ribs with breathing
- restlessness and lots of saliva
- irritability
- blueness of the lips or face.

What to do:
- Create a warm humid atmosphere – take the child into the bathroom and run the hot taps to create steam; or spray the hot shower against the sides of a bath, making sure the baby is safe from scalding. Alternatively, use a kettle to boil water continuously. When the attack has subsided, put the child back in bed and try to create a moist atmosphere in the bedroom – for example, by draping a very damp towel near a hot radiator.
- If the symptoms persist and the child shows signs of cyanosis or difficulty in breathing, **call the doctor**.
- Give paracetamol syrup and plenty of warm drinks.
- Cuddle and reassure the child, who is usually very frightened.

General care:
- Any baby with croup should be seen by the doctor to exclude **epiglottitis**, which is potentially fatal (see page 201).
- Sometimes the attack of croup is a one-off event; however, at the first signs of a cold, humidify the child's bedroom. Vaporisers can be bought from pharmacies and are very effective. ➲

➲ Croup continued

- Karvol capsules or Olbas oil may be used in a vaporiser.

Possible complications:
- Children with asthma are prone to attacks of croup and may require special asthma preventer drugs at the first signs of a croup attack.

Failure to thrive

What is it? Failure to thrive is the general description used for a baby who does not gain weight at the expected rate – that is, according to the centile charts. To thrive means to grow well.

Causes: There are many possible reasons for failure to thrive. These include:
- **Genetic factors**. Small parents generally have babies who are small and who grow into small children.
- **Under-feeding**. Babies need 150 mls of milk per kg of their body weight every day. If they receive less than the required amount, they will not gain weight satisfactorily. Some reasons for under-feeding include:
  - First-time parents who are feeding their baby 'on demand' may not give enough food as babies do not always cry when they are hungry and may appear satisfied.
  - Babies of low birth weight actually need more calories than those of normal birth weight. (They need to make up for losing out on the valuable nutrients provided in the womb.)
  - Some premature babies tire easily when feeding and may sleep for longer periods.
  - Some babies have sucking difficulties caused by cleft lip and palate.
- **Difficulties with absorbing food**. Certain disorders interfere with the absorption of vital nutrients from food. These include:
  - Cow's milk intolerance (see page 97).
  - Cystic fibrosis (see page 154).
  - Coeliac disease (see page 95).
- **Physical disorders**. Although rare, certain physical conditions may result in failure to thrive. These include:
  - Heart disorders.
  - Pyloric stenosis (see page 106).
- **Infection**. Any infectious illness can temporarily affect the baby's ability to thrive. These include:
  - Infections of the ear, nose and throat.
  - Gastro-enteritis.
  - Urinary tract infections.
  - Whooping cough.
- **Emotional and social factors**. The provision of a safe, secure and happy home environment is essential to a child's health and well-being. Difficulties include:
  - *Neglect*. This may be intentional – a form of child abuse – or unintentional, for example, resulting from poor parenting skills or lack of support, such as the mother or main carer making up the feeds incorrectly.
  - *Difficult mother–baby relationship.* **Bonding** and **attachment** may be poor, or the mother may experience post-natal depression.
  - *Financial problems.* Parents living in poverty may find it difficult to meet all the needs of a young baby. ➲

➲ Failure to thrive continued

– *Lack of stimulation.* A baby who is left alone for long periods will probably also be under-fed and will lack the stimulation and loving attention needed for healthy growth and development.

Signs and symptoms:
- Failure to thrive is usually noticed by health visitors and doctors at the child health clinic. Health visitors may visit the home to check on a child's health if the parent does not attend the clinic.

What to do:
- Determine the cause of the baby's failure to gain weight as expected. Find out the answers to the following questions:
  – Is the baby developing according to the accepted norms of holistic development – physically, intellectually, emotionally and socially?
  – How big are the baby's parents – and grandparents?
  – Was the baby born prematurely or termed 'light-for-dates'?
  – How often – and how much milk – is the baby taking each day?
  – Has the baby been diagnosed with any digestive disorder or infectious illness?
  – What are the nappies like – for example, is the baby producing 'abnormal' stools?
  – What is the relationship like between the baby and the primary carers?
  – Has the mother or main carer any difficulties in the relationship with the baby?

General care:
- Once the cause for the condition has been determined, appropriate care will be offered.
- Regular monitoring of the baby's weight will be carried out at a child health clinic.
- Dietary problems are discussed and advice given to maintain a nutritionally balanced diet.
- Any physical condition or illness will need to be treated; for example, a baby diagnosed with cow's milk protein intolerance will be offered substitute milk.
- Health visitors regularly monitor the growth and development of babies who fail to thrive.
- Social workers will provide extra support for families and carers who are experiencing difficulties.

Possible complications: If the baby's failure to thrive is caused by an underlying medical or physical problem, then the complications of that condition may occur. If the problem is due to physical or emotional neglect, an investigation will be started by the Child Protection Team of the Social Services Department.

Gastro-enteritis

What is it? Gastro-enteritis is inflammation of the stomach and intestines, causing diarrhoea and/or vomiting.

Cause: In babies, the usual cause is a virus – transmitted through the air or by contact with infected faeces. Bacteria in food or drinks can also cause gastro-enteritis.

Signs and symptoms:
- Diarrhoea.
- Vomiting.
- Reluctance to feed.
- Abdominal pain: the baby may draw the knees up.
- Fever.
- Generally unwell and lethargic. 

➲ Gastro-enteritis continued

What to do:
- Call a doctor immediately if the baby is under three months old, and you suspect gastro-enteritis. Vomiting and diarrhoea in a young baby can lead to dehydration (see page 83).
- Prevent dehydration by giving the baby a **rehydrating solution**. You can make this by adding two level teaspoons of sugar to 200 ml of boiled water that has been allowed to cool. Babies who are entirely breastbed should be given rehydrating solution before the breast feed.
- If there is no improvement within 24 hours, call the doctor.

General care:
- Gradually introduce the baby's normal diet as the symptoms subside.
- Ensure that principles of hygiene are strictly followed (see pages 44–48).

Possible complications:
- Dehydration due to loss of body salts through vomiting and diarrhoea is a serious complication in babies – and can be fatal.

Heat rash

What is it? Heat rash is a rash of very tiny clear or red bumps on the skin. It is most common in babies and very young children, but can occur at any age.

Cause: Heat rash is caused by over-heating, such as wearing too many clothes in warm weather. The pores leading to the sweat glands become blocked. With an increase in heat and humidity, the sweat glands attempt to provide sweat as they would normally, but because of the blockage, this sweat is held within the skin and forms little red bumps – or occasionally small blisters – in babies.

Signs and symptoms:
- An itchy rash usually appears on the baby's chest or back, or other areas of heavy perspiration, for example the neck, face and skin folds; the rash may look like:
  - lots of small red bumps, or
  - clusters of fluid-filled skin blisters.

What to do:
- Cool the baby by removing layers of clothing.
- Offer frequent tepid baths – this can be very soothing.

General care:
- Apply Calamine lotion or cream to relieve the itching.
- Dress the baby in appropriate clothing for the weather and the room temperature – several light layers are better than one warm layer.

Possible complications:
- The rash should disappear within a few hours.
- If the rash persists after cooling the baby down, then seek medical aid to rule out other possible causes.

Hypothermia

What is it? Hypothermia is low body temperature – below 35 °C (95 °F). In babies, it is sometimes called neonatal cold injury.

New-born babies are particularly susceptible to chilling for the following reasons:
- In relation to body weight they have an unusually large surface area from which to lose heat.
- The surface of the body is wet at birth and heat will be lost by evaporation if there is any delay over drying the baby. ➲

➲ Hypothermia continued

- In both pre-term and light-for-dates babies, the layer of insulating fat immediately under the skin is insufficient to prevent heat loss.
- Shivering is one of the body mechanisms for maintaining or raising the body temperature. The new-born baby does not have this adaptive mechanism.
- It takes several days for the baby's metabolism and heat production to function adequately.
- Some new-born babies tend to be drowsy and inactive during the early days of life. Activities such as feeding, crying and limb movements normally increase heat production.

Hypothermia can occur in older babies and young children too – usually following exposure to extreme cold weather or falling into cold water.

Cause: There are many causes for a baby losing body heat:

- A cold room.
  - New-born babies require a room temperature of 24 °C (75 °F);
  - During the first few weeks, the room temperature should be maintained (day and night) at a temperature of 20 °C (68 °F).
- Bathing a baby in a cool room
- Not wearing a hat in cold weather: babies lose a lot of body heat through the head.

Signs and symptoms:

- Skin feels cold to the touch; often this is first noticed when the baby comes into contact with the mother's cheek or breast.
- Feet and fingers are often cooler than the rest of the baby, but in hypothermia the tummy, limbs and even the nape of the neck feel cold to the touch.
- The baby may *look* healthy, with rosy cheeks and red hands, so it is important to touch the nape of the neck to determine the temperature.
- May be quiet and difficult to rouse from sleep.
- Difficult to feed.
- Hands and feet may be swollen; occasionally the baby's eyelids may also be swollen.

What to do:

- Call the doctor.
- Warm the baby *gradually*:
  - Raise the temperature of the room as quickly as possible.
  - Cuddle the baby close to you, so that your warmth is transferred to the baby.
  - Put a hat on the baby's head.
  - Wrap the baby loosely in a warm blanket; avoid putting too many layers on the baby as these will only insulate the baby from the surrounding warmth.
  - Encourage the baby to feed.

NOTE: Never apply heat directly to the baby. For example, if you use a hot water bottle to heat the baby's cot, remove it before putting the baby in.

General care:

- Prevention of hypothermia.
  - Keep room temperature constant at around 20 °C. A wall thermometer is useful.
  - Dress the baby in appropriate clothes for the weather; a hat should always be worn outside in cold weather.
  - Always bath the baby in a warm room and dry and dress them quickly afterwards.

Possible complications:

- Severe hypothermia (a body temperature of below 32 °C) can lead to unconsciousness and even death.

Lactose intolerance

What is it? Lactose intolerance is an intolerance to lactose – the sugar found in milk. It is *not* an allergy.

Cause: Lactose intolerance is caused by an inability to break down the lactose in the small intestine, because of a deficiency of the necessary enzyme. It can also develop as a complication of gastro-enteritis or coeliac disease. Some permanent lactose intolerance is genetic in origin and is common in people of African or Asian descent.

Signs and symptoms:
- Diarrhoea and/or vomiting soon after drinking or eating foods containing lactose.

What to do:
- See the doctor. He or she will give the baby a test dose of lactose and then examine the faeces to see whether an excessive amount of the sugar has passed through the intestines without being absorbed.

General care:
- A dietician will devise a lactose-free diet for the baby. This may include certain fermented milk products , such as yoghurt, but will exclude milk itself.

Possible complications:
- If not diagnosed early, lactose intolerance can result in **failure to thrive**.

Meningitis

What is it? Meningitis is an inflammation of the lining of the brain. It is a very serious illness, but if detected and treated early, most children make a full recovery.

Cause: Meningitis is usually caused by an infection that can be bacterial or viral. The bacteria are carried quite harmlessly at the back of the throat by about 1 in 10 of the general population (and as many as 1 in 4 teenagers). It is spread via tiny droplets of fluid we breathe or cough out into the air around us.
Bacterial meningitis can occur at any time of year, but the less serious viral meningitis (affecting mostly children *over* five years old) tends to peak in winter.

Signs and symptoms: In babies under 12 months look for the following:
- Tense or bulging fontanelles.
- Blotchy or pale skin.
- High temperature.
- Refuses feed.
- A stiffening body with involuntary movements, or a floppy body.
- A high-pitched, moaning cry.
- The baby being difficult to wake.
- Red or purple spots (anywhere on the body) that do not fade under pressure – do the 'Glass Test'. See page 104.

In older children, look for the following symptoms:
- Headache.
- Fever.
- Neck stiffness and joint pains; the child may arch the neck backwards because of the rigidity of the neck muscles.
- Inability to tolerate light.

One or more of the following symptoms may indicate **septicaemia**:
- High temperature – above 39 °C/102.2 °F, which becomes difficult to control with fluids and infant paracetamol (suitable from three months). ➲

➲ Meningitis continued

The 'Glass Test'

Press the side or bottom of a glass firmly against the rash – you will be able to see if the rash fades and loses colour under the pressure. If it *doesn't* change colour, summon medical aid immediately.

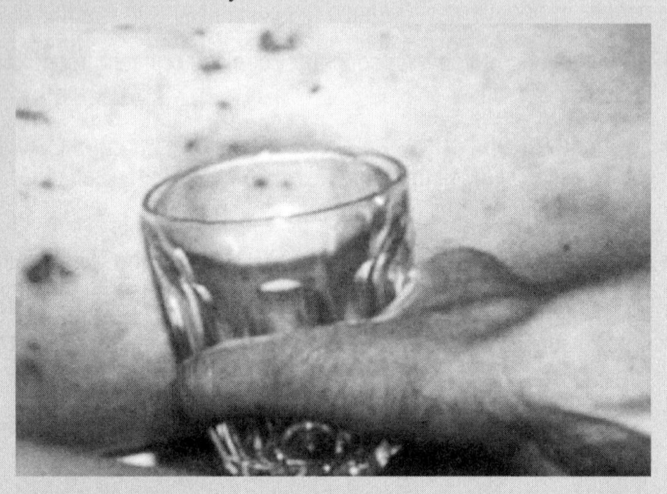

NOTE: If spots are appearing on the baby's body, this could be septicaemia, a bacterial infection described as the 'meningitis rash'.

- Severe or repeated vomiting.
- Pain in joints and muscles.
- Cold hands and feet.
- Drowsiness, irritability and agitation.
- Rapid breathing.
- Blank and staring expression.
- **The meningitis rash**. A pin-prick red rash, that doesn't disappear under the glass tumbler test, and develops into purple bruises. These marks can spread very quickly. **Summon medical aid immediately**.

What to do:

- **Call an ambulance immediately** if you notice these signs or symptoms, or take the child to the nearest hospital accident and emergency department – whichever is quicker.
- If you call the GP in less serious cases, describe the signs and symptoms in full. You may be asked to go straight to the surgery or to the nearest hospital accident and emergency department.
- While waiting for the ambulance or doctor, comfort and reassure the child in a darkened room and try to reduce the fever (see page 81).
- The most immediate form of treatment is antibiotics given in high dosages.

General care:

- The child will be admitted to hospital urgently and given antibiotics **intravenously**.
- A **lumbar puncture** will determine the cause of the infection. (If it is found to be viral meningitis, the antibiotics will be discontinued.)
- Family members and anyone else who has been in close contact with the child may also be offered antibiotics to kill any bacteria being carried and to prevent the disease spreading. ➲

➲ Meningitis continued

Possible complications:
- Children who contract bacterial meningitis and are promptly treated usually recover fully.
- In a minority of cases, deafness or brain damage may occur.
- Rarely the illness may prove fatal, even when treated promptly.
- Viral meningitis does not require any specific treatment and usually clears up within a few weeks.

Prevention of meningitis:
- The Hib vaccine is given routinely as part of the immunisation programme. It protects against the *haemophilus influenzae* strain of the disease.
- A recent addition to the immunisation programme is the vaccine against *Meningitis C* – the strain that causes septicaemia (see page 103).
- Even with these immunisations, there are many other forms of meningitis that cannot yet be eradicated.

Milk spots

What are milk spots? Milk spots (or **milia**) are seen frequently in new-born infants. They appear as pearly white bumps on the cheeks, nose, and chin. They are not itchy and do not worry the baby at all.

Cause: Milk spots are caused when the sebaceous glands in the new-born baby's skin become blocked; this is because the glands are immature.

Signs and symptoms:
- Tiny, white-headed bumps on the face of a new-born baby.

What to do and general care:
- None needed. Milk spots are quite normal and disappear within a few weeks.

Possible complications:
- On rare occasions milk spots may become infected and require further treatment from the GP.

Nappy rash

What is it? Any rash on the skin area covered by a nappy.

Cause: It is usually caused by prolonged contact with moisture, bacteria, and ammonia. The ammonia and other skin irritants are made by the action of bacteria from bowel movements on certain chemicals in the urine. Bouts of diarrhoea cause rashes in most children.

Signs and symptoms:
- A sore nappy area.
- Red, raw spots in the nappy area.
- Blisters and weals in the nappy area.
- A strong smell of ammonia when you change the baby's nappy.
- The baby cries when the nappy is dirty or when being changed.

What to do: Call a GP or health visitor immediately *if*:
- a fever occurs with a bad-looking nappy rash
- the rash isn't almost better in 2–3 days
- the nappy rash becomes bright red or raw
- pimples, blisters, boils, sores, or crusts develop
- the baby appears very unwell
- you have other concerns or questions. 

➲ Nappy rash continued

General care: The key to successful treatment is keeping the area dry and clean so that it can heal itself.

- **Check the nappy about every hour**. If it is wet or soiled, change it immediately. Exposure to faeces causes most of the skin damage. Make sure that the baby's bottom is completely dry before fastening the fresh nappy.
- **Increase air exposure**. Leave the baby's bottom exposed to the air as much as possible each day. Practical times are during naps or after bowel movements. Put a towel or nappy under the baby.
- **Avoid airtight plastic pants for a few days**. When the nappy is on, fasten it loosely so that air can circulate between it and the skin. If you use disposable nappies, punch holes in the plastic layer to allow air to circulate.
- **Rinse the skin with warm water**. Washing the skin with soap after every nappy change will damage the skin. Use a mild soap *only* after bowel movements. The soap will remove the film of bacteria left on the skin. After using a soap, rinse well. If the nappy rash is quite raw, use warm water soaks for 15 minutes three times a day.
- **Night-time care**. At night use the new disposable nappies that are made with materials that lock wetness inside the nappy and away from the skin. Avoid plastic pants at night. Until the rash is better, wake at least once during the night to change the baby's nappy.
- **Using creams and powders**. Most babies don't need any nappy cream. However, if the baby's skin is dry and cracked, apply an ointment to protect the skin after you wash off each bowel movement. A barrier ointment is also needed whenever the baby has diarrhoea. Avoid talcum powder because of the risk of pneumonia if the baby inhales it.

Prevention of nappy rash:

- Changing the nappy *immediately* after the baby has a bowel movement and rinsing the skin with warm water are the most effective things you can do to prevent nappy rash.
- If you use towelling nappies and wash them yourself, you will need to use bleach to sterilise them. During the regular cycle, use any detergent. Then refill the washer with warm water, add 1 cup of bleach, and run a second cycle. Unlike bleach, vinegar is not effective in killing germs.

Possible complications:

- With proper treatment nappy rashes are usually better in 3 days.
- If they do not respond to the initial treatment, a yeast infection (Candida) has probably occurred. Suspect this if the rash becomes bright red and raw, covers a large area, and is surrounded by red dots. A special anti-fungal cream will be prescribed.

Pyloric stenosis

What is it? Pyloric stenosis is the narrowing of the outlet (pylorus) from the stomach into the small intestine. It is an uncommon condition that occurs in babies less than two months old and results in allowing only a small amount of feed to enter the intestine – the remainder being vomited.

Cause: The cause is unknown, but the condition occurs more often in boys than girls in a ratio of five to one.

Signs and symptoms:

- In most cases, babies will begin by bringing up small amounts of milk after feeds; this will gradually get worse, until the baby can no longer keep any milk down.
- Persistent projectile vomiting – the baby will vomit the feed *several metres* across the room. ➲

➲ Pyloric stenosis continued

- The baby is constantly hungry and will often want to feed again immediately after vomiting.
- Constipation or infrequent bowel movements.
- Weight loss and general signs of **failure to thrive**.
- Dehydration due to the fluid not being absorbed in the intestine.

What to do:
- Contact the doctor, who will examine the baby (while feeding) to feel for the thickened pylorus; this can be felt as a small, hard lump on the side of the abdomen.
- Offer small amounts of feed to prevent over-filling the stomach.

General care:
- If pyloric stenosis is suspected, an ultrasound examination will be performed in hospital and the baby will be admitted for surgery.
- A minor surgical operation relieves the obstruction by widening the pylorus; intravenous fluids are given if the baby is dehydrated.

Possible complications:
- There are usually no ill-effects after an operation and normal feeding is generally re-established within 2 to 3 days. The condition does not recur.

Squint

What is it? A squint is when the eyes do not look in the same direction at the same time.

Cause: Babies under the age of 3–4 months often squint because the mechanism that co-ordinates the eyes is not fully developed. A squint in older children is often due to long-sightedness.

Signs and symptoms:
- When the baby is looking directly at an object, you notice:
  - an eye that turns too far in – a convergent squint
  - an eye that turns too far out – a divergent squint
  - an eye that turns up or down – a vertical squint.

What to do:
- See a doctor if the baby is older than 4 months and you notice a squint.
- Be aware that a baby with a wide bridge to the nose can appear to have a squint when there is none.

General care:
- If a squint is diagnosed, the baby will be referred to an ophthalmologist, who may prescribe:
  - eye exercises
  - patching the unaffected eye to encourage use of the squinting (or 'lazy') eye
  - an operation to correct the squint surgically.

Possible complications:
- As long as treatment is provided soon after a squint appearing, the baby's vision should develop normally.

Sticky eyes

What is it? Sticky eyes is the name given to **conjunctivitis** in young babies. It is a mild inflammation of the conjunctiva – the membrane covering the eyeball – and is just like having a cold in the eye. It can affect one or both eyes.

Cause: Sticky eyes is usually caused when the narrow tear ducts are underdeveloped or blocked, providing a warm, moist area for bacteria to flourish. It can also result from the spread of infection from the mother's cervix during birth. ➲

➲ Sticky eyes continued

Signs and symptoms:
- There may be a thick white or yellow discharge from the eyes.
- The baby's eyes are often stuck together in the morning.
- There may be redness around the eye area.
- If the tear ducts are blocked, then the eyes will be constantly watering.

What to do:
- Bathe the eyes in warm water or saline to wash away the discharge and remove any crusts on the eyelids. Use a fresh cotton swab for each eye, and wipe from the inner to the outer corner of the eye. Try using a weak saline solution made by dissolving one teaspoon of regular cooking salt in 600 ml/1pt of warm previously boiled water.
- If both eyes are affected, consult the doctor, who may prescribe antibiotic drops or cream. The baby's eyes should clear up within a day, but continue to use the cream for 24 hours after the eyes have cleared. If, after two or three days, there is no improvement, go back to the doctor.

General care:
- If the condition results from a blocked tear duct, the doctor will recommend frequent massaging of the affected duct (see below).
  - Using the tip of a very clean forefinger, gently massage the tear duct at the inner part of the eyelid, by the bridge of the nose. Repeat four to five times a day.

Possible complications:
- Blocked tear ducts which persist after the first year of life will need treatment (under anaesthetic) by an ophthalmic surgeon.

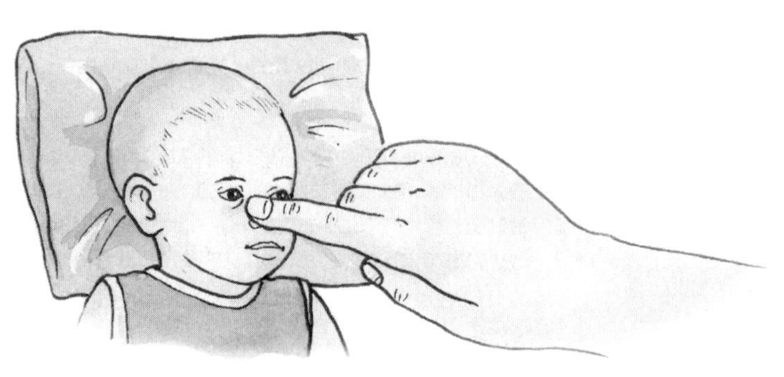

Massaging an affected tear duct

Sudden infant death syndrome (SIDS)

What is it? The sudden, unexplainable death of a baby under 1 year old is called sudden infant death syndrome (SIDS). It is also known as 'cot death.'
Typically, a death from SIDS happens without warning between midnight and 8 a.m. when a baby is thought to be asleep, and the baby dies very quickly, without any apparent suffering. Ninety per cent of SIDS deaths involve babies under 6 months old. The most vulnerable age appears to be between 2 months and 4 months old. Male babies are at slightly greater risk.

Cause: The exact cause of SIDS is not known. Experts think it probably results from the combination of at least one inborn factor with other factors. Researchers are investigating several theories:

1 One theory involves prenatal events, such as implanting of the placenta low in the uterus or separation of the placenta before birth, which may damage the part of the infant's brain that controls breathing during sleep. ➲

➲ Sudden infant death syndrome (SIDS) continued

2 Another possible cause is an abnormality of the baby's immune system and a **metabolic** disorder.
3 Some researchers believe it may be due to a stomach 'bug', such as helicobacter pylori.
4 Another theory is that compression in a baby's neck arteries may lead to breathing trouble and, thus, to SIDS; a baby may suffer from artery compression when he or she moves during sleep to try to clear bedding or other material from their nose. This may help explain why sleeping on their stomach increases infants' risk of SIDS. Arterial compression may also be caused by a change in blood flow due to overheating, or exposure to cigarette smoke.

Risk factors:
- Placing a baby to sleep on his or her back **reduces** the risk.
- Exposing a baby to cigarette smoke or overheating a baby **increases** the risk.

How to prevent sudden infant death syndrome

- Always place a baby on the back or side to sleep.
- Don't smoke and avoid smoky atmospheres.
- Don't let a baby get too hot and don't overheat the room (18–20 °C).
- Keep a baby's head uncovered in bed. Place the baby's feet at the end of the cot to prevent the baby wriggling under the covers (see below).
- If you think the baby is unwell, contact the doctor.

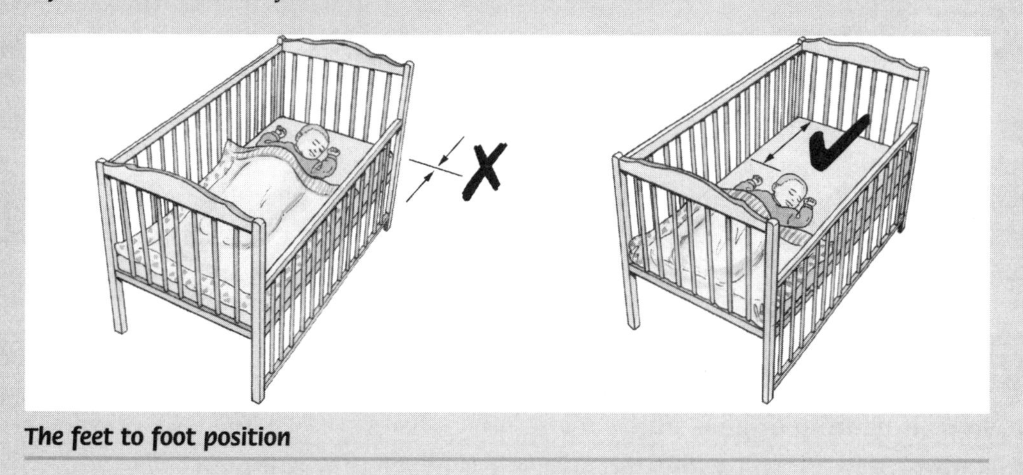

The feet to foot position

Other safety tips:
- Avoid plastic sheets or bumpers, ribbons and bits of string from mobiles. If they're anywhere near the baby, he or she could get tangled in them.
- If the baby is a natural tummy sleeper, keep turning him or her over and tuck in securely with blankets (as long as the weather is not too hot); a musical mobile may help to keep the baby happy while lying on the back.
- If the baby is snuffly or has a blocked nose, place a small pillow under the head end of the mattress, but make sure the baby does not slide down under the covers to the end of the cot.
- Make sure there's no gap between the cot mattress and the sides of the cot through which the baby's body could slip. This is particularly important if you replace the ➲

Sudden infant death syndrome (SIDS) continued

mattress with a new or second-hand one. If you *do* use a second-hand mattress, make sure that it is firm, clean and dry, well aired and generally in good condition.

- Remove any loose plastic covering from the mattress that could come off and smother the baby.
- Don't put the baby to sleep on a bean bag, water bed, sheepskin mattress or other materials that may interfere with the baby's breathing — such as pillows, blankets, comforters, quilts, fluffy bedding or stuffed toys — and don't put such materials on or around the baby.
- Don't give a baby under the age of one a pillow.
- Don't let anyone fall asleep nursing a baby.
- Don't let the baby fall asleep propped up on a cushion on a sofa or armchair.

Controlling the temperature/preventing overheating

- Small babies cannot control their own temperature. It's just as important to avoid them getting too hot as it is to avoid them getting chilled. Overheating is known to be a factor in cot death.
- If the room is warm enough for you to be comfortable wearing light clothing (18–20 °C), then it is the right temperature for the baby. A simple wall thermometer can help (see below).
- Give the baby one light layer of clothing (or bedding) more than you're wearing. If the room is hot for *you*, keep the baby's clothes or bed covering light.
- Do not use duvets (quilts) until the baby is one year old. They get too hot.
- Although it is fine to take the baby into your bed for comfort, a baby falling asleep under your duvet may get too hot.
- Keep the baby's head uncovered indoors (unless it's *very* cold) because a baby needs to lose heat from his or her head and face.
- Never use a hot water bottle or electric blanket. Babies have a delicate skin, which can scald, or burn, easily.
- Ill or feverish babies don't need any extra bedding. In fact they usually need less.
- Remove hats and extra clothing as soon as you come indoors or enter a warm car, bus or train, even if it means waking the baby.

Urgent medical attention is needed if the baby:

- **Stops breathing or goes blue**
- **Is unresponsive and shows no awareness of what is going on**
- **Has glazed eyes and does not focus on anything**
- **Cannot be woken**
- **Has a seizure or fit**

DIAL 999 AND ASK FOR AN AMBULANCE

Further information: If a baby in your care ever stops breathing, you should call for emergency help and perform **cardiopulmonary resuscitation (CPR)**. Learn and practise on a special baby resuscitation mannequin how to perform artificial ventilation and cardiac massage (see colour section after page 236). ➲

Sudden infant death syndrome (SIDS) continued

While there is no treatment for the victims of SIDS, there *is* support for the grieving parents and family. If a baby in 'your' family dies from SIDS, you will probably need a lot of emotional support. The sudden death of a baby can be especially hard simply because it is so unexpected and you do not have time to prepare for it or to say goodbye. Finding the baby after he or she dies can be very traumatic, too.

Many parents feel guilty about their baby's SIDS death. Often they experience disbelief, denial, numbness and anger. Some become depressed. All these emotions can be compounded by the need for investigations into the cause of death.

Many parents who lose a child to SIDS fear that someone else in the family is in danger. This may lead them to be especially protective of their other children or to be fearful that SIDS will happen again in their family. But SIDS is a **rare medical problem** – it will not necessarily occur again in the same family, and it does not affect older children. In families that have lost a baby to SIDS, it can be important to reassure the baby's siblings that SIDS can't happen to them.

The CONI support scheme

CONI (Care of the Next Infant) is a scheme developed by the **Foundation for the Study of Infant Deaths** to provide organised support for families who have suffered a loss of a child through cot death. Families who have suffered the loss of a baby in this way feel greater anxiety when expecting their next baby; the CONI programme ensures that their baby will be under increased surveillance during the first few months of life and that extra support will be given if there is a problem. Parents are offered:

- weekly visits from their health visitor
- the loan of an apnoea monitor, which records the baby's breathing movements or electronic scales for daily weighing – whichever they prefer
- tuition in resuscitation skills and the significance of temperature, smoking and positioning the baby on the back
- a daily diary to record symptoms
- additional support from their family doctor (GP) and paediatrician.

CONI is usually offered to parents for a minimum of six months, or two months longer than the age at which their baby died.

Coping with sudden infant death in a day nursery

Most typically the baby is found dead at home, either first thing in the morning or after a period, often very brief, of being left alone in their cot or pram. Unfortunately, sudden infant death does sometimes occur while babies have been sleeping in their day nursery cot or while in the care of a nanny or childminder. You need to know how to deal with such an event, and in particular how to respond to parents. If a baby is pale and unresponsive when you attempt to rouse him or her from a nap:

- check for breathing and pulse and if they are absent:
- **start cardio-pulmonary resuscitation (CPR) immediately** – see colour section after page 236
- call an ambulance
- ask a colleague to remove all other children to an area well away from the ill child
- contact the parents and explain that the baby is very ill and that the ambulance has been called. Suggest that they go directly to the hospital.

If you are a nanny or childminder working on your own, start CPR, and carry the baby **continuing resuscitation** while you wait for the ambulance to arrive.

When any baby (or adult) dies suddenly and unexpectedly, a post mortem has to be carried out to find the cause of death. Police are automatically contacted by the ambulance staff and will need to take evidence from the home or nursery, including taking statements from the people directly involved. ➲

Sudden infant death syndrome (SIDS) continued

Support for child care workers Anyone directly involved in the death of a baby will be severely affected. It is important to share your feelings with other staff members, so that you can work through your grief together. People on the outside often don't appreciate the depth of the loss you have experienced and expect you to get over it fairly quickly. The Foundation for Sudden Infant Deaths and The Child Bereavement Trust can help by providing counsellors.

Thrush

What is it? Thrush is an infection that commonly develops in the mouth of babies and young children. It sometimes appears around the anus, buttocks and thighs.

Cause: Thrush is caused by a yeast-like fungus called *Candida albicans*. It lives naturally on the skin and in the vagina, mouth and bowel, alongside other bacteria that the body needs. This natural balance can be disturbed when illness or a course of antibiotics affects the body's immune system. This allows the candida to flourish, and once this happens it quickly multiples, damaging mucus membranes and causing inflammation.

Signs and symptoms:
- Spots inside the baby's cheeks that look like the remains of milk which, when wiped gently with a tissue, reveal a sore red patch beneath.
- White spots on a red rash starting around the anus, which spreads to the buttocks and inner thighs.
- A bright red nappy rash that isn't helped by normal creams.
- The baby may refuse feeds.

What to do:
- Consult the doctor, who will prescribe:
  - An anti-fungal gel or liquid to be dropped into the baby's mouth after every feed. The sores should start to improve within a day or two.
  - An anti-fungal cream for the mother's nipples if she is breastfeeding. This should always be washed off before breastfeeding.
  - An anti-fungal cream for the bottom area if the baby has nappy rash. The sores should start to clear up within two or three days.

General care:
- If the baby finds it painful to feed from a bottle or finds it hard to suck from the breast, try feeding by spoon.
- Wash your hands scrupulously after nappy changes and before feeds.
- If the thrush develops during a course of antibiotics, finish the treatment but use anti-fungal medication at the same time.
- An alternative treatment for oral thrush is the homeopathic remedy Borax 6c at the first sign of infection. Give it four times a day for up to five days.

Possible complications:
- If none of the anti-fungal treatments work, consult the GP again because a secondary bacterial infection may have set in on top of the thrush.

Umbilical hernia

What is it? An umbilical hernia is a protruding navel that bulges with crying or straining.

Cause: It is caused by a weakness in the abdominal wall allowing a small loop of intestine to protrude through at the navel.

Signs and symptoms:
- A soft swelling either at the navel or slightly above the navel; it usually appears within a few weeks of birth. (See below.) ➲

➲ Umbilical hernia continued

- The bulge may not be present in the morning, but may reappear during the day; it may also disappear when the baby is quiet.
- The bulge is more noticeable when the baby cries or tenses the abdomen.
- It is completely painless.
- If you feel the area with your finger, you will find a small round opening in the muscles of the abdominal wall. The hernia passes through this ring.

What to do:
- Umbilical hernias are very common. No immediate treatment is required and the hernia usually disappears by the baby's first birthday.

General care:
- Crying does not make hernias any bigger or last any longer. They are not painful and they never break.
- The opening in the muscles usually closes spontaneously by school age. Half of the persistent ones close by adolescence.
- No treatment is needed unless the hernia persists beyond the age of 5 or 6 years. At that age, outpatient surgery can be performed to close the defect if the child is concerned about how it looks or if the muscle defect is more than 2 centimetres (about 1 inch) across.
- Taping a hernia closed does not speed healing and can lead to a skin rash or infection.

Possible complications:
- The only complication (which occurs in far less than 1 per cent of cases) is getting a loop of intestine stuck in the opening. If you think this has happened (if, for instance, the hernia becomes hard and tender and cannot be pushed back in), call the doctor immediately. (This rare condition is a strangulated hernia.)

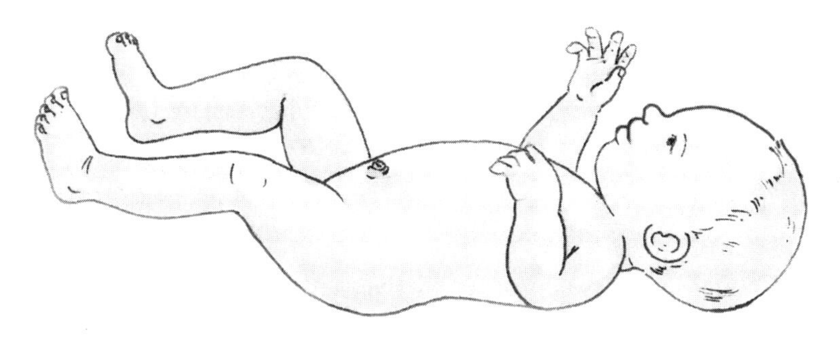

The swelling of the navel is a sign of umbilical hernia

Revision questions

1. What is heat rash – and how can it be prevented?
2. Describe the signs and symptoms of croup. How can you care for a child with croup?
3. What does 'failure to thrive' mean?
4. What is hypothermia and how may it be prevented? Why should babies and children with hypothermia be warmed very slowly?
5. List four measures which may help to prevent SIDS.

Chapter 6: The main conditions affecting children 1–8 years old

◆ *Blood and circulatory disorders* ◆ *Digestive tract and dietary disorders* ◆ *Ear disorders* ◆ *Emotional and behavioural problems* ◆ *Eye disorders* ◆ *Genetic disorders* ◆ *Infectious diseases* ◆ *Life-threatening conditions* ◆ *Muscle, bone and joint disorders* ◆ *Nervous system disorders* ◆ *Respiratory tract disorders* ◆ *Skin disorders* ◆ *Urinary tract disorders*

Blood and circulatory disorders

◆ *Anaemia* ◆ *Congenital heart disease* ◆ *Henoch-Schonlein purpura* ◆ *Thrombocytopoenia*

What are blood and circulatory disorders?

Disorders of the blood may affect the transport of oxygen around the body or the blood clotting mechanism. Most serious blood disorders are now treatable, even those such as **leukaemia**, which was once fatal. Congenital heart disorders are the most common serious birth defects. While many of these defects clear up naturally over time without treatment, others can be life-threatening and require surgery to repair the heart.

Anaemia

What is it? The term anaemia describes a shortage of the red blood cells (haemoglobin) that carry oxygen around the body. Anaemia is the most common of all the blood disorders.

Cause: The most common cause of anaemia in children is an insufficient amount of iron in the body to create adequate supplies of haemoglobin.

Signs and symptoms: A child may have no symptoms if the anaemia is mild. In more severe cases, symptoms include:

- Pale skin. **NOTE:** A dark-skinned child may appear paler around the mouth and lips and the conjunctiva of the eyes.
- Lack of energy.
- Shortness of breath on exertion.
- Brittle fingernails.
- Sore mouth or tongue.
- Headaches and occasional dizziness.

What to do:

- Consult a doctor, who will test the child's blood to confirm the diagnosis and its severity.
- If the cause is iron deficiency, the doctor will recommend a diet rich in iron – plenty of lean meat, liver, eggs and green vegetables.
- Babies will be given a milk formula enriched with iron.
- Iron may be prescribed in medicine form. ➲

General care:
- Encourage the child to eat a diet rich in iron.
- If the child does not eat meat, ensure that he or she is given plenty of green vegetables and see the doctor about iron supplements.

Possible complications:
- If left untreated, anaemia can lead to impaired mental development

Congenital heart disease

What is it? Congenital heart disease is a general term that is used to refer to a group of different heart abnormalities that a baby can be born with. The different abnormalities have different effects, but the kind of problems that they can lead to include a slow growth rate, difficulties with feeding and an abnormal breathing pattern.

Cause: Heart defects occur when something goes wrong with the development of the baby's heart in the first few weeks after conception. In the majority of cases, this is due to a combination of genetic and other factors (such as the mother having an infection in early pregnancy). Some heart defects can be detected antenatally by ultrasound scanning.

Types of heart defect: The most common types of congenital heart defect are:

1 **Ventricular septal defect**. A hole between the right and left ventricles which may close spontaneously.
2 **Aortic stenosis**. A narrowing between the left ventricle and the aorta.
3 **Atrial septal defect**. A hole between the right and left atrium. There are various types of this defect and some may close spontaneously.
4 **Patent ductus arteriosus**. The ductus arteriosus (a blood vessel that acts as a bypass in a baby's circulation before birth) does not close as it should in the first few weeks of life.
5 **Pulmonary stenosis**. A narrowing of the pulmonary valve opening.

Other rare defects, which result in more serious problems include:
- **Coarctation of the aorta**. A narrowing of the main artery.
- **Transposition of the great arteries**. The aorta and pulmonary artery are transposed so deoxygenated blood is circulated to the body and oxygenated blood back to the lungs.
- **Tetralogy of Fallot**. This is a combination of a hole between the two ventricles and narrowing between the right ventricle and pulmonary artery.

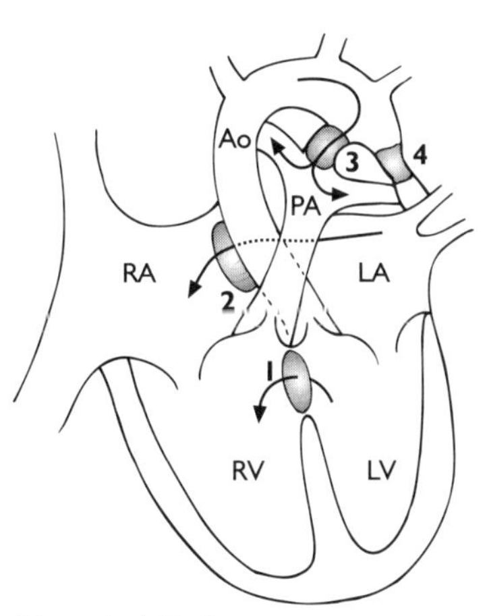

Abbreviations:
RA – Right atrium
LA – Left atrium
RV – Right ventricle
LV – Left ventricle
PA – Pulmonary artery
Ao – Aorta

Heart abnormalities illustrated:
1 – Ventricular septal defect
2 – Atrial septal defect
3 – Patent ductus arteriosus
4 – Coarctation of the aorta

Congenital heart defects

➲ Congenital heart disease continued

Signs and symptoms: Symptoms of congenital heart disease vary according to the nature and severity of the defects. Problems with the heart may be detected during routine medical examination of the new-born baby. Some defects are not diagnosed until later in childhood or even until adult life. Symptoms in children include:

- A heart murmur (abnormal heart sounds). This can be heard when the doctor listens to the baby's heart through a stethoscope. Most murmurs do not indicate congenital heart disease.
- Feeding problems and loss of weight in babies.
- Shortness of breath on exertion.
- Become tired very easily.
- Being particularly prone to infections.

What to do:

- Consult the doctor if you notice any of the symptoms listed above.
- Call the doctor immediately if you are aware that the child has congenital heart disease and notice any of the following symptoms: fever, lack of energy or a poor appetite – these could mean the child has an infection called bacterial endocarditis.

General care:

- Some defects do not need any treatment at all, while others can be treated medically (i.e. by giving drug therapy or medicines).
- The child will probably need to have an operation (surgery) to repair the defect. This is usually done during infancy, although in some cases it is not carried out until the child is older. Rarely, an operation needs to be done shortly after birth.
- The child will be monitored by a paediatrician or by a paediatric cardiologist (a children's heart specialist) and will also be assessed in hospital from time to time.
- Unless the defect is very complex, usually only *one* operation is needed.
- Try not to be too over-protective; many parents and carers find it difficult not to be over-protective, but it's actually better for the child if they are treated as normally as possible and are not too restricted in what they are allowed to do.
- Always ensure that the child completes any course of antibiotics because of the risk of bacterial endocarditis.
- Make sure that the child always carries a card (obtained from the doctor) stating that he or she has congenital heart disease.

Possible complications:

- In most cases ventricular septal defects close up on their own before the child is five years old.
- In cases where there is an affected child there is a slightly increased risk that future children may be affected. If two children are affected the future risk increases.
- In cases of specific syndromes – e.g. **Marfan's syndrome** or Down's syndrome (see page 154) – inheritance patterns will depend on the cause of the condition.

Further information:

- Children with congenital heart disease usually develop normally, but they may do certain things like sitting, crawling and walking later than other children.

Henoch-Schonlein purpura

What is it? Henoch-Schonlein purpura is a type of vasculitis – an inflammation of the blood vessels. The disease is fairly common in children between the ages of 2 and 10 years, and is not usually serious. ➲

➲ Henoch-Schonlein purpura continued

Cause: The cause of Henoch-Schonlein purpura is unknown. It often follows a viral respiratory infection and appears to be some kind of allergic reaction to the virus. It has also been seen following a streptococcal throat infection, prescription medicines, bee stings, chemical poisons, cold exposure, and food allergies. It can occur in epidemics and occurs most commonly between November and February.

Signs and symptoms: Tiny blood vessels in the skin swell and then haemorrhage (or bleed), giving rise to the characteristic rash of Henoch-Schonlein purpura.

The rash:

- usually begins with red bumps, which can appear anywhere on the body, but especially on the legs and buttocks
- is made up of swollen blood vessels, or bruises, that do not fade when pressed.
- is often itchy, because of the allergy
- consists of tiny bruises that heal and turn to a rust colour, and then fade. Each spot lasts for about five days
- often comes in several crops, and a single child may have a rash of a variety of different colours
- clears up leaving no trace.

Other symptoms include:

- Joint pain and swelling, particularly the knees and ankles.
- Abdominal pain, with vomiting and diarrhoea.
- Blood in the faeces.
- A low-grade fever, and just not feeling well, often accompanies it.

What to do:

- Consult a doctor within 24 hours of the onset of symptoms.
- The doctor may prescribe anti-inflammatory drugs to relieve the symptoms of abdominal pain.
- If symptoms are mild, no treatment is necessary and the child usually makes a complete recovery within 2 or 3 days.

General care:

- If the child is experiencing joint pain or abdominal pain, give paracetamol.
- Encourage the child to rest when feeling unwell.

Possible complications:

- Relapses may occur up to a year later (particularly after the child gets another cold or is re-exposed to the offending agent).
- The kidneys can remain inflamed for up to two years.

Further information: The order in which the symptoms appear varies. A child might have unexplained abdominal pain, or knee pain, or bloody stools, or blood in the urine for a week before other symptoms appear to bring the correct diagnosis into focus.

Thrombocytopoenia

What is it? Thrombocytopoenia is a condition where there is an abnormally low number of platelets in the blood. Platelets are essential for blood clotting.

Cause: The cause of thrombocytopoenia is unknown, but it usually develops within two weeks following a viral infection.

Signs and symptoms: The symptoms of this condition are caused by abnormal bleeding and include:

- A widespread flat, purple rash caused by bleeding into the skin; the rash does not disappear when pressed. ➲

➲ Thrombocytopoenia continued

- Nosebleeds.
- Bleeding in the mouth.
- Blood in the urine, resulting from bleeding in the kidneys; the urine may show blood clearly or may appear dark and smoky.
- Bruising from very slight pressure.

What to do:
- **Call the doctor immediately**.
- The child will probably be admitted to hospital for tests to exclude any other condition.

General care:
- The condition usually requires no treatment, but clears up on its own within a few weeks.
- Avoid any strenuous activity.
- Comfort and reassure the child.
- In severe cases, where there is persistent bleeding in the mouth or from the nose, children may be treated in hospital with corticosteroid drugs or gamma-globulin.

Possible complications:
- Most children make a full recovery within a few weeks.
- Rarely, the symptoms may persist for up to six months.

Revision questions

1 What are the signs and symptoms of iron-deficiency anaemia?
2 Describe a suitable diet for a child with nutritional anaemia.
3 What is thrombocytopoenia?
4 How can you tell if there is blood in the urine?
5 Describe the rash of Henoch-Schonlein purpura (HSP). What are the complications of HSP?

Digestive tract and dietary disorders

◆ *Appendicitis* ◆ *Constipation* ◆ *Diabetes mellitus* ◆ *Gastro-enteritis*
◆ *Hepatitis A* ◆ *Infestations affecting the digestive tract – Threadworms – Toxocara*
◆ *Rickets* ◆ *Toddler's diarrhoea*

What are digestive tract and dietary disorders?

Problems affecting the digestive system are very common as causes of illness in childhood. One of the most common signs that something is wrong with the digestive system is diarrhoea, when the bowel movements are abnormally frequent, fluid and copious. Other symptoms of infection or illness are vomiting and abdominal pain. While these symptoms are often distressing for both the parent or carer and the child, they are rarely a serious threat to health. Other digestive disorders are less common, but some may cause chronic illness which can affect the child's growth and development if not treated. Dietary disorders may occur as a result of poor nutrition. Eating disorders, such as obesity and anorexia, used to be associated with the teenage years but are becoming more common in younger children.

Appendicitis

What is it? Appendicitis is an infection of the appendix, a tube-like glandular structure attached to the beginning of the large intestine (colon). It is uncommon below two years of age and most common in the late teens and early twenties. It is more common in males than in females.

Cause: There is no known cause for sudden inflammation of the appendix.

Signs and symptoms: Sometimes the condition is difficult to recognise as it affects children differently. It may begin with mild discomfort that comes and goes (this is known as a grumbling appendix). The following are more definite symptoms:

- Crampy, colicky-like pain in the centre of the abdomen – around the navel – spreading to the lower hand side of the abdomen after a few hours.
- The child may have sharper pains when moving or taking deep breaths.
- Loss of appetite.
- Nausea (feeling sick) and may vomit.
- Constipation *or* diarrhoea.
- Bad breath and a dry coated tongue.
- Raised temperature.

What to do:

- Call the doctor and parents immediately.
- If the pain has been continuous for more than six hours, call an ambulance or take the child to a hospital accident and emergency department.
- If appendicitis is confirmed, the child will be admitted for surgical removal of the appendix. **Do not give the child anything to eat or drink.** Do not give paracetamol – it might mask the nature of the pain and delay correct diagnosis.

General care:

- Reassure the child – a hot water bottle wrapped in a towel and held against the site of the pain can help.
- The child will usually be discharged from hospital after 3 or 4 days and can take a normal diet.
- Any strenuous physical activities should be avoided for about a month after the operation.

Possible complications:

- If the appendix bursts (perforates), peritonitis (inflammation of the lining of the abdomen) will occur. This causes acute, intense pain over the whole abdominal area and is a medical emergency. **Call an ambulance immediately**.

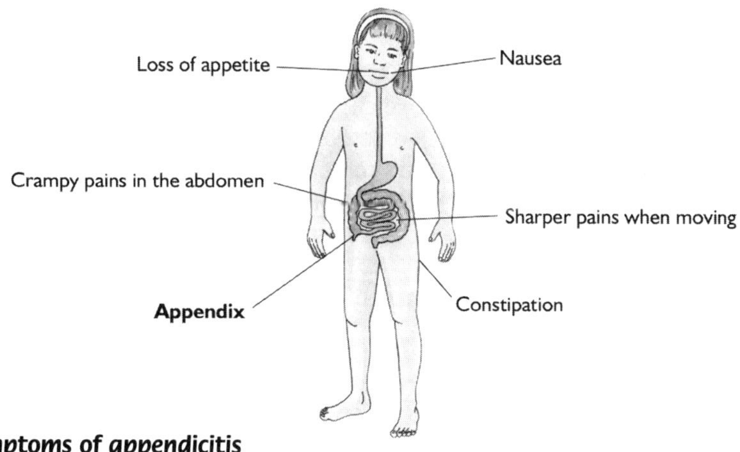

Signs and symptoms of appendicitis

Constipation

What is it? Constipation occurs when there is pain and difficulty in passing faeces or stools, and they emerge as hard, dry lumps; it is associated with infrequent bowel movements. Occasionally, bright red blood may be passed with hard stools. This blood comes from a slight tear in the skin around the anus, which happens when a constipated child struggles to pass an abnormally large and hard bowel movement.

NOTE: Infrequency of passing stools alone is *not* constipation. Children differ greatly in their bowel habits – from 3 or 4 motions a day to one motion every 3 or 4 days.

Cause: Constipation may be *short-term* or *chronic* (lasting a long time).

Short-term constipation may be caused by:

- Dehydration – resulting from any illness involving vomiting, diarrhoea or fever.
- Insufficient fibre in the child's diet.
- Certain medicines that have a constipating effect.
- Changes made to a child's diet, for example the change from breast or formula milk to cow's milk.

Chronic constipation may be caused by:

- Withholding of faeces. Children who are toilet training may become constipated; they may then start to withhold their faeces and refuse to go to the toilet and this will create further constipation problems. This can happen if the child starts training too early or if there are emotional problems.
- The pain resulting from a small break or tear around the anus that develops as a result of passing hard stools; the child will avoid going to the toilet because of the fear of pain.
- Lack of fibre or liquid in the diet.
- Food intolerances.
- Inadequate toileting facilities in early years settings.

Signs and symptoms:

- Passing hard dry stools.
- Infrequent motions.
- Pain when passing stools.

In chronic constipation:

- Liquid faeces trickle out of the anus, sometimes mistaken for diarrhoea; this is known as impaction and is caused by the hard dry stools becoming stuck in the rectum, resulting in a watery overflow.
- Excessive straining and pain when passing stools.
- Blood on the faeces.
- Blood or soiling on the underwear.
- Loss of appetite.

What to do:

- Give the child plenty to drink – fruit juices are best.
- Children over six months should eat dietary fibre, found in wholegrain bread and cereals, fruit and vegetables, as part of their balanced diet.
- Find out the cause of the child's constipation and deal with it appropriately.
- Consult a doctor if:
  - the child is constipated *and* has severe abdominal pain, fever, and/or a swollen abdomen
  - the child has severe constipation that lasts longer than one week in spite of a change in diet and exercise.

General care:

- In most constipated children, you can help just by changing their diet to one that is rich in fibre and with plenty of fluids, and by encouraging them to exercise more. Regular exercise stimulates the bowels. ➲

➲ Constipation continued

- Avoid giving children more than 500 ml (1 pint) of milk per day as it can have a constipating effect.
- For older children, you could try giving them prunes and prune juice, bran cereal, spinach, carrots and raisins. If dietary changes are not enough, some doctors recommend stool softeners or laxatives. Only give these if the doctor advises them.
- Do not give enemas or suppositories.
- If the child is toilet-trained, you can encourage him or her to sit on the toilet for about 10 minutes every morning after breakfast; this is the best time of day for the bowels to be stimulated – food stimulates the gastro-colic reflux.

Possible complications:

- If no *physical* causes can be found for the constipation and treatments do not relieve it, the child may be referred to a paediatrician or a child psychiatrist for further investigation.
- Constipation in childhood has *not* been found to increase the risk of bowel problems in later life.

Further information:

- Constipation is fairly common in babies just starting on solid foods. Try using prunes, apricots, pears, beans, plums and decrease foods like rice cereal, bananas or rice. Occasionally, a change of formula may be helpful, but always talk to the doctor before making a change.
- Constipation is more common in the summer months, when children are not keeping up fluid intake to compensate for increased fluid losses from sweating in the heat.

Diabetes mellitus

What is it? Diabetes mellitus is a common condition in which the amount of glucose (sugar) in the blood is too high because the body is unable to use it properly. This is because the body's method of converting glucose into energy is not working as it should. Diabetes happens either where there is a shortage of insulin, a hormone produced by the pancreas, which is needed to move glucose from the bloodstream into the body's cells where it is converted into energy, or when the body's insulin doesn't work properly. This in turn causes an excess of glucose in the blood (**hyperglycaemia**).
The term 'diabetes mellitus' – Greek for 'fountain of sugar' – derives from ancient physicians' observation that the urine of people with diabetes was sweet.

Cause: Diabetes develops when there is a severe lack of insulin in the body because most or all of the cells in the pancreas that produce it have been destroyed. Nobody knows for sure *why* these cells have been damaged but the most likely cause is an abnormal reaction of the body to the cells. This may be triggered by a viral or other infection. The type of diabetes affecting young children is an auto-immune condition. That is, the immune system, which exists to protect the body against infection and disease, turns against itself, destroying the insulin-producing cells in the pancreas. This results in a complete deficiency of insulin
Although the condition can occur at any age, it is rare in very young children and becomes more common as children get older.

Signs and symptoms:

- Increased thirst.
- Frequent passing of urine – especially at night; children who have previously been dry at night may start to wet the bed (**enuresis**); this is caused by the body trying to rid itself of excess glucose.
- Breath smells of pear drops (acetone). ➲

➲ Diabetes mellitus continued

- Extreme tiredness – caused by reduced energy as a result of the body being unable to move glucose into the cells.
- Loss of appetite and weight; the amount of weight lost can be quite dramatic – up to 10 per cent of the child's total body weight can be lost in as little as two months; this is caused by the body breaking down protein and fat stores as an alternative source of energy.
- Genital itching caused by excess glucose irritating the genital area. This may lead to the development of the yeast infection, thrush.
- Blurred vision; this is caused by abnormally high blood glucose levels changing the shape of the lens which affects focus.

If the condition is not recognised swiftly, the condition can lead to:

- Rapid breathing and signs of distress.
- Increased drowsiness.
- Loss of consciousness or coma. When fat and muscle is broken down by-products called **ketones** form and the child may fall into a coma. This sort of coma is more common in childhood diabetes because there is an absolute shortage of insulin.

What to do:

- Contact the doctor as soon as possible after noticing the symptoms.
- The doctor will test the urine for sugar and may also take a blood sample.
- The child will be admitted to hospital for further tests and treatment.

General care: Although there is no cure for diabetes, the condition can be successfully managed by insulin injections and a special diet; the aim of treatment is to normalise blood glucose levels and prevent complications caused by persistently raised blood glucose levels.

- Children need injections (under the skin) of insulin for the rest of their lives; insulin cannot be taken by mouth because it is destroyed by the digestive juices in the stomach. Children may need to take 2 to 4 injections every day. The sites for injecting the insulin are varied each day to prevent damage to the skin.
- The child's hospital specialist may prescribe the use of an insulin pump. This is a device that delivers a constant supply of insulin through a needle placed in the skin of the abdomen.
- They also need to eat a healthy diet that contains the right balance of foods; this will be monitored by a specialist nurse or dietician. Glucose drinks may be given to maintain energy levels when a child loses his or her appetite.
- Families and carers become skilled at balancing the daily nutritional needs – measured in carbohydrate portions.
- Blood glucose levels are measured daily; the child's finger is pricked using an automatic device. The drop of blood obtained is applied to a special strip that shows the blood glucose level.

Possible complications. One dangerous complication of insulin treatment is

- **hypoglycaemia**, which must be treated promptly to avoid possible brain damage from prolonged low blood sugar levels.

Other complications may occur in later life if the condition is not controlled with insulin and diet. These include:

- A higher risk of heart disease and stroke.
- Kidney failure.
- Eye disease.
- Foot ulceration. 

➲ Diabetes mellitus continued

Further information: **Blood glucose levels.** When sugar and starchy foods have been digested, they turn into glucose. If somebody has diabetes, the glucose in their body is not turned into energy, either because there is not enough insulin in their body, or because the insulin that the body produces is not working properly. This causes the liver to make more glucose than usual, but the body still cannot turn the glucose into energy. The body then breaks down its stores of fat and protein to try to release more glucose, but still this glucose cannot be turned into energy. This is why children with untreated diabetes often feel tired and lose weight. The unused glucose passes into the urine, which is why children with untreated diabetes pass large amounts of urine and are extremely thirsty.

Meeting the needs of a child with diabetes in an early years setting

Children with diabetes should be treated as any other child. Diabetes is not an illness and children should be encouraged to take part in the daily routine and activities of the setting. Guidelines for supporting the child with diabetes and their family are:

- Ensure that all contact records are up to date – that is, home contact numbers, GP, diabetic specialist nurse, etc.
- Always contact parents immediately if the child becomes unwell and keep them informed of the child's progress.
- Ensure there is always a supply of glucose tablets or sweet drinks in the care setting.
- When on outings, take a supply of sweet drinks or glucose tablets with you.
- Allow the child to take glucose tablets or snacks when required – most children with diabetes carry glucose tablets with them.
- Make sure you and all other members of staff know how to recognise and deal promptly with a child who has a hypoglycaemic attack.
- Always stay with the child if he or she feels unwell and allow privacy if blood glucose level testing is necessary during the day.
- Observe the child carefully during any vigorous exercise, such as swimming or climbing.
- Be understanding if the child shows emotional or behaviour problems caused by the necessary restrictions to their routine.
- Inform the child's parents if you are planning an activity which might involve extra strains and excitement.
- Ensure that the child eats regularly and that cooks are consulted about the child's dietary needs.

Hypoglycaemia

Recognising a hypoglycaemic attack

Often a hypoglycaemic attack is triggered by too much insulin, not enough food, illness or unusually strenuous exercise. Signs include:

- Weakness or hunger.
- Confused or aggressive behaviour.
- Loss of concentration or co-ordination.
- Rapid, shallow breathing. ➲

- ◆ Sweating.
- ◆ Dizziness.

Managing a hypoglycaemic attack

- ✓ Stay with the child.
- ✓ Sit the child down and reassure him or her.
- ✓ Give the child a sugary drink or sweet food.
- ✓ If the child recovers quickly after a sweet drink or food, give some more and allow the child to rest.

If the child does not recover quickly or becomes unconscious, **call an ambulance immediately** and put the child in the recovery position. Always inform the parents of any hypoglycaemic attack, so that adjustments can be made to the treatment.

Gastro-enteritis

What is it? Gastro-enteritis is an infection of the stomach and intestines that causes cramps and diarrhoea.

Cause: Gastro-enteritis can be caused by:

- **Viruses**. Many types of viruses are responsible for gastro-enteritis. The most common one is rotavirus – often responsible for severe gastro-enteritis in babies and young children. Viruses are transmitted through the air or by contact with infected faeces, usually because of poor hand-washing techniques.
- **Bacteria**. Bacteria such as shigella, E.coli and salmonella are transmitted through food and drink.

Signs and symptoms: About 1 to 5 days after infection, the following symptoms appear:

- Diarrhoea – loose, watery faeces.
- Vomiting.
- Loss of appetite.
- Raised temperature – especially with rotavirus infection.
- Often abdominal pain or discomfort.
- Looking and feeling generally unwell and listless.

What to do:

- Call the doctor if there are signs of dehydration (see page 83) or if vomiting and diarrhoea continue for more than 24 hours.
- Replace lost fluids by giving frequent drinks of cooled, previously boiled water – or rehydrating solution (available from chemists).

General care:

- Keep the child at home to prevent the spread of infection.
- After 2–3 days, introduce the child's normal diet gradually.
- Practise high standards of hygiene; wash bowls used for vomit straightaway and always wash your hands after disposing of any waste.
- Reassure the child, who may feel frightened and wretched when vomiting.
- Clean the child's anal area carefully and apply a barrier cream to prevent soreness.
- Encourage the child to have plenty of rest.
- Watch out for any signs of dehydration – see page 83.
- Always inform the child's parents if a child develops gastro-enteritis while in your care.

Possible complications:

- Dehydration is the most common complication; if left untreated it can lead to kidney damage and heart irregularities.
- If the child is severely dehydrated, he or she will be admitted to hospital for intravenous feeding with rehydrating solutions. ➲

➲ Gastro-enteritis continued

Further information:
- Gastro-enteritis caused by virus infection cannot be prevented, but the child will be immune to the particular virus after infection.
- Bacterial infection can often be prevented by following strict hygiene routines when handling and preparing food.
- Children will be infectious to others until the bouts of diarrhoea have completely stopped, and may still be mildly infectious for several weeks afterwards, so attention to hygiene is very important.

Hepatitis A

What is it? Hepatitis A is an infection of the liver.

Cause: It is caused by the virus called hepatitis A. It is caught by eating or drinking something which has been contaminated by infected faeces. Food prepared or washed with contaminated water can easily transmit the infection. It is the commonest cause of liver infection in the UK, and around the world is estimated to affect up to ten million people each year.

Signs and symptoms: The incubation period before symptoms develop is between 2 and 6 weeks, and how severely someone is affected varies from person to person. Some people may not have any symptoms at all and others just mild symptoms similar to those of a 'flu-like' illness. This is particularly common when infants and young children are infected.
Possible symptoms include:
- Weakness.
- Headache.
- Fever.
- Loss of appetite.
- Nausea and vomiting.
- Abdominal pain, particularly in the upper right area of the tummy where the liver is situated.
- Diarrhoea.

These may all occur for a week or more before the **jaundice** appears.
- **Jaundice** is when the skin and the whites of the eyes become yellow. This occurs in hepatitis infection because the liver is unable to perform one of its tasks of removing a substance called bilirubin from the blood. Bilirubin is a pigment and as it builds up in the blood it causes the yellow colouring.
- Dark-coloured urine.
- Pale faeces.

What to do:
- See the doctor within 24 hours of the onset of symptoms. There is no drug treatment for hepatitis A. Usually the child can be cared for at home, but, rarely, may need hospital care if the condition is severe.
- Prevent **dehydration** by giving hourly drinks and allow the child to stay in bed if he or she wishes.

General care:
- Jaundice may last for up to two weeks, but the child may need to be kept at home to recover for a few weeks more.
- Prevent the spread of hepatitis by scrupulous hand-washing and boiling cooking utensils.
- All family members should be immunised against hepatitis A to control the spread of the infection.

Possible complications:
- Very rarely there is permanent damage to the liver. Usually the child develops immunity after the first attack. ➲

➲ Hepatitis A continued

Further information: The majority of people from the UK who become infected with hepatitis A contract it abroad when travelling. It is common in Africa, northern and southern Asia, Central America, and southern and eastern Europe. If travelling to high-risk countries:
- avoid eating raw or inadequately cooked salads, vegetables, and shellfish
- check whether tap water is safe to drink before you go
- make sure that all family members are immunised against hepatitis A before travelling.

Infestations affecting the digestive tract

Threadworms

What are they? These are minute parasites that look like very fine threads of white cotton up to 1 cm in length. It is a very common condition in children and many are infected without realising it. Threadworms spread by producing large numbers of tiny eggs which cannot be seen with the eye. The eggs are present in dust and stick to food, carpets, towels, bed linen and toilet seats. Because they are so small and widespread they get on fingers and under fingernails and are easily swallowed. In the bowel they hatch into worms, which lay eggs around the child's bottom. At first the eggs are coated with a sticky substance which wears off and then the eggs disperse into the air.

Cause: Children catch threadworms by sucking objects or eating food that has been contaminated with the eggs. If the eggs are swallowed, they develop into adults while in the intestines. In cool moist conditions the eggs remain infectious for 6 to 8 weeks. If the child scratches her or his bottom, the eggs are caught under the fingernails; if the fingers are then put in the mouth, the eggs are ingested to develop into more threadworms.

Signs and symptoms:
- Itching in the anal region, particularly at night when the worms lay their eggs.
- In girls, an itchy vulva.
- Inflammation and soreness of the anus due to scratching.
- Thin white threads may be seen wriggling in the child's faeces.
- Pain when urinating caused by a urinary tract infection.
- Sleep may be disturbed because of the intense itchiness.
- Sometimes children begin to wet the bed.

What to do:
- If you suspect the child has worms, contact your doctor who may ask you to collect some of the eggs for microscopic examination. (This can be done by pressing a piece of sticky tape onto the child's anus first thing in the morning, before the child washes or uses the toilet. The sticky tape will collect any eggs.)
- The doctor will treat the *whole family* with oral anti-parasitic drugs, even if they do not display any symptoms. The treatment is usually repeated 10 days later to ensure all parasites are killed.

General care:
- Vacuum play areas, bedrooms and the bathroom at the beginning of treatment.
- Ensure that everyone showers or bathes thoroughly in the morning.
- Keep the child's towels and flannels separate.
- Bath the child or wash around the bottom each morning.
- Make sure everyone in the family washes their hands and scrubs their nails before every meal and after going to the toilet.
- Disinfect the toilet seat, toilet handle or chain regularly.
- Pregnant or breastfeeding mothers and parents of children under the age of two should consult the doctor for alternative treatment methods. ➲

➲ Threadworms continued

- All bedding and clothes should be washed and dried to ensure there are no remaining eggs.

Preventing threadworms:
- Ensure the child washes his or hands after going to the toilet. Your hands should be washed carefully after changing nappies.
- Keep the child's nails short.
- Children should wear underwear or pyjamas at night.
- Ensure that strict hygiene rules are followed in any early years setting, for example cleaning toys and any objects which children put in their mouths, and washing all fresh food before eating.

Further information: Threadworms are most common in urban environments and particularly affect children between the ages of 5 and 9 years. Children do not suffer any long-term harm and parents and carers should be reassured that the condition is nothing to be ashamed of – it is a very common condition.

Toxocara

What is it? Toxocara is the common roundworm that lives in the intestines of almost all new-born puppies and in some adult dogs and foxes. Dogs which harbour adult worms pass the toxocara eggs into the environment in their faeces. In humans a minute larval worm hatches out in the intestine; it immediately burrows though the wall of the intestine into the bloodstream and then passes into the tissues of the body. It can then cause inflammation in various organs, for example the lungs, brain, eyes, kidneys and muscles.

Cause: People catch toxocara by accidentally swallowing tiny mature toxocara eggs. **Very young children** are most at risk because:
- they play on the ground and tend to put their fingers and playthings in their mouths
- they may be licked on the face by puppies.

Dog breeders and their families are also at risk if hands are not carefully washed after handling young puppies.

Signs and symptoms: Diagnosis is often difficult because the signs and symptoms depend on where the larva is sited; some or all of the following symptoms may be noticed:
- Vague aches, dizziness and nausea.
- Anaemia – pale skin and conjunctiva, tiredness and lethargy.
- Loss of appetite and weight.
- Loss of vision or blurring of vision, caused by the passage of the toxocara larva through the eye.
- Cough and wheezing.
- Epileptic seizures are rare but do occur.

What to do:
- Consult a doctor if you notice any of the symptoms of toxocara infection.
- The doctor will take blood samples to check for the toxocara antibodies and for anaemia.
- Specific anti-parasitic drugs are prescribed and antibiotics may be given to treat any infections.

General care: *Toxocariasis is largely preventable if you take these steps:*
- Remember to worm your dogs.
- Dispose of their faeces promptly and carefully.
- Wash your hands before handling food. 

➲ *Toxocara* continued

- Wash children's hands after they have been handling dogs or soil.
- Watch out for toddlers eating soil and try to prevent it.

If left untreated, symptoms eventually die down as the child's immune system and natural defences against disease overcome the infection within 1 year to 18 months.

Possible complications:
- It takes just one single larva in the eye to cause some degree of permanent visual impairment or even blindness.

Further information:
- Toxocara worms also live in the intestines of cats.
- There are between 100 and 200 new cases of toxocaral eye disease diagnosed annually in the UK.
- In the UK about half the most serious cases of toxocara infection, such as blindness, occur in families who have never owned a dog or a cat.
- With an estimated population of about six million dogs in the UK producing 1000 tons of faeces daily, dog fouling in parks and playgrounds is a serious problem. Some toxocara eggs can survive in soil for up to three years.

Rickets

What is it? Rickets is a rare bone growth disorder that produces a variety of symptoms in children.

Cause: Rickets is caused by a lack of vitamin D. Vitamin D is formed in the skin when it is exposed to sunlight. It may also be obtained from some foods, such as fish and eggs. Lack of vitamin D affects the kidneys and disrupts the calcium and phosphorus metabolism in the body. This in turn affects the deposition of calcium in the bones, resulting in deformity.

Signs and symptoms:
- Babies with rickets are usually restless, grow more slowly than normal, and do not crawl or walk until older than normal.
- If the condition continues, the ends of the long bones become enlarged. When the child starts to walk, the legs may bend, resulting in either **bow legs** or knock-knees.
- The chest may also be deformed, producing a pigeon breast, and small knobs may develop on the ends of the ribs.

What to do:
- Consult a doctor who will arrange tests to confirm the diagnosis.
- Rickets is treated by giving a concentrated supply of vitamin D in addition to an adequate diet. Calcium supplements may also be prescribed to help restore the normal calcium metabolism.

General care:
- Ensure that the child is exposed to sunlight.
- Follow the dietary advice given by the doctor or dietician.

Further information:
- Any deformities usually disappear if the condition is treated in the early stages.

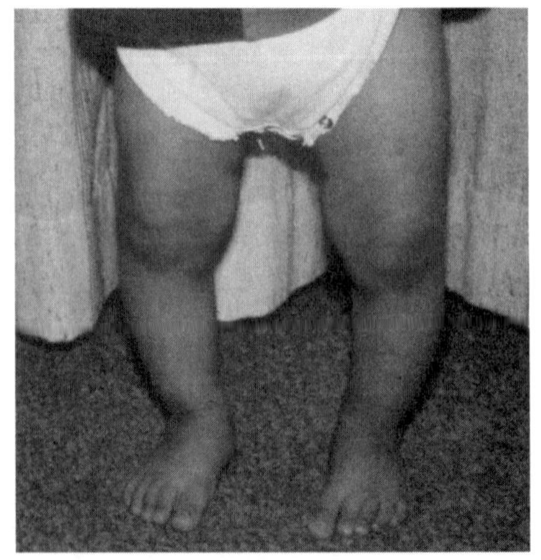

Bowing of the legs in a child with rickets

Toddler's diarrhoea

What is it?	Toddler's diarrhoea occurs when an otherwise healthy child (between the ages of 1 and 3) passes loose, watery faeces.
Cause:	The cause of toddler's diarrhoea is uncertain, but is thought to be the result of poor chewing of food.
Signs and symptoms:	• Loose, watery faeces often containing recognisable pieces of food, for example raisins, corn, carrots and peas. • Nappy rash if the child is in nappies.
What to do:	• Consult a doctor to exclude other causes of diarrhoea, such as an infection.
General care:	• Encourage the child to chew foods thoroughly. • Mash or liquidise foods which are difficult to chew and digest.
Possible complications:	• Children generally grow out of toddler's diarrhoea by three years of age. As it is not an infectious condition, there is no need for the child to be kept away from friends or from nursery or school.

Revision questions

1. What are the main signs and symptoms of gastro-enteritis? How could you help to prevent the spread of gastro-enteritis in a nursery or school?
2. Where is the pain of appendicitis felt?
3. What is diabetes mellitus? What is hypoglycaemia and how would you recognise it?
4. How is hepatitis A transmitted from one person to another? What is bilirubin and how would you recognise that a child has jaundice?
5. Why are threadworms a common infection in young children? How can you help to prevent threadworms?

Ear disorders

◆ *Ear infections: Otitis media – Otitis externa* ◆ *Foreign bodies in the ear*
◆ *Glue ear*

Hearing problems in childhood

About one child in every 1000 is born with permanent hearing loss. This is mainly due to damage to the **cochlea**, or auditory nerve, and occasionally to defects in the middle or outer ear. About 150 more children *acquire* permanent hearing loss each year, mostly as a result of meningitis. In addition, most children suffer spells of 'glue ear', when fluid builds up behind the eardrum, causing temporary hearing problems, but generally this clears up without treatment. Childhood hearing tests are designed to detect permanent hearing problems so that they can be treated early. (These tests are described on pages 285–286.)

Ear infections

Ear infections are one of the most common health problems in children under the age of three and they can lead to hearing problems. Any section of the ear can become infected, but middle ear infection (otitis media), where the normally air-filled space becomes filled with pus, is the most common.

Otitis media

What is it? The best way to define otitis media is to look at what the words mean. They are actually made up of three parts: *oto* meaning 'ear' *-itis* meaning 'inflammation', and *media* meaning 'middle', or more exactly, 'middle ear'. So, otitis media means 'inflammation of the middle ear'. The inflammation occurs as a result of a middle ear infection and can occur in one or both ears. Middle ear infections are common in young children because they have narrow, short Eustachian tubes that lie horizontally rather than sloping downwards as steeply as in adults. This not only makes it easy for viruses and bacteria to travel from the nose and throat to the middle ear, but mucus tends to build up rather than drain away.

Cause: Acute otitis media is caused by bacteria (or viruses) that enter from the nose or throat and ascend the Eustachian tube to reach the middle ear. This occurs when the Eustachian tube is not functioning properly, often because it is inflamed from a cold, sinus or throat infection, or an allergy attack. Infection in the middle ear causes earache, a red inflamed eardrum, and a build up of pus and mucus behind the eardrum.

Signs and symptoms:

- The sudden appearance of runny wax in the ear canal can be a sign of otitis media.

Babies and very young children cannot describe or localise the pain of earache. They may:

- be miserable and go off their feeds
- be feverish, sleep badly or rub the side of their face or pull at their ear
- also have diarrhoea and vomiting.

Older children may:

- complain of a sharp, throbbing pain or ache in the ear
- be miserable and lose their appetite
- have a fever, vomiting and diarrhoea
- have some hearing loss – usually only temporary.

NOTE: If the pain stops suddenly, the eardrum may have ruptured and pus streaked with blood may ooze out of the ear.

What to do:

- Contact the parents if the child is not at home, or if you are in sole charge at the child's home.
- **Consult the doctor immediately** if:
  - the child complains of earache
  - the child has a raised temperature.
- The doctor will look inside the child's ears, using an instrument called an **otoscope**. With the otoscope inserted in the ear, the doctor can check for redness and fluid behind the eardrum and see if the eardrum moves in response to air pressure. A mobile (vibrating) eardrum is normal.
  The GP may prescribe antibiotics, which will help a bacterial infection but not a viral one.
- Gently remove any sticky or crusty discharge on the ear lobe with cotton wool soaked in warm water. **Do not attempt to clean inside the ear**.
- If the child has a temperature, give children's paracetamol (always with the parent's consent). ➲

➲ *Otitis media* continued

- To relieve any pain, put a warm soft cloth on the child's sheet or pillow and place the affected ear against the cloth. Lying flat often increases the pain, so try propping the child up on pillows.
- For older children, use a thickly covered hot water bottle. Never leave a baby with a hot water bottle as they cannot push it away if it feels too hot.

General care:
- In most cases, earache subsides within 24 hours.
- Until the ear infection has cleared, the child should not be allowed to swim, and care must be taken to ensure water does not enter the ear when washing the child's hair.
- Have the child's ears checked a couple of weeks later to ensure that the fluid has completely cleared and that hearing is back to normal.

Possible complications:
- Left untreated, middle ear infections can damage the cavity or bones within it and cause permanent hearing loss.
- Rarely, a burst – or perforated – eardrum may result in permanent scarring which can affect the child's hearing.
- Glue ear (see page 132). In some children the fluid in the middle ear persists after the initial infection and glue ear results.

Further information: Children who cannot describe earache may simply tug or rub the affected ear. Do not give ear drops unless the doctor prescribes them. Follow the guidelines on page 250.

Alternative remedies: If the child is allergic to dairy products, he or she may be more susceptible to ear infections. Dairy foods encourage the production of mucus which can cause a build up of fluid in the middle ear. Think about swapping to soya or goat's milk, but check with the doctor or health visitor first. A nutritional therapist will be able to confirm which allergies are at the root of the problem.

Otitis externa

What is it? Otitis externa is an infection of the external ear canal – the passage which leads from the ear flap (the pinna) to the eardrum.

Cause: Otitis externa may be caused by:
- A foreign body in the ear.
- A skin disorder such as eczema or seborrhoeic dermatitis.
- A boil in the ear canal.
- Damage to the skin by over-vigorous cleaning or scratching.

The infection is more common in children who swim a great deal and is sometimes called 'swimmer's ear'.

Signs and symptoms:
- Pain and itchiness in the ear – a baby may pull at the ear and cry.
- Redness and tenderness of the ear flap and external ear canal.
- Discharge of pus or blood from the ear.
- Partial hearing loss – particularly if the ear canal is blocked by wax.
- An itchy, dry, scaly ear.

What to do:
- Inform the parents who should consult a doctor as soon as possible; the doctor will examine the child's ear with an otoscope and may then clean the ear out with a ➲

➲ *Otitis externa* continued

probe. He or she will probably prescribe antibiotic ear drops or tablets to treat the infection. (See page 250 for how to give ear drops to a child.)
- Comfort and reassure the child.
- Give children's paracetamol to relieve the pain (with the parent's consent).

General care:
- Don't interfere with the child's external ear canal. Wash around the ear flap but never poke cotton wool swabs into the area to clear wax, for example – otherwise you risk pushing the wax further in to the ear canal and causing further infection.
- To relieve any pain, put a warm soft cloth on the child's sheet or pillow and place the affected ear against the cloth. Lying flat often increases the pain, so try propping the child up on pillows.
- For older children, use a thickly covered hot water bottle. Never leave a baby with a hot water bottle as they cannot push it away if it feels too hot.
- Take care when washing the child's hair not to get water into the ear; use a shower cap when bathing – or try sponging the hair instead.
- The child should not go swimming until clear of infection.

Possible complications: Otitis externa can lead to otitis media if not treated promptly. Children with eczema and dermatitis may suffer from recurrent infections.

Foreign bodies in the ear

The most common foreign bodies to become stuck in a child's ear are small objects, like beads, pushed in by the child or by a playmate. Rarely, a small insect may fly into the ear and become trapped there. If it cannot be easily removed it may cause an infection of the external ear canal (otitis externa) or damage the eardrum.

Glue ear

What is it? Glue ear occurs when the middle ear becomes filled with a thick, sticky mucus that is produced by the middle ear lining. The eardrum and the small bones in the middle ear are unable to vibrate efficiently and transmit sound to the inner ear.

Cause: Glue ear is caused by an excess of mucus which accumulates in the middle ear. This is particularly so if the Eustachian tube (the narrow canal that connects the middle ear to the back of the throat) is blocked by inflammation. Glue ear often follows infections such as otitis media, tonsillitis and sinusitis.

Signs and symptoms: Hearing loss caused by glue ear may be permanent or may come and go. This can result in any or all of the following:
- The child may complain of partial deafness.
- The child may be inattentive and slow at learning.
- A young child may not quieten or smile at the sound of your voice.
- At seven months, the child may not turn to a noise made outside of their line of vision.
- By the age of nine months the child may become distressed when you are out of sight and they may be startled when you appear suddenly.
- They may turn the television volume too loud.
- The child may find it difficult to sit still and concentrate in a group.
- Older children may complain of a stuffy or full feeling in the ear. 

➲ Glue ear continued

What to do:
- Take the child to the doctor, who will examine the ears by looking into them with an otoscope. If glue ear is diagnosed, the GP may:
  – refer the child to an ear, nose and throat (ENT) specialist
  – in mild cases, prescribe antibiotics to clear up the infection and special medicines to reduce the swelling in the Eustachian tubes.

General care:
- If the child is between 6 and 18 months, a distraction test may be carried out whereby the baby is distracted by a person holding a toy in front of them while a second person makes noises from behind to establish the baby's response.
- From 18 months to 2½ years a hearing performance test will be conducted in which the child is given simple instructions from behind a screen.
- For children over this age, tests which involve a range of sounds played through headphones are carried out. (See also pages 285–286 on hearing tests.)
- In some cases, the child may need an operation under general anaesthetic in which a hollow needle may be used to withdraw fluid from the middle ear. Many children have a tiny plastic tube, called a **grommet**, inserted in the eardrum which allows the air to flow in and out of the middle ear. This grommet usually stays in place for about nine months, and children are advised not to dive or swim underwater whilst it is in place.
- If the child has difficulty with pronouncing sounds or if there is language delay, they will be referred to a speech therapist.

Possible complications: Permanent hearing loss.

Revision questions

1 Why are ear infections fairly common in young children?
2 How can you tell the difference between otitis media and glue ear?
3 How would you support a child with a hearing impairment in a nursery or school?
4 How can you help a child who has earache?
5 Why should a child's hearing be tested after an ear infection?

Emotional and behavioural problems

Children often show emotional and behavioural problems at certain times. Usually these problems disappear quite quickly without treatment and may be the result of temporary stress or upset. Other specific conditions cause long-term difficulties for children and their families. The conditions included in this section are the ones you are most likely to encounter within an early years education setting.

Attention deficit hyperactivity disorder (ADHD) ◆ Autism or autistic spectrum disorder (ASD) ◆ Developmental dyspraxia ◆ Eating disorders: Anorexia nervosa – Obesity – Food refusal ◆ Enuresis (Bedwetting) ◆ Soiling or encopresis

Attention deficit hyperactivity disorder (ADHD)

What is it? ADHD is a condition which affects between 1 and 2 per cent of children in the UK. In general, children with ADHD are impulsive and restless, and have difficulty in maintaining attention and concentrating on the task in hand.

Cause: The cause of ADHD is not known, but some believe it is caused by insufficient levels of dopamine in the brain. This hormone causes the electrical impulses which control all that we do to misfire, and results in uncontrolled, impulsive behaviour and often poor co-ordination (**dyspraxia**) and other learning difficulties (which may include **dyslexia**). It is thought that the condition is hereditary, and many families can look back and recall that a family member showed the features of ADHD before the condition was 'discovered'. Sometimes these symptoms go unnoticed until the child starts school and is compared with other children.

What to do: Consult a doctor if you suspect the child has ADHD. He or she may refer you to a consultant paediatrician, a psychologist or psychotherapist for advice and treatment.

General care: Depending upon the needs of the individual child and the severity of the condition, a combination of medical, teaching and behavioural help can be given:

- **Ritalin** is a drug which, although a stimulant, seems to have a calming effect on two-thirds of children with ADHD; it enables the child to concentrate better and to behave in a calmer way.
- Effective **teaching techniques** include establishing clear boundaries and creating predictable routines; a child with ADHD benefits from having the school day organised into a recognisable structure.
- Dealing with the child's unwanted behaviour at once; choose one or two particularly difficult behaviour traits to work on first and remember to ***praise*** the child when improvements occur.

Possible complications: Children with ADHD are more likely to:

- Be depressed or anxious.
- To behave in a confrontational and antisocial way – for example arguing with and defying adults.
- Have speech and language problems.
- Have co-ordination problems.
- Have poor self-esteem and difficulty with developing social skills.

Support for the child with ADHD and the family:

1. Behaviour management approaches often start by teaching parents and carers the A-B-C approach.
   - **A = Antecedents**. Identify the events or circumstances which seem to lead to difficult behaviour or trigger specific problems. These are known as *antecedents*.
   - **B = Behaviour**. Describe the actual *behaviour* in detail (what does the child do, for how long, what don't they do).
   - **C = Consequences**. Observe the *consequences* of this behaviour (what happens to the child, how other people react, what sort of attention is given).

   Carers are then shown how to gradually change the child's behaviour, concentrating on small changes at a time and giving praise for any small step in the right direction.
2. Children taking stimulant medication need to take their tablets regularly, as the effects of medication only last for four to five hours. As a parent or carer you need to ensure that anyone looking after the child is aware of this. Children should also be seen regularly by a specialist to monitor their progress and check for any side-effects. For example, some children develop sleep problems, lose weight, or may even become depressed. ➲

➲ Attention deficit hyperactivity disorder (ADHD) continued

Further information: Most children with ADHD improve with treatment as they get older. A few go on to display more anti-social behaviour later in childhood.

Signs and symptoms

A child with ADHD may show some or most of the following signs and symptoms:

□ Fidgeting with hands and feet and squirming in their seat; the child acts as if 'driven by a motor' and seem to be on the go the whole time.	□ Difficulty in awaiting their turn in games or group situations; the child finds it hard to socialise from an early age.
□ Difficulty in playing quietly.	□ Talking incessantly and unable to listen without interruption; the child might appear to want to take over and be the centre of attention.
□ Inability to finish tasks.	□ Often blurts out answers to questions.
□ Difficulty following instructions.	□ Difficulty sustaining attention.
□ Often shifts from one incomplete activity to another.	□ Often interrupts or intrudes on others.
□ Often does not seem to listen.	□ Often has difficulty organising things; the child may lose things or be oblivious to mess.
□ Often engages in physically dangerous activities without considering the consequences, e.g. running into the road without looking for traffic.	

Sometimes these symptoms go unnoticed until the child starts school and is compared with other children.

CASE STUDY

Our son, Jack – though highly intelligent – was difficult from birth. His problems showed themselves early on in the complete refusal to do as he was told. He seemed happy enough, but if we asked him to do something, he invariably ignored us or did the complete opposite! He seemed unable to get along with the other children we met – at home or at the local playgroup. Sometimes he was so bossy and domineering with his friends that they began to refuse to come and play with him. Jack also seemed very clumsy; for instance, he frequently fell over when walking or running, and couldn't draw or colour like the other children. He could not, and still cannot, ride a bike.

By the time he started school he was showing real behaviour problems and we were becoming increasingly aware that something was very wrong. His teacher said that he ➲

never seemed to sit still and finish an activity. This was exactly the way he behaved at home; he'd start playing with something, and then would be distracted by the phone or some other sound and would just leave whatever he was doing and start rushing around like a mad thing. He was wearing us out and nobody seemed to know how to help him. We were eventually referred to a child psychologist, a physiotherapist and an occupational therapist (he was only 4½ years old at the time!). The child psychologist told us the difficulties were caused by the huge discrepancy between his verbal and non-verbal skills and the occupational therapist suggested he was **dyspraxic**. No-one even mentioned ADHD as a possibility. None of this really addressed our problems. Behaviour at home and at school was increasingly difficult. Jack was beginning to fail to learn – and for a child like him this was tearing him and me apart.

Questions

1 Why is it so difficult to decide whether or not a child has ADHD?

2 How can nursery managers, teachers and carers help a child like Jack to reach his full potential?

3 Find out all you can about ADHD and methods of behaviour therapy.

Autism or autistic spectrum disorder (ASD)

What is it? Autism is a life-long developmental disability affecting social and communication skills. Children with autism often have accompanying learning disabilities but, whatever their general level of intelligence, they will share a common difficulty in making sense of the world in the way most people do. In most children with autism some types of skills will be better than others so that their development will not only be slower than usual but will also be uneven and different from most children with other learning disabilities.

Causes of autism: There is no known cause but because about one-quarter of children with autism have neurological symptoms, many specialists now believe there may be a physical and/or genetic factor. One theory is that autism may be related to abnormal levels of essential fatty acids in the blood, or to an abnormal blood flow through the brain. It is *not* due to emotional problems or emotional deprivation. Onset of autism is almost always before the age of three years.

It affects four times as many boys as girls, and has no class or racial barriers.

Features of autism: The degree to which children with an autistic spectrum disorder are affected varies, but all those affected have what is known as a *triad of impairments*. This triad affects:

- **Social interaction** (difficulty with social relationships).
- **Social communication** (difficulty with verbal and non-verbal communication).
- **Imagination** (difficulty in the development of play and imagination).

In addition to this triad, repetitive behaviour patterns are a notable feature and a resistance to change in routine.

A child with autism may show some or many of the following characteristics:

- Lack awareness of other people.
- Avoid eye-to eye contact.
- Prefer to play alone.
- Over-sensitive to certain sounds.
- Extremely resistant to change and become obsessed with one particular topic or idea. ➲

➲ Autism or autistic spectrum disorder (ASD) continued

- Have difficulty in understanding and using normal speech patterns. Echolalia – an automatic repetition of what is said to him or her – is common.
- Develop obsessions, with attachment to or collections of one particular type of thing.
- Have delay in speaking, which may be 'robot-like' when it does happen.
- Show repetitive behaviour, rocking, walking on tip toe, etc.
- Show abnormal body movements, for example arm flapping, flicking fingers for hours on end, grimacing, rocking and charging in different directions at great speed.
- Have sudden screaming fits; may injure themself.
- Show an isolated special skill, for example drawing, music or an outstanding rote memory. Extreme examples of such skills include an 18-month-old who could sing a whole opera, and a two-year-old who can read. Such individuals are known as idiots-savants.

Diagnosis: A diagnosis of autism is not usually made until the child is two years old, although parents may have noticed a general lack of curiosity in their child with poor sleeping and feeding patterns and general unresponsiveness in the first year.

Support and education for the child with autism: There is no known effective treatment apart from medication to control the associated problems of epilepsy and hyperactivity. Many therapies are being tried, for example:

- Holding therapy, in which parents group together for long periods of time and try to foster emotional responsiveness by firm holding techniques.
- Behaviour therapy, with reward and discouragement for acceptable and unacceptable behaviour.
- Daily Life Therapy – developed by Dr Kitahara in the Boston Higashi school in the USA – offers a programme of physical education and age-appropriate lessons in a residential setting.
- The National Autistic Society's Early Bird Programme. This combines group training sessions for parents with individual home visits, when video feedback is used to help parents apply what they learn when they are working with their child. Parents ➲

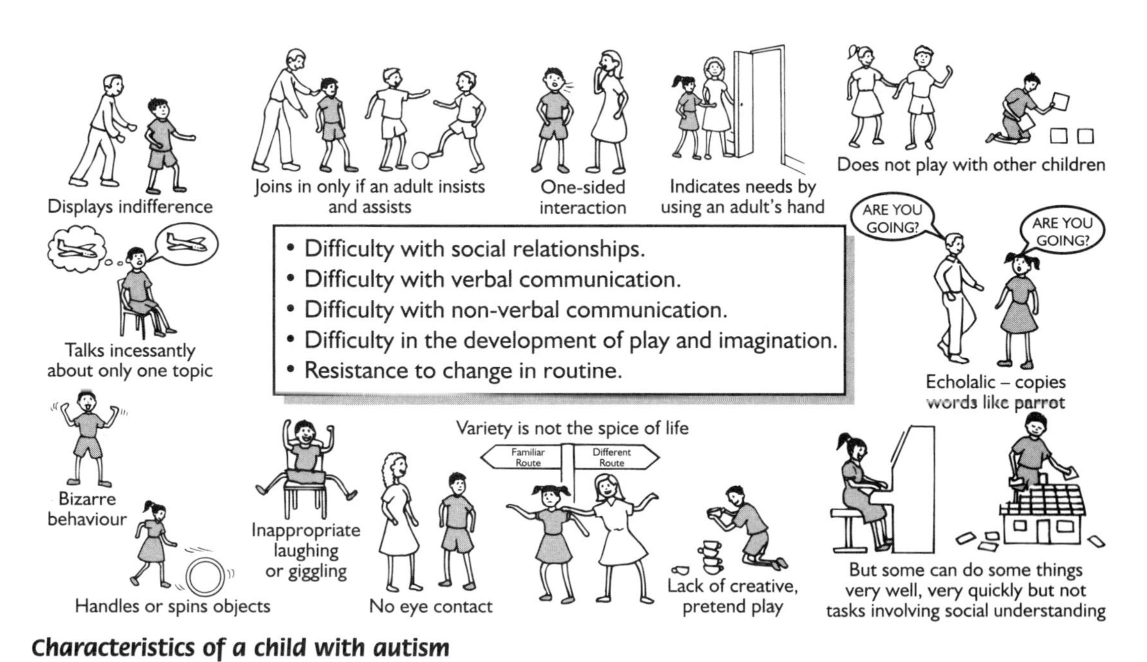

Characteristics of a child with autism

➲ Autism or autistic spectrum disorder (ASD) continued

have a weekly commitment to a three-hour training session or a home visit, and to ongoing work with their child at home, during the three-month long programme.

- Lovaas method – developed by Professor Lovaas in California, USA – offers an intensive programme of therapy using behaviour modification techniques.

The child with severe autism will need constant one-to-one care, requiring considerable patience and skill on the part of all family members. Any changes to the person's routine must be carefully planned.

Education: Early childhood education, for example at a nursery or playgroup, will help the family integrate into the community. Most children with severe autism attend local schools for children with severe learning difficulties; others require residential care – the National Autistic Society runs several schools which offer day, weekly or termly facilities.

The teaching of **self-help skills** is an essential aspect of education for any child with autism, as these can help them to achieve maximum independence and make life easier for everyone. Because the child with autism *looks* 'normal', parents often have difficulty alerting others to the fact that he or she has special needs. To an extent, parents may often have to take on the role of educator, sometimes even with professionals, for example GPs, teachers and health visitors.

There are other ways in which parents may choose to help their pre-school child, such as:

- using *picture symbols* to develop communication
- trying a gluten and/or casein-free diet, or
- using educational software on a home computer.

Asperger syndrome: Most children with Asperger syndrome represent the other end of the autistic spectrum. Language delay is not as common as in autism, but there are often problems with communication and the child with Asperger syndrome is usually aware of his disability. Features of the syndrome are:

- Social naiveté or simplicity.
- Good grammatical language, using language only for own interests.
- Very specialised interests, often highly academic, for example movement of the planets, railway timetables.
- Lack of common sense arising from unawareness of their environment.

ACTIVITY

1 Find out if there is any special provision for children with autism in your local area.
2 Find out about the work of the National Autistic Society.
3 List the **social skills** required to participate fully in daily activities in a reception class. Try to describe the difficulties a child with autism may have in integrating.
4 What help and support is available to the family with a child with autism?
5 What might the effects be on siblings of living with a child with autism?

Developmental dyspraxia

What is it? Dyspraxia is an immaturity of the brain which results in messages not being properly transmitted to the body. Children with dyspraxia can be of average or above intelligence, but are often immature in the way they behave. They may try very hard ➲

➲ Developmental dyspraxia continued

to fit in and be accepted at school but often throw tantrums when at home. Dyspraxia is also called Clumsy Child Syndrome and affects at least 2 per cent of the population to some extent; 70 per cent of children affected are boys.

Cause: There is no known cause for dyspraxia

Signs and symptoms: During the child's first three years, the following signs may indicate that a child has dyspraxia: ➲

The child may:

- ☐ be irritable and difficult to comfort – from birth
- ☐ have delayed early motor skill development; sitting unaided, rolling from side to side, do not go through the crawling stage
- ☐ be delayed in toilet training
- ☐ have sleeping difficulties
- ☐ have delayed language development; single words not obvious until the age of three
- ☐ have feeding difficulties: colic, milk allergies, etc.
- ☐ constantly move arms and legs
- ☐ be sensitive to loud noises
- ☐ avoid simple construction toys, such as jigsaws and Duplo™
- ☐ be highly emotional and easily upset

Later on, the child may:

- ☐ be clumsy: constantly bumping into objects and falling over
- ☐ often flap their hands when running or jumping
- ☐ be messy eaters; prefer to use fingers to eat and often spill liquid from drinking cup
- ☐ not be able to hold a pen or pencil properly and be confused about which hand to use
- ☐ have difficulties throwing or catching a ball
- ☐ be slow to learn to dress or to feed themselves
- ☐ be very excitable, becoming easily distressed and having frequent temper tantrums
- ☐ prefer adult company, feeling isolated in their peer group
- ☐ have speech problems, be slow to learn to speak or speech may be incoherent
- ☐ may be unable to hop, skip or ride a bike
- ☐ have very high levels of motor activity: always swinging and tapping feet when seated, clapping hands and unable to sit still
- ☐ be sensitive to touch: they may find some clothes uncomfortable; may also dislike high levels of noise
- ☐ have reading and writing difficulties
- ☐ have poor short-term memory; they often forget tasks learned the previous day
- ☐ be unable to answer simple questions even though they know the answers
- ☐ show a lack of imaginative play – e.g. not enjoying dressing up or playing inappropriately in the home corner
- ☐ have phobias or show obsessive behaviour
- ☐ be intolerant to having hair or teeth brushed, or nails and hair cut
- ☐ have a poor sense of direction

➲ Developmental dyspraxia continued

Not all of these will apply to every child with dyspraxia, and many of these problems can be overcome in time, but also could be met by more problems.
Older children are usually very verbally adept and converse well with adults. They may be ostracised by their own peer group because they do not fit in. They may cleverly avoid doing those tasks that are difficult or even impossible for them.

Assessment: These is no *cure* for dyspraxia but the earlier a child is treated then the greater the chance of improvement. Assessment involves obtaining a detailed developmental history of the child, and using developmental tests or scales to build up a learning ability profile.

Support for the child and family: Occupational therapists, physiotherapists and extra help at school can all help a child with dyspraxia to cope or overcome many difficulties.

Eating disorders in childhood

What are eating disorders? Eating disorders are a way of coping with painful feelings that are difficult to talk openly about. The eating disorder is an unconscious attempt to avoid these feelings, or to keep them under control. During the process of growing up the body undergoes many changes, both physically and emotionally. Slowing down or stopping these changes can be seen as a way of trying to regain control of this changing person. It is a way of avoiding all the demands of growing up and the issues that it brings.

Causes: There are many reasons why a child may develop an eating disorder. Often there is no single cause, but a whole chain of events which makes the child feel unable to cope with his or her life. Research has shown that some people are genetically susceptible to developing an eating disorder, which is triggered by factors such as life events and personal or family situations.

Anorexia nervosa

What is it? Anorexia means loss of appetite. Anorexia nervosa is an eating disorder that makes children become intensely afraid of being overweight. Because of this fear, they cut down on their food intake, and increase their activity levels, so that they stay underweight by 15 per cent or more. It usually affects adolescent girls, but is becoming more common in younger children.

Cause: There is no known single cause of anorexia nervosa.

Signs and symptoms: The child with anorexia nervosa:

- has a distorted body image
- is clearly underweight and often emaciated, but still worries about being 'too fat'
- watches what she eats, is always 'on a diet,' and even denies being hungry when she's really starving
- avoids food and family mealtimes
- may have fine hair growing on the face and body (lanugo) – a sign of starvation

What to do:

- Anorexia nervosa is a dangerous illness that needs to be treated by a doctor. Treatment often includes behaviour therapy and psychotherapy, along with diet changes to make up for long periods of poor nutrition. ➲

➲ *Anorexia nervosa* continued

General care:
- The child with an eating disorder can be helped by a psychiatrist, who may prescribe antidepressants or other medications. The psychiatrist may also suggest that the child's entire family be seen for family psychotherapy.
- When a child with an eating disorder has started to have medical complications that seriously affect her heart, blood, digestive system or other organs, she may need to be treated in a hospital. Once she is stable enough to return home, other types of therapy can start. A careful regimen of re-feeding rather than rapid weight gain is advised.

Possible complications: As a child with anorexia nervosa gets thinner, her poor nutrition begins to affect many body organs. The child may:
- begin to have postural hypotension (her blood pressure drops and she feels like passing out if she stands up too fast)
- develop an abnormally slow heart rate, as low as 20 beats per minute
- suffer from anaemia and constipation, appear unusually pale, and may always complain of feeling 'cold'.

If left untreated, anorexia nervosa can mean that the child can literally starve to death.

Further information: Anorexia is most common in teenage girls, especially at about age $14\frac{1}{2}$ years and again at age 18. However, it has been diagnosed in children as young as five years of age.

Obesity

What is it? Obesity literally means fatness, but it is now recognised as an eating disorder that results in the child being overweight. Obesity in children is on the increase. Not only is this a health hazard while they are young, but it also sets a pattern for later life.

Cause: Obesity is caused by a mixture of factors, and each will contribute to obesity:
- **Lack of exercise:**
  - Cycling or even walking to school is not as safe as it was. Parents are now more likely to run their children to school by car.
  - Non-physical playing. Television and computer games compete with games that involve physical activity.
- **Inappropriate diet:**
  - Children eat more sweets and crisps and drink more fizzy drinks, partly because of advertising, but also because they are more available.
  - Change in meals. Fast food is overtaking traditionally prepared meals. Many convenience meals involve coating food with fatty creams or batters.
  - Poor fresh fruit consumption. Despite it being more readily available, many children do not eat enough fresh fruit, preferring processed varieties that often contain extra sugar and fat products.

Signs and symptoms:
- Upper arms and thighs have rolls of fat which strain the sleeves and legs of clothes that otherwise fit well.
- When the child's weight is plotted on a **centile chart**, the child weighs 20 per cent more than expected for the norm for their age, sex and height. ➲

➲ *Obesity* continued

What to do:
- Consult the doctor, who will examine, measure and weigh the child, and exclude any underlying medical condition.
- An effective diet will be planned for the child and support given by the health visitor or community dietician.

General care:
- Offer a healthy, well-balanced diet to prevent further weight gain.
- Give children low-fat snacks for their breaks and meals at school.
- Get children out of the house as much as possible by linking in computer games with physical activity games.
- Limit their use of computer games and watching TV. Encourage exercise such as swimming.
- Make exercise a family activity, so that children learn that exercise is fun, not a chore.
- Promote physical exercise.
- Avoid sugary snacks and fizzy drinks which are high in calories.
- Do not give sweets and crisps as rewards.
- Be a good role model – offer healthy foods and help the child to exercise more by joining in their active play.
- Aim for a broad range of food rather than excluding or severely restricting foods. Occasional burgers, sweets and chips are fine as long as they are balanced by other less fattening foods.
- Avoid 'dieting' in children. It may lead to obsessive eating behaviours such as anorexia nervosa and bulimia. Obesity in childhood may also lead to obesity in adulthood.

Possible complications: Being overweight can lead to problems such as:
- Recurrent chest infections.
- Heart disease.
- Problems with weight-bearing joints.
- Poor self-esteem.

Further information:
- Excess weight can creep up slowly, just as it can with adults. It can also happen very quickly if the child's level of activity drops suddenly, after moving house to where there is less area to play outside, for example.
- Obese children don't just have a struggle to contain and manage their *physical* problem; they also have to deal with people's *attitudes*. Those attitudes can range from disrespect, through mockery, to bullying and prejudice. It is not just other children who hold these attitudes – adults unwittingly pass on their ideas about 'fatness' and personality.
- Children who are teased and mocked because of their appearance often develop psychological problems, which can be very hard to resolve.

ACTIVITY

Obesity is a chronic disorder, just as diabetes and asthma are chronic disorders. And just like diabetes and asthma, it requires skilled, knowledge-based and sensitive management from child care professionals to help children who are affected to lead safe, meaningful and enjoyable lives.

1 Consider the word 'obesity'. What images come to mind? Make a list of the positive, and the negative, images that arise. ➲

2 Compare your list with a friend's list. You have probably found far more negative images than positive ones. The vast majority of people consider obesity not just to be a negative *condition*, but also a negative *word*.
3 Now list the disparaging terms and labels you have heard used to describe obese people and compare these with a friend's list.
4 How could you help a child who is overweight to have good self-esteem? Think of ways in which nursery and school settings could encourage a child with obesity to adopt a healthy attitude towards eating.

Food refusal

What is it? Food refusal is a consistent and repeated refusal to attempt to eat, chew or swallow food.

Cause: Food refusal is fairly common amongst toddlers – often because they are too busy playing and exploring their world to make time for meals. Frequent refusal to eat can result in mealtimes becoming a battleground, with parent and child testing each other's patience to the limit.

Signs and symptoms:
- The child refuses to eat at family mealtimes.
- The child may eat snacks and 'junk food' at other times.

What to do:
- First, check the child's weight against the growth charts to exclude any cause for concern; consult the doctor to exclude any medical disorder.
- If the child is obviously well and growing normally, offer regular meals in small, attractively presented portions.

General care:
- Allow the child to eat according to appetite.
- Offer small snacks (or mini-meals) of nutritious food, such as fruit, cheese cubes or milk drinks; active toddlers *need* to eat between the normal three meals a day to keep up their energy levels.
- Try not to let family mealtimes become a battleground. Encourage the child to take control and to learn that eating is an active, rather than a passive process.
  - Allow the child to eat by any method or combination of methods – fingers and fists as well as with spoons. Tolerate any mess!
  - Don't scoop the food into the child's mouth; if the child asks for help, load the spoon with food and encourage them to take the spoon to feed themself.
  - Let him or her eat in any order or combination – for example, don't insist that they eat all their main course before having any dessert.
  - Keep the meals simple and offer food you know they are likely to eat; any leftovers should be removed without fuss.
  - Try to keep mealtimes enjoyable and a sociable experience; serve treats as part of mealtimes rather than as snacks between.
  - Don't ever use food as a reward, punishment, bribe or threat. Keep the child's eating separate from issues of discipline.

Possible complications: Serious eating disorders may develop in later childhood if the problem of food refusal is not successfully managed.

Enuresis (Bedwetting)

What is it? Enuresis – the medical name for bedwetting – is the involuntary passing of urine and the most common form of bedwetting among children is nocturnal enuresis (wetting the bed at night).

Cause: Most children who wet the bed have done it all their life, and in many cases no reason can be found. Often it is passed on through the family. Bedwetting also happens, or has happened, to a close relative in up to 85 per cent of cases. Fifty-seven per cent of children who wet their beds either have a brother, sister or a parent who has experienced the same problem. One explanation could be that these children are heavy sleepers who do not wake up when their bladder is full. Also, some children develop bladder control later than others.

At night, some children produce too little of the anti-diuretic hormone (ADH) which controls the production of urine.

Enuresis may also have a *medical* or *psychological* cause such as cystitis, diabetes, problems at school, at home, the arrival of a new baby in the home or the divorce of the child's parents.

Signs and symptoms:

- A child younger than six years old regularly wets the bed.

NOTE: Frequent bedwetting is common in children up to the age of six. Approximately 15–20 per cent of all five-year-olds and six-year-olds wet the bed and most of those are boys.

What to do: Consult the doctor if:

- the child still wets the bed after the age of six
- the child suddenly starts wetting the bed without having done so earlier
- the child's urine has a strong smell, or if the child says that it hurts during or after urination
- the child starts to wet her or himself during the day
- the child urinates more than usual, day or night
- the child has constipation or defecates in his or her pants.

The doctor will start by asking questions about the child, such as when they learnt to go to the toilet in the daytime. They will probably also ask if someone else in the family has had the same problem. After this, the doctor will examine the child, feeling their stomach and abdomen. Often, the doctor will ask for a urine sample in order to rule out a bacterial infection or cystitis. The doctor may also take a blood sample.

General care:

- Protect the bed by using a waterproof mattress, or a fitted waterproof mattress cover under the bottom sheet. This must be fastened securely to prevent any danger of suffocation. Place clean night clothes and sheets next to the bed so the child can change if she or he wakes up.
- Don't make the bedwetting a big issue in the family. Most children are embarrassed about wetting the bed, so it will help if the family support the child and show a positive attitude.
- Don't get angry with the child or punish them if they wet their bed. This could only make matters worse.
- Let the child know that many other children do it too. If someone in the family has had the same problem, tell the child about it. Knowing that others have been affected in the same way will help a child deal with the problem.
- If the child is in agreement, keep a calendar or diary and mark Dry Nights with a star.
- Praise the child when he or she wakes up in the morning without having wet the bed. Encouragement is often the most helpful way of dealing with the problem. ➲

➲ Enuresis (Bedwetting) continued

- Don't put a nappy on the child at night as this will make the child less aware of the problem and not teach them to notice when they need to urinate.

If methods using praise and encouragement don't work:

- Try using a **bedwetting alarm** that makes a ringing or buzzing sound or vibrates if the child wets the bed. (These are successful in curing the condition in 70 per cent of cases.)
- The alarm is often very effective because it makes the child wake up as soon as the first drop of urine hits the underwear or the sheet. The child is thus made aware that he or she is urinating and what it feels like when their bladder is full. (**NOTE:** Don't use a bedwetting alarm if the child objects to it.)
- Don't be embarrassed to discuss further options with the GP or health visitor if none of the above suggestions appear to be effective.

Further information:

- Many parents have been told to wake the child in the middle of the night and make them go to the bathroom. Studies show that the positive effect of this is almost non-existent, since the child does not wake up by him or herself because of the need to urinate.
- It may take weeks or months before there is any change. Training a child will take time, so patience is required from all involved. Most children naturally stop wetting the bed eventually.

Soiling or encopresis

What is it? When a child who is older than four regularly has stool or bowel movement accidents, the condition is called encopresis. Chronic **constipation** often leads to encopresis. The stools may be firm, soft, or liquid. Most children achieve bowel control by the age of three years and the occasional accident after the child has been toilet trained is not a problem. Encopresis is a persistent soiling in inappropriate places.

Cause: Chronic constipation is the most common cause of encopresis. Hard, dry stools accumulate in the bowel and loose, watery motions trickle out past them. The problem often starts as the result of some emotional disturbance in the child's life, for example the arrival of a new baby. It may also be a reaction to over-fussy toilet training.

Signs and symptoms: A child with encopresis:

- has stool accidents or liquid stools at times other than during an illness.
- complains about clothing that is too tight around the waist. If you press gently around the edges of the child's stomach or abdomen, you may find a mass that feels almost like the links of a sausage. The mass will have the shape of a large, upside down U that runs up one side of the abdomen, across the top and down the other side.
- complains of pain related to having a bowel movement. Sometimes a child will tell you that he or she can't go to the toilet because it hurts too much.
- has a poor appetite.
- complains of a stomach ache, heartburn, or cramps; may feel too full to eat; or may vomit.

What to do:

- Check if the child is affected by stress, for example caused by a new baby, moving house or starting school.
- Try to determine whether the child is constipated – ask them when they last had a bowel movement. ➲

➲ Soiling or encopresis continued

- **Consult a doctor** as soon as possible, if you think the child has chronic constipation. The doctor might prescribe a mild laxative and either the GP or health visitor will advise you on how to reduce the constipation in future. If there are thought to be emotional causes for the encopresis, the GP or health visitor may refer the child to a **psychotherapist**.

General care:

- Include as many natural, unprocessed foods as possible in the child's diet, including some fibre in the form of wholegrain (e.g. wholemeal bread) and fresh fruit and vegetables.
- Make sure the child is drinking plenty of fluids.
- Don't punish the child or show disgust if he soils his pants; this could make the condition worse.

If the encopresis becomes a long-term, chronic problem, a **treatment plan** may include:

- The use of enemas to clean out the colon and rectum. When this has been done, the child will need to regularly take laxatives to soften stools and promote bowel movements.
- In addition, the child will need to use a regular toileting schedule. After each meal and at bedtime, the child must sit on the toilet and try to have a bowel movement. This goal is to establish a pattern of regular bowel movements. It is easier to have a bowel movement after meals because of the **gastrocolic reflex** that occurs when we eat. As food goes to the stomach to begin to be digested, this reflex makes the intestines contract to move the stool along so that there will be room for more digested food.
- As part of toileting, a child will need to practise a special technique: holding his breath while tightening his abdominal muscles and bearing down to have a bowel movement.

Encopresis cannot be cured overnight. The child and the family will need to be patient. It is important that the child isn't blamed or teased about this condition, which he or she cannot control. Instead, the child should be praised as each step of the treatment is successfully carried out.

Possible complications: Untreated encopresis can lead to several conditions that threaten a child's health; these conditions include:

- **Megacolon.** This is a disorder in which the colon gets bigger because of the large amount of faeces that stay in the bowel. As the colon gets bigger, its muscles and nerves lose the ability to signal the need for a bowel movement.
- Bleeding and cracking of the skin, called fissures, may occur around the rectum as the result of passing large, hard, dry stools. This can be very painful.
- Blood may appear in the stool, due to the irritation of the colon lining caused by hard, dry, compacted faeces.
- Children may develop urinary tract infections and wetting accidents when the overloaded colon presses on the bladder, or prevents the bladder from emptying completely.

Further information: Fortunately encopresis is rare, but it is a condition that requires very sensitive treatment. More than half of children who soil also wet their beds (see page 144 on enuresis).

Revision questions

1. What is autism or autistic spectrum disorder (ASD)?
2. What is attention deficit hyperactivity disorder (ADHD)?
3. What is developmental dyspraxia? How could you help a child with dyspraxia in a child care setting?
4. Why is obesity on the increase in children? How could you help a child to follow a sensible, healthy eating plan?
5. What is encopresis? How could you minimise the embarrassment for a child who soils himself in the nursery setting?

Eye disorders

◆ *Blepharitis* ◆ *Bruised eye* ◆ *Conjunctivitis* ◆ *Foreign bodies in the eye* ◆ *Squint* ◆ *Stye*

Blepharitis

What is it? Blepharitis is a common inflammation of the eyes, and is often associated with skin conditions such as eczema.

Cause: Blepharitis can be caused by an infection, or become inflamed by flakes of **cradle cap** or dandruff irritating the eye. It is sometimes caused by an allergic reaction to pollen, cat fur, cosmetics or cigarette smoke. It is not serious but it can be infectious. It also tends to recur.

Signs and symptoms:

- The eyelid has a crust around the rim.
- In the morning, the child's eyes may be crusted together.
- There may be white flakes of skin between the eyelashes.
- Yellow greasy scales at the roots of the lashes in seborrhoeic forms of blepharitis.
- One eye or both eyes may look pink, as in **conjunctivitis**.
- Eyelashes may be growing in the wrong direction, or may fall out.

What to do

- If the lids become unusually inflamed, they may be infected: **consult the doctor immediately** for advice. The doctor will prescribe an antibiotic cream or ointment.

General care:

- If the child wakes up with encrusted eyes, hold a warm wet tissue over each eye. Repeat until the crusts are soft enough to enable the child to open his or her eyes. Wash your hands thoroughly afterwards.
- Aim to keep the eye from becoming encrusted: Try:
  - bathing the eyelids with clean cotton wool and warm water, saline or cooled chamomile tea
  - clearing away any scales; use a piece of cotton wool dipped into the boiled and cooled water and wipe the child's eyes one at a time, from the inner to outer corner. Do this two or three times a day, making sure to wash your hands afterwards.
- If possible, persuade the child not to rub the eyes. ➲

➲ Blepharitis continued

- At night, you could apply soft white paraffin, aloe vera gel or aqueous cream to the child's eyelids to keep them from crusting together overnight.
- Keep the child's towels and face cloth separate from the rest of the family's until the condition has cleared up.

Alternative remedies: Gently wash the eyelids in a saline solution, made by dissolving one teaspoon of cooking salt in 600 ml/1pt of warm water. Then apply calendula ointment

Possible complications:

- Where blepharitis is obviously associated with **seborrhoeic dermatitis** or dandruff, the problem may keep recurring; keeping dandruff under control helps prevent flare-ups. Use a shampoo, for example Nizoral TM, sold only in pharmacies for the control of dandruff.

Bruised eye

What is it? A bruised eye is commonly known as a black eye. It is a collection of old blood beneath the skin around the eye.

Cause: Any injury to the soft skin around the eye area causes bleeding beneath the skin which drains towards the eyes. The injury can be:

- **Accidental injury**. Most children instinctively put out their arms when falling, but an accident such as walking into a door handle or knocking against a sharp corner of a table can cause a bruised eye.
- **Non-accidental injury**. This means that the child has been injured by someone else rather than by an accident.

Signs and symptoms:

- At first the skin around the eye takes on a yellow tinge, then the skin turns a dark blue or purple – before fading after a few days.
- Swelling may cause the eye to partially close.
- A darker-skinned child will have an area of much darker skin around the eye.

What to do:

- Comfort and reassure the child.
- Check the eye to see if there is a foreign body present.
- Apply a cold compress – a wad of gauze or lint soaked in water – to the eye to provide comfort.
- Try to find out how the child acquired the bruise.
- If the injury has occurred in an early years setting, complete the Accident Book immediately and inform the parents or carers.

General care:

- If the bruising is severe, the child should be seen by a doctor to make sure that there is no damage to the eye itself.

Possible complications:

- If the blow has struck the area between the eyes or the nose, both eyes may be bruised. The child should be seen by a doctor as permanent injury could result.

Further information: When a child has repeated bruised eyes, you will need to investigate further. In an early years setting, always report any concerns to the person in charge, who will talk to the parents, contact the health visitor or inform the social services department.

Conjunctivitis

What is it? Conjunctivitis is the most common infectious disease of the eye that affects children. The conjunctiva – the transparent membrane that lines your eyeball and your eyelid – can become inflamed for various reasons.

Cause: There are three main causes:

1 **Bacteria**. Bacterial conjunctivitis, commonly known as **pinkeye**, is spread by hand-to-eye contact.
2 **Virus**. Viral conjunctivitis is often caused by the viruses associated with colds, sore throats and measles. Viral conjunctivitis sometimes occurs in epidemics, spreading rapidly through nurseries and mother and baby groups.
3 **Allergy**. Allergic conjunctivitis; some children react to allergens such as pollen, but this is more common in adults.

Signs and symptoms:

- The whites of one or both eyes look pink.
- The eyelids swell up, almost closing the eye.
- The child may rub the eyes if they are itchy.

The different types of conjunctivitis produce different symptoms:

1 **Bacterial conjunctivitis** usually infects both eyes and produces a heavy discharge of mucus.
2 **Viral conjunctivitis** is usually limited to one eye, causing copious tears and a light discharge.
3 **Allergic conjunctivitis** produces tears, itching and redness in the eyes, and sometimes an itchy, runny nose.

What to do:

- Bathe the child's eye or eyes in warm water or saline to wash away the discharge and remove any crusts on the eyelids. Always wipe from the inner to the outer corner of the eye.
- Try using a weak saline solution made by dissolving one teaspoon of regular cooking salt in 600 ml/1pt of warm (previously boiled) water.
- If *one* eye is affected, check eyes to see whether an eyelash or a speck of grit on the inner eyelid could be causing the inflammation. If so, wipe it away with a clean piece of tissue.
- If *both* eyes are affected, consult the doctor, who may prescribe antibiotic drops or cream.

The child's eyes should clear up within a day, but continue to use the cream for 24 hours *after* the eyes have cleared. If, after two or three days, there is no improvement, go back to the doctor.

General care:

- Wash your hands *and* the child's hands with soap and water frequently, and whenever the child touches the infected eyes.
- Keep the child's towel and face cloth separate from the rest of the family's.
- Most cases of conjunctivitis run a predictable course, and the inflammation usually clears up in a few days.

Possible complications:

- Although conjunctivitis *can* be highly contagious, it is rarely serious and will not damage the child's vision if detected and treated promptly.

Alternative remedies: Herbalists recommend using eyebright, raspberry or calendula to soothe the eye and clear the infection. Homeopathy, Chinese herbalism (TCM) and acupuncture can also be helpful in clearing the condition.

Foreign bodies in the eye

If a foreign body such as a speck of dust or grit enters the child's eye, the eye will water and the child will not want to open the eye. If you can see something moving loosely over the white part of the eye, you can try to remove it. **If, however, the object is embedded in the eyeball, or is in the coloured part of the eye (the iris), don't touch it.**

Small specks of dust or grit are not serious as they are washed out naturally by the tears. However, if the child's eyeball is scratched, if an object has pierced it, or there is a cut on the eyeball or eyelid, this is serious and should be treated as an emergency.

Squint

What is it? Also known as **strabismus**, a squint is an inability to move both eyes in the same direction at the same time. It is the most common vision problem in children. There are different types of squint:

- The most common type of squint is the **convergent squint**, which occurs when one eye looks inwards towards the nose. Long-sighted children may develop a convergent squint as they strain to focus when looking at close objects.
- A **divergent squint** is when one eye looks outwards away from the nose and occurs when the muscles attached to the eyeball are not balanced.

If a child has either of these squints, they may have double vision.

Some babies may appear to have a squint that is not a true squint. It is called 'epicanthus' and is caused by folds of skin on a wide nose. Epicanthus does not exclude the possibility of a squint being present, and so you should always seek an expert opinion.

Cause: A squint occurs when the muscles attached to an eye are not correctly balanced, so one eye converges or diverges from the other. Some babies are born with a squint, which is inherited. Young babies are not able to always co-ordinate their eye muscles and one eye may occasionally turn. By three to four months however, the eye muscles will strengthen and the baby should look straight with both eyes. Children with good sight in one eye only, can develop a squint if the weaker eye is not treated.

Signs and symptoms:

- The eyes do not look in the same direction.
- When a light is shone into the eyes, the reflection from the pupils is not symmetrical.
- When sitting, the child may twist oddly to focus on something.
- The child may close or cover the affected eye because he or she is experiencing double or blurred vision in that eye.

What to do:

- Check that the child has a squint by holding a bright toy about 20 cm from the face and slowly move it from side to side. At four months, the baby should follow the toy with both eyes. If an eye flickers or drifts, this suggests the child may have a squint.
- Contact the doctor, who will refer the child to an **optometrist** for tests. If the squint cannot be corrected with eye exercises or glasses, the child may be referred to an eye surgeon.

General care: Squints can be treated in several ways: 

➲ Squint continued

- The child may be given a patch to wear over the good eye for a certain period of time each day. This will force the child to use the weaker eye.
- Unequal vision between the eyes may need to be corrected with glasses.
- Older children will be shown exercises to tone the eye muscles.

Most squints can be successfully corrected by these methods, but in some cases surgery is required to realign the eye muscles. After the operation, the eye will be bloodshot and swollen and healing will be gradual. The full effect of surgery may take a few weeks to assess.

Possible complications: If left untreated a squint can result in:
- Sight becoming worse in the affected eye.
- The child being teased about his or her appearance.
- If at some later point the sight in the better eye is lost, for example by accident, the squinting eye could not compensate and the child would be visually impaired.

Further information:
- About 1 in every 4 children will have a squint some of the time up to the age of six months.
- Squint is a common condition which may become apparent shortly after birth or become more visible once the child starts nursery or school.
- By the age of five years, the child should have normal vision and any defects that develop should be dealt with rapidly.

Caring for children who wear glasses

✓ Encourage a child to wear their glasses at all appropriate times.

✓ Make sure that you provide positive images of children wearing glasses in early years settings – for example by posters, displays and books.

✓ Encourage children to take responsibility for their glasses – for example wiping them with a soft lens cloth and always putting them in their case when not being used.

✓ Check that glasses are comfortable and of the right prescription; watch for signs that the child needs to have the prescription re-checked – for example if a child is constantly screwing up his or her eyes while wearing glasses or trying to look round the corner of the lenses.

Stye

What is it? A stye is a pus-filled swelling (a boil) on the margin of the eyelid.

Cause: It is caused by the inflammation of one or more of the hair follicles from which the eyelashes grow, and it almost always appears on the lower eyelid.

Signs and symptoms:
- A red, swollen eyelid.
- A yellow head of pus on the eyelid around the base of an eyelash.
- Pain or tenderness to the touch.

What to do:
- If the spot on the eyelid is merely red and sore, leave it alone and discourage the child from touching it.
- If the stye is pus-filled and painful, apply a warm compress – or a wad of cotton wool squeezed out in hand-hot water – several times a day, removing it each time when it is cold. ➲

➲ Stye continued

- If you can see the eyelash at the centre of the stye, try to pull it out gently with a pair of tweezers. Get someone else to hold the child's head still if you do attempt this, to prevent damaging the eye with the tweezers if the child suddenly moves.
- If the eyelash won't come out, leave it and continue with the warm compresses.

General care:
- If the home treatment does not clear up the stye within 4 or 5 days, consult the doctor, who may prescribe an antibiotic ointment or eye drops.
- Always wash your hands carefully before and after treating the stye, as the infection can be passed around the family.

Possible complications:
- Blepharitis.

Revision questions

1. What is conjunctivitis? How could you help to prevent the spread of conjunctivitis in a nursery or school setting?
2. List the different types of squint. How would you recognise a squint?
3. What is a bruised eye? How would you treat a child who bruises an eye whilst in your care?
4. How can you care for a child who wears glasses?
5. What would you do if a child has a foreign body in the eye?

Genetic disorders

◆ *Cystic fibrosis* ◆ *Down's syndrome* ◆ *Duchenne muscular dystrophy* ◆ *Fragile X syndrome* ◆ *Haemophilia* ◆ *Phenylketonuria* ◆ *Sickle cell anaemia* ◆ *Thalassaemia*

What are genetic disorders?

All children inherit certain characteristics from their parents. The study of inherited characteristics is called **heredity. Genetics** is the branch of biology concerned with heredity and individual characteristics. Specific conditions and rare disorders may have a genetic basis. Where this is the case there will be a variety of causes. For example, the causes may include a **single abnormal gene**, a **chromosomal abnormality** or a **genetic predisposition allied to other factors**.

Genes

Humans, like every other organism, are made up of cells. We all start off as just one cell at the time of fertilisation. This cell contains two sets of genes, one from our mother and one from our father. Genes are formed from **DNA**, the substance in cells that provides the blueprint for growth in every living organism. For ease of storage and access, the genes are packaged up into 46 protein parcels called **chromosomes**. As the single cell divides, the genes are copied so that every new cell possesses the full complement of genetic material.

Genetic disorders

Genetic disorders occur when the DNA sends out a wrong message. They are inherited in different ways, depending on whether the defective gene is **dominant** or **recessive**:

- **Dominant gene**. When the gene is dominant, the baby needs to receive the defective gene from only one parent to have the condition.

  Examples of dominant gene disorders:
  - Tuberous sclerosis (a disorder affecting the nervous system).
  - Achondroplasia (once called dwarfism).
- **Recessive gene**. When the gene is recessive, both parents must be carriers.

  Examples of recessive gene disorders:
  - Cystic fibrosis (see page 154).
  - Sickle cell anaemia (see page 159).
  - Phenylketonuria (see page 159).
  - Thalassaemia (see page 159).
  - Tay-Sach's disease (a rare disorder of the nervous system).

  There is also a gender-linked route, called **X-linked** inheritance.
- **X-linked inheritance**. In this gender-linked inheritance, the mother is a carrier and unaffected, but may pass on a serious genetic abnormality to her sons. Her daughters will be unaffected but run a 50 per cent chance of being carriers of the condition .

  Examples of X-linked disorders:
  - Haemophilia (see page 158).
  - Fragile X syndrome (see page 158).
  - Duchenne muscular dystrophy (see page 156).

Table 6.1 A summary of genetic defects and their pattern of inheritance

Dominant gene defects	Recessive gene defects	X-linked gene defects
Tuberous sclerosis Achondroplasia Huntingdon's chorea Neurofibromatosis Marfan's syndrome	Cystic fibrosis Friedreich's ataxia Phenylketonuria Sickle cell anaemia Tay-Sachs disease Thalassaemia	Haemophilia Christmas disease 'Fragile X' syndrome Muscular dystrophy – Duchenne type

Unaffected parent	Affected parent	Unaffected parent (carrier)		Unaffected parent (carrier)		Carrier mother		Unaffected father	
○○	○△	○△		○△		⊗●		Ⓨ⊗	
Unaffected child	Affected child	Unaffected child	Unaffected child	Unaffected child	Affected child	Unaffected boy	Affected boy	Unaffected girl	Unaffected girl (carrier)
○○	○△	○○	○△	○△	△△	⊗Ⓨ	●Ⓨ	⊗⊗	●⊗
1 in 2 chance	1 in 2 chance	1 in 4 chance	1 in 4 chance	1 in 4 chance	1 in 4 chance	1 in 4 chance	1 in 4 chance	1 in 4 chance	1 in 4 chance

Key: △ = defective gene ○ = normal gene ● = defective x chromosome ⊗ = normal x chromosome Ⓨ = Y chromosome

- **Chromosomal defects** vary considerably in the degree to which they affect the individual. About 1 in every 200 babies born alive has a chromosomal abnormality, that is, the structure or number of chromosomes differs from normal. Many embryos with chromosomal defects do not survive – they are usually lost during the first few months of pregnancy through miscarriage.

  Examples of chromosomal defects:
  - Down's syndrome. This is the most common chromosomal defect (see page 154).
  - Turner's syndrome. Girls have a webbed neck, are short in stature and may not develop sexually; they may also have heart abnormalities.
  - Cri du chat syndrome. A very rare condition in which a portion of one particular chromosome is missing in each of the affected individual's cells.

Cystic fibrosis

What is it? This is a serious condition which causes recurrent chest infections and an inability to absorb **nutrients** from the intestines. Although cystic fibrosis is present from birth, the condition may not become apparent for many months or years and when it *is* detected, damage to the lungs may have already begun.

Cause: Cystic fibrosis is caused by a faulty gene inherited from both parents who may be carriers but not display any symptoms. The abnormal gene causes sticky secretions of mucus which clogs the airways, leading to the child developing chest infections. The gene also affects food digestion leading to diarrhoea.

Signs and symptoms:
- Failure to grow normally, due to malabsorption (failure to thrive).
- A cough which gradually gets worse.
- Recurrent chest infections.
- Severe diarrhoea with pale, foul smelling faeces.

What to do:
- Consult the doctor who may refer the child to the hospital for tests. Children with cystic fibrosis will have a higher salt content in their sweat; therefore a sample of the child's sweat will be taken and analysed. Genetic tests will also be carried out.

General care:
- If the child is diagnosed with cystic fibrosis, vitamin supplements and pancreatin will be prescribed for the child to take with meals. This will help in the proper digestion of food.
- A high energy diet (a diet high in calories) will be recommended.
- Parents and carers will be shown how to give physiotherapy to clear phlegm from the lungs.
- Children with this condition are susceptible to lung infections and antibiotic treatment is very important in protecting the lungs.

Possible complications: One child in 2000 is affected by cystic fibrosis.
There is no cure for cystic fibrosis but earlier diagnosis and new methods of treatment mean that most people survive into adulthood.

Down's syndrome

What is it? Down's syndrome is a genetic condition occurring when there is an extra chromosome number 21. Why this abnormality occurs still isn't known – even though it is the most common cause of learning disability and is estimated to affect around 1 in 1000 babies born. ➲

➲ Down's syndrome continued

Cause: The most common type of Down's syndrome occurs because of an unusual cell division which has produced either an egg or sperm with 24 chromosomes instead of 23. When this egg or sperm fuses with an ordinary egg or sperm, the first cell of the developing baby has 47 chromosomes instead of 46, and all the baby's cells will have 47 chromosomes.

Down's syndrome is normally suspected soon after birth because of certain distinguishing characteristics; chromosome tests are then carried out to confirm the diagnosis.

Characteristics of children with Down's syndrome:

- Eyes that slant slightly upwards and outwards; there is also often an **epicanthic** fold – a fold of skin that runs vertically between the two eyelids at the inner corner of the eye.
- A small round face and full cheeks.
- A flat back to the head.
- A relatively large, sometimes protruding, tongue in a relatively small mouth.
- Hands that are broad, with short fingers and a little finger that curves inwards; the palm may have only one crease running across it.
- A deep groove between the first and second toe that extends as a long crease on the side of the foot.
- **Hypotonia** – reduced muscle tone which results in floppiness. This improves without treatment as the child gets older.
- Slow physical development.
- A below average weight and length at birth.

Between 40 per cent and 50 per cent of children with Down's syndrome also have a heart defect.

Children with Down's syndrome develop and learn in the same way as children without the condition, but at a slower rate.

Care needs of children with Down's syndrome: These will obviously vary from one child to another and the needs will also be different according to family circumstances and any associated physical health problems. Most of these care needs are the same as for any developing child; it is usually only the *time scale* that is different. Some children with Down's syndrome are within the normal intelligence range; others have a range of learning difficulties. Some special care needs are:

- Help with bodily functions.
- Supervision to ensure safety: some children take a relatively long time before they can recognise and avoid common dangers, so they will need closer supervision both inside and outside the home.
- Stimulation to maximise potential achievement.

Supporting the child with Down's syndrome in an early years setting:

1 **Promoting motor skills**
Children with Down's syndrome tend to have lax muscle tone and so need additional help in developing their **motor skills**; they will benefit from a wide variety of materials such as:
- special spring-loaded scissors, extra thick chunky pencils, large knob inset puzzles, etc.

They also benefit from a wide range of multi-sensory activities.

2 **Promoting independence**
Developing self-help skills is important in order to prepare the children as much as possible for the demands of school, especially as other children may 'mother' them. So they may need *additional* help in areas such as:
- toilet training and dressing themselves 

➲ Down's syndrome continued

- feeding and drinking independently, and, for example, unwrapping a packed lunch.

Skills should be taught through a 'small steps' approach. Liaison between pre-school and home is particularly important in order to maximise consistency.

3 Promoting speech and language development

Most children with Down's syndrome have some degree of speech and language impairment. Most will start to speak between the age of 2 and 3 years old. However, the vast majority manage to communicate extremely well from an early age with very little or no use of spoken language.

- Children with Down's syndrome can be taught to use signs and gestures (such as **Makaton** or **Signalong**); these are a real aid to both a child's understanding and ability to communicate. Signs and speech are used together; as the child becomes more able to say the words, the signs are dropped, often by the age of five.

4 Hearing

Many children with Down's syndrome have some degree of hearing loss, even if only a fluctuating one. This will also affect the development of their speech to some extent.

5 Ability to concentrate

Many children have **shorter concentration spans** than their peers. They also have more difficulty processing input from more than one sense at a time (e.g. copying and listening), which inhibits their ability to focus. These difficulties are particularly apparent in the early years and many young children with Down's syndrome may be easily distracted, flitting from one activity to another.

Complications:

- 40 per cent of children with Down's syndrome have **heart problems** at birth, half of which are serious and require surgery.
- More than half of children with Down's syndrome have significant hearing problems and problems with vision are even more common.
- It is likely that up to 30 per cent of people with Down's syndrome may develop thyroid disease.
- More minor complaints, such as dry skin and coughs and colds, are also more common.

Further information: Down's syndrome occurs in families from all social, economic, cultural, religious and racial backgrounds.

Duchenne muscular dystrophy

What is it? Duchenne muscular dystrophy is the most common form of muscular dystrophy in children. The main features of the disorder are progressive weakness and wasting of muscle.

Cause: The disorder is caused by an X-linked gene (i.e. the gene is on the X chromosome; girls have two of these and boys only one). This means that only boys are affected but that their mothers are often carriers. Each subsequent son of a carrier has a 50:50 chance of being affected and each daughter has a 50:50 chance of being a carrier herself.

Signs and symptoms:

- Most affected boys develop the first signs of difficulty in walking at the age of 1 to 3 years.
- By about 8 to 11 years (rarely earlier or a little later) they become unable to walk.
- Frequent falling and difficulty in getting up after a fall: the child may try to stand up by rolling over onto his front and using his hands to 'walk' up his legs. This is due to the weakness of the leg muscles.
- Waddling gait. 

➲ Duchenne muscular dystrophy continued

- Inward curvature of the lower spine.
- The calf muscles may appear larger because the muscles are replaced by fat.

What to do:

- Consult a doctor if a male toddler has decreased ability to walk or climb stairs or has difficulty lifting his arms above his head.
- Often early years workers and teachers are the first to notice the difficulties experienced by a child with muscular dystrophy. Any concerns should be reported to a senior member of staff who can discuss them with the child's parents.
- Diagnosis is usually made after hospital tests; all affected boys have very abnormally high levels of an enzyme called creatine kinase in their blood.
- Unfortunately no cure has yet been discovered. Much can be done to help limit the effects of the muscular dystrophy but no treatment is yet known which affects the actual *loss* of muscle cells.

General care: The family of a child diagnosed with Duchenne muscular dystrophy will require a great deal of support. The main areas to consider are:

- **Maintaining mobility and independence**. Physiotherapy, hydrotherapy and the use of orthopaedic aids, such as splints, can all be used. Walking sticks, powered wheelchairs and other rehabilitative devices can also help children maintain mobility and independence. Surgery can sometimes relieve muscle shortening. Respiratory care, deep breathing and coughing exercises are often recommended.
- **Support for the child and their family**. Parents, carers and teaching staff will need to discuss aspects of the child's progress, and to ensure that the child's needs are met within home and school. This may entail the child being the subject of a statement of **Special Educational Needs** (see page 298). Parents and other family members will experience a wide range of emotions when hearing of the diagnosis. They can obtain support from various voluntary support groups, including the Muscular Dystrophy Association.
- **Genetic counselling**. Because there is a risk of any future children being affected by the particular gene responsible for the disorder, it is important to seek genetic advice and appropriate tests for those members of the family who are at risk of being carriers.

Possible complications:

- The child's muscle weakness increases and gradually spreads to affect more muscles, including the respiratory muscles.
- Boys become increasingly susceptible to chest infections and generally need to use a wheelchair by the time they reach puberty. Life expectancy is generally not above the early twenties.

Further information: About 100 boys with Duchenne muscular dystrophy are born in the United Kingdom each year. There are about 1500 known boys with the disorder living in the UK at any one time. For the general population the risk of having an affected child is about 1 in every 3500 male births.

ACTIVITY

Find out all you can about one of the more common genetic disorders – e.g. Down's syndrome, cystic fibrosis or haemophilia. Prepare a fact sheet that includes the following information:

- ☐ A brief description of the disorder, with cause and incidence.
- ☐ The effects on the child and on their family.
- ☐ The support services available to families – both **statutory** and **voluntary**.

Fragile X syndrome

Fragile X syndrome is the most common *inherited* form of learning difficulty. It gets its name from a gene on the X chromosome. The range of effects on the individual child is very wide; the table below lists some of the main characteristics which may be associated with Fragile X syndrome; however, it is rare for *all* the features listed to be present.

Table 6.2 Some characteristics associated with fragile X syndrome

Behaviour	
Overactivity	Unable to settle for long to any one activity: always rushing around
Demanding attention	Demands for attention are persistent and insistent
Hand-flapping	Usually at times of anxiety or distress
Excitability	Acting without thinking first, responding impulsively to first perceptions
Speech and language	
Dysarthria	Difficulty in articulating sounds
Dysphasia	Difficulty in selecting the words with which to speak
Echolalia	Compulsive repetition of the last word or phrase spoken to them
Palilalia	Compulsive repetition of their own words or phrases
Lack of fluency	Speech is often rapid and digresses from subject
Emotional and social development	
Emotional lability	Tendency to react emotionally to relatively minor upsets
Sensitivity	Extra sensitive to any perceived criticism
Security	Need for constant reassurance; often appears to need a routine
Reaction to environment	Displays variability in reactions to 'busy' environments; appears overwhelmed if a lot is going on around them, particularly in noisy settings
Cognitive development	
Verbal skills	Verbal skills are better than reasoning skills
Abstract reasoning	Tendency to be diverted by attention to irrelevant aspects of tasks and events
Understanding of maths	Difficulty with number concepts and basic arithmetical processes
Vocabularly	Relative strengths in vocabulary and associated verbal areas

Haemophilia

Haemophilia is one of the commonest disorders of the blood clotting system, occurring in 1 in 10,000 people. Haemophilia is caused by a deficiency of factor VIII (normally produced in the liver), the gene which is on the X sex chromosome.

Just how easily or badly children with haemophilia bleed will depend on the severity of the deficiency. The mildest sufferers will only have abnormal bleeding after major injury, whereas those most affected will have spontaneous haemorrhages, particularly into joints but also skin, muscle and organs, causing extensive tissue damage. Haemorrhages into the brain are particularly difficult and can be fatal.

Phenylketonuria

Phenylketonuria is a very rare metabolic disorder, which prevents the normal use of protein food. If untreated, it usually damages the nervous system and leads to mental retardation. It affects around 1 in 10,000 babies in the UK. All babies born in the UK are routinely tested for phenylketonuria (PKU) by means of a simple blood test – the **Guthrie Test**. A small blood sample is taken from the baby's heel when about 7–11 days old and is sent for analysis to a central laboratory. Early diagnosis is vital and treatment involves a special formula protein diet which has to be followed throughout the person's life.

Sickle cell anaemia

Sickle cell anaemia is an inherited condition caused by an abnormal form of haemoglobin in the blood. The red blood cells (normally round) become sickle-shaped (or crescent-shaped). The cells clump together and lodge in the smaller blood vessels, preventing normal blood flow and resulting in anaemia (lack of haemoglobin).
In Britain it is most common in people of African or Caribbean descent, but may also occur in people from India, Pakistan, the Middle East and the Eastern Mediterranean.

Features of sickle cell anaemia: Children with sickle cell anaemia can almost always attend a mainstream school but are subject to *crises* which may include the following:

- **Pain** – often severe, occurring in the arms, legs, back and stomach – due to the blockage to normal blood flow.
- **Infections** – children are more susceptible to coughs, colds, sore throats, fever and other infectious diseases.
- **Anaemia** – most children are anaemic; only if it is severe will they feel lethargic and ill.
- **Jaundice** – may show as yellow staining of the whites of the eyes.

Treatment Blood transfusions may be necessary. Infections should be treated promptly and immunisation against all the normal childhood diseases is recommended.

Caring for a child with sickle cell anaemia:

- **Know how to recognise a crisis**. If the child suddenly becomes unwell or complains of severe abdominal or chest pain, headache, neck stiffness or drowsiness, contact parents without delay – the child needs urgent hospital treatment.
- **Make sure the child is always warm and dry**. Never let a child with sickle cell anaemia get chilled after PE or swimming.
- **Make sure the child does not become dehydrated** – allow him or her to drink more often and much more than normal.
- **Make sure that the child is fully immunised** against infectious illnesses and any prescribed medicines (e.g. vitamins and antibiotics) are given.
- **Help with schoolwork**. If badly anaemic, the child may find it difficult to concentrate and regular visits to the GP or hospital may entail many days off school.
- **Give support** – the child may find it difficult to come to terms with the condition; make allowances when necessary.

Thalassaemia

Thalassaemia is a group of inherited blood disorders in which there is a fault in the production of haemoglobin. Many of the red cells produced are fragile and rapidly broken up, leading to anaemia. Thalassaemia is prevalent in the Mediterranean region, the Middle East, and South East Asia, and in families originating from these areas. ➲

➲ Thalassaemia continued

Cause: Thalassaemia is only a risk when both parents carry the faulty gene, as the baby inherits one copy of the gene from each parent. If one parent is normal then the child will receive one normal gene and is only at risk of being a carrier.

Features of thalassaemia: Children with thalassaemia are healthy at birth but later show the following symptoms:
- Pale, irritable and weak.
- May not feed properly.
- Fail to thrive.

They are unable to make blood properly and become very anaemic.
The difficulties experienced by children with thalassaemia are similar to those of sickle cell anaemia.

Further information: Treatment consists of regular blood transfusions throughout life. Regular blood transfusions can lead to accumulation of iron in the body and other complications.
It is possible to cure thalassaemia with a bone marrow transplant but it is difficult to find a good match and there may be risks and complications.
Preventing thalassaemia is possible through **genetic testing**, but this can then lead to the dilemma of whether to terminate a pregnancy.

Revision questions

1 What is Down's syndrome? What are the characteristic features of a child with Down's syndrome?
2 What is Fragile X syndrome? What sort of health problems might a child with this syndrome have?
3 What is cystic fibrosis? How is it diagnosed and what are the child's long-term health needs?
4 What is sickle cell anaemia? How can a sickle cell crisis be prevented?
5 What is Duchenne muscular dystrophy? How can the condition be recognised and what support is available to the family?

Infectious diseases

◆ *Chickenpox* ◆ *Diphtheria* ◆ *Fifth disease (Erythema infectiosum)* ◆ *Hand, foot and mouth disease* ◆ *Kawasaki disease* ◆ *Measles* ◆ *Mumps* ◆ *Polio* ◆ *Roseola infantum (3-day fever)* ◆ *Rubella (German measles)* ◆ *Scarlet fever* ◆ *Tetanus* ◆ *Tuberculosis* ◆ *Whooping cough (Pertussis)*

What are infectious diseases?

Infections are still a major cause of illness in children, and they range from a mild attack of the common cold to a life-threatening illness such as meningitis. Children are particularly susceptible to infection because their immune systems have not yet built up resistance. Most common childhood infections are not serious and clear up quickly. Some serious viral infections, such as measles and rubella, are less common now because of routine immunisation. Bacterial infections can usually be cured rapidly by antibiotics.

Chickenpox

What is it? Chickenpox is one of the common childhood infections. It is highly infectious and affects mainly children under the age of 10 years. It is usually a mild illness. However, in adults and children with weakened immune systems, chickenpox can cause serious complications and even death. Chickenpox is sometimes called **varicella**.
The *incubation period* is 2–3 weeks.

Cause: Chickenpox is caused by a virus – herpes zoster – which also causes **shingles** in older people. The chickenpox virus spreads from person to person by direct contact with fluid from broken chickenpox blisters. It also spreads through the air by coughing or sneezing.

Signs and symptoms:

- Mild fever or headache which precedes the rash.
- Generally unwell.
- A rash, which has the following features:
  - Small, dark red spots, which occur in batches on the chest and back.
  - These rapidly turn into an extremely itchy outbreak of blisters – these are clear fluid-filled blisters with red bases; they occur in successive crops all over the body and face.
  - The blisters dry and become scabs in 4–5 days.
  - Spots at various stages of development are usually present at the same time.

See colour section after page 220.

What to do:

- Reassure and comfort the child.
- Contact the parents.
- There is no need to consult the doctor unless you are unsure whether it *is* chickenpox, or if the child is very unwell and/or distressed.
- Paracetamol will help bring down a temperature. (See also page 81 for how to reduce a raised temperature).

General care:

- Give plenty of liquids to drink.
- Give the child comforting baths; you could try adding a handful of bicarbonate of soda to the bath water.
- Dress the child in loose comfortable cotton clothes.
- Use calamine cream or lotion to ease the itchiness. The doctor may prescribe anti-histamine cream or medicine if the itching is severe.
- Discourage the child from scratching the spots.
  - Keep their fingernails short.
  - Explain why they must try not to scratch the spots and try to distract them with simple activities.
  - Very young children can wear cotton mittens to prevent them from scratching.
- The doctor may prescribe antibiotics to treat spots that become infected with bacteria.
- You should also inform the school/nursery in case other children are at risk.
- *Never* give aspirin to a child with chickenpox or any other viral illness, because of the risk of **Reyes syndrome**.

NOTE: Keep the child away from anyone who is, or is trying to become pregnant. If the child was with anyone pregnant before he/she became unwell, let that woman know about the chickenpox and tell her to see her GP.

Possible complications: The most common complications of chickenpox are:

- Scarring from scratched spots.
- Skin infections – such as **impetigo** (which can be treated by antibiotics). ➲

➲ Chickenpox continued

Other rarer complications are:
- Pneumonia.
- Encephalitis (inflammation of the brain).
- Hepatitis (inflammation of the liver).

Chickenpox can also lead to severe problems in pregnant women, causing stillbirths, birth defects, or infection of the new-born during childbirth.

Further information:
- Chickenpox is so contagious in its early stages that an exposed person who has not had chickenpox has a 70–80 per cent chance of getting the disease.
- Although people cannot get chickenpox twice, the same virus causes **shingles**. A person with shingles can spread the virus to an adult or child who has not had chickenpox, and that person can develop chickenpox.
- An infected child is contagious from 1 to 2 days before the rash appears and until all the blisters have dried out and formed scabs. Once the scabs have dried, the child can return to school if they feel well enough.
- In the USA, a vaccine is offered to prevent chickenpox, but there is no vaccine available in the UK.

Diphtheria

What is it? Diphtheria is an acute and highly contagious bacterial infection that mainly affects the nose and throat. It is extremely rare now in the UK because of the success of immunisation programmes. The incubation period for diphtheria is 2–4 days, although it can range from 1 to 6 days.

Cause: Diphtheria is caused by bacteria and spread by droplet infection.

Signs and symptoms: In its early stages, diphtheria can be mistaken for a **bad sore throat**. The degree of severity varies widely but the following are all characteristic signs:
- Generally unwell.
- Very sore throat.
- Headache.
- A low-grade fever.
- Swollen neck glands.
- A thick coating – or membrane – in the nose, throat, or airway. This coating is usually whitish-grey and can cause:
  - breathing problems, and
  - difficulty in swallowing.

In more advanced stages, the child may have:
- great difficulty breathing or swallowing
- may complain of double vision
- have slurred speech
- show signs of going into shock (pale, cold skin; rapid heartbeat; sweating; and an anxious appearance).

What to do: Call the doctor immediately if you suspect diphtheria.

General care: Children with diphtheria are treated in a hospital.
- After a doctor confirms the diagnosis through throat culture and blood counts, the child is given:
  - a special anti-toxin to neutralise the diphtheria toxin already circulating in the body; the anti-toxin is given through injections or intravenously. The child is ➲

➲ Diphtheria continued

closely observed while the anti-toxins are given because the solution, which is made from horse serum (blood), may cause an allergic reaction.
  – antibiotics to kill the remaining diphtheria bacteria.
- The child must be isolated. Family members who have not been immunised, or who are very young or elderly, must be protected from contact with the child.
- After the antibiotics and anti-toxin have taken effect, the child will need prolonged bed rest (4–6 weeks, or until full recovery).
- Bed rest is particularly important if the child's heart has been affected by the disease.

Possible complications: In advanced cases, diphtheria toxins (or poison) spread through the bloodstream and can lead to potentially life-threatening complications:
- Heart failure: the toxins can cause tissue damage that affects the heart's ability to pump blood.
- Further chest infections such as bronchopneumonia.
- Damage to the kidneys.
- Nerve damage, eventually leading to paralysis.

Further information:
- Diphtheria is *highly* contagious. It is easily passed from the infected person to others through sneezing, coughing, or even laughing. It also can be spread to others who pick up tissues or drinking glasses that have been used by the infected person.
- Children under five years old and adults over 60 are particularly at risk of contracting diphtheria, as are those living in crowded or unsanitary conditions, the undernourished, and children and adults who do not have up-to-date immunisations.
- People who have been infected by the diphtheria bacteria can infect others for up to four weeks, even if they don't have any symptoms.

Prevention: Preventing diphtheria depends almost completely on immunising children with the combined **diphtheria/tetanus/ pertussis vaccine (DTP)**. Although most children tolerate it well, the combined DTP vaccine sometimes causes mild side-effects such as redness or tenderness at the injection site, a low fever, or general irritability. Severe complications, such as an allergic reaction or seizures, are very rare.
Most cases of diphtheria occur in children who have not received the vaccine at all or who have not received the entire course.

Fifth disease (Erythema infectiosum)

What is it? Fifth disease is a mildly to moderately contagious viral infection common among school-age children, particularly in the winter and spring.

Cause: Fifth disease is caused by a virus. It is spread by airborne droplets – through coughing or sneezing – or through blood infected with the virus.

Signs and symptoms:
- It usually begins with the distinctive, sudden appearance of bright red cheeks that look as though the child has been slapped. It is also known as **slapped-cheek syndrome**.
- Raised temperature.
- A rash with the following features:
  – Flat or raised red rash, usually on the thighs and upper arms, which appears 1–4 days after the reddened cheeks.
  – It may be itchy and may last from 2 to 10 days.
  – The rash fades from the centre of red areas toward the edges, giving it a lacy appearance. ➲

➲ Fifth disease (Erythema infectiosum) continued

– The rash can recur with exercise, warm baths, rubbing the skin or emotional upset. See colour section after page 220.
- Less commonly, headache, sore throat and joint pains.

NOTE: Not all children with fifth disease develop the rash.

By the time the rash appears, children are no longer contagious and may attend school or day care. The incubation period (the period between infection and signs or symptoms of illness) is usually 4 to 14 days but can be as long as 21 days.

What to do:
- Call the doctor if the child has any form of anaemia, especially sickle cell anaemia or thalassaemia, as fifth disease can cause severe illness in these children.

General care:
- No treatment is necessary. The distinctive rash is harmless and fifth disease causes no symptoms that require medical treatment.
- Comfort and reassure the child.
- Offer plenty of fluids and give paracetamol to reduce the temperature.

Possible complications: If a pregnant woman is infected in the first half of her pregnancy, there is a small risk of severe anaemia in the foetus.

Further information: Fifth disease got its name many years ago when it was the fifth disease recognised among several childhood illnesses which have similar rashes; the others are measles, rubella, scarlet fever and chickenpox. It is also called Erythema infectiosum and slapped-cheek disease.

Hand, foot and mouth disease

What is it? Hand, foot and mouth disease is a mild viral infection, mainly affecting children between 1 and 4 years in **epidemics**; it occurs chiefly in the summer and early autumn. It is highly contagious and the *incubation period* is usually 3–5 days.

Cause: Hand, foot and mouth disease is caused by a virus.

Signs and symptoms:
- Slightly raised temperature.
- Tiny raised blisters appear on the inside of the mouth; these sometimes develop into ulcers on the inside of the cheeks and the tongue.
- Reluctance to eat.
- After 1 or 2 days, flat, whitish blisters with a red ring around them appear on the hands and feet. These are more common on the backs of the hands and on the fingers and on the upper surface of the feet.
- The blisters are not usually itchy or painful.

See colour section after page 220.

What to do:
- Relieve the symptoms by:
  – giving liquid paracetamol for painful mouth ulcers and to reduce temperature
  – offering plenty of bland fluids, such as water or milk; do not give fruit juices which contain acids and may make the pain worse.

General care:
- Relieve the soreness in the child's mouth by rinsing the mouth out every hour with $\frac{1}{4}$ teaspoon of bicarbonate of soda dissolved in 100 ml of warm water.
- Try using a straw for drinks.
- Offer a diet of soft foods, such as soup and ice cream, while the mouth is sore.
- Keep the child away from school or nursery until the blisters have disappeared – usually they go within 3 or 4 days. ➲

➲ Hand, foot and mouth disease continued

Possible complications:
- There are no long-term effects of the illness and a single attack provides lifelong immunity.

Kawasaki disease

What is it? Kawasaki disease is an inflammatory condition that affects multiple organ systems. It occurs mainly in children under the age of five years and causes fever, rash and swelling of the lymph nodes.

Cause: The exact cause of Kawasaki disease is unknown, but researchers believe that viral illness precedes the condition. Epidemics of the disease seem to occur every two to three years.
The incubation period for Kawasaki disease is not known.

Signs and symptoms:
- A fever, lasting more than five days; within three days of the abrupt onset of fever, the following symptoms appear:
- Swollen glands (lymph nodes) in the neck, usually on one side and singular.
- Red, blotchy rash over the entire body.
- Swelling and redness of the hands and feet that interferes with walking.
- Red, dry, cracked lips.
- Swollen, sore, red, cracked-appearing tongue, commonly called 'strawberry tongue'.
- Conjunctivitis: bloodshot eyes with no discharge.
- Extreme irritability, vomiting and severe abdominal pain.
- During the second week of the illness, there will be peeling and flaking of the skin from the hands and feet.

What to do:
- Call the doctor immediately.
- The child may be admitted to hospital for diagnostic tests and treatment. If the child is diagnosed with Kawasaki disease, he or she will probably be given:
  - **Gammaglobulin** by injection. Gammaglobulin consists of **antibodies** which reduce inflammation and appear to protect against injury to the heart's arteries.
  - **Aspirin**. Aspirin helps to thin the blood and prevent blood clots. It also helps to reduce inflammation in the body.

NOTE: Never give aspirin to a child because of the risk of Reyes syndrome. Kawasaki disease is the only childhood condition for which aspirin is the recommended treatment, but it *must* be given by a doctor.

General care:
- Children are usually acutely ill for about 10 days.
- Most children recover completely within 5 to 6 weeks, and the disease is unlikely to affect the same child twice.

Possible complications: The most serious complications of Kawasaki disease are its potential effects on the heart and coronary arteries, which occur in roughly 20 per cent of children who are diagnosed.
- Inflammation of the heart muscle, a condition called **myocarditis**. However, the degree to which the heart and blood vessels are involved varies from child to child.
- Inflammation of the coronary arteries; they can then develop **aneurysms** (weakening and bulging of the artery wall). This increases the risk of a blood clot forming in this weakened area blocking the artery and could possibly lead to a
- **heart attack** (myocardial infarction). ➲

Kawasaki disease continued

Further information:

- Kawasaki disease was named after Tomisaku Kawasaki, the Japanese doctor who first identified this disease in 1967.
- Studies have shown that treating Kawasaki disease within 10 days of its onset can greatly reduce the risk of heart-related complications. Usually, any heart problems that may have been observed disappear within 5 or 6 weeks, and there is no lasting damage.
- In a small percentage of cases, though, coronary artery abnormalities persist.

Measles

What is it? Measles is a highly infectious illness. It mainly affects babies under the age of one, when they are too young to be vaccinated, and adolescents who have not been vaccinated. Babies less than eight months old are rarely affected because they have acquired some immunity from their mothers.

Cause: Measles is caused by a highly infectious virus, which is spread by airborne droplets coughed or sneezed by an infected person. It takes between 8 to 14 days for symptoms to appear (the *incubation period*). Measles was once quite common, but is now much rarer in the UK because of national immunisation programmes.

Signs and symptoms: Measles starts with the child feeling generally unwell, before developing the following:

- a fever
- runny nose
- red, watering eyes; the child often avoids bright light because the eyes feel sore
- a dry cough.

The following characteristic signs and symptoms then appear.

- You may notice tiny white spots, called **Koplik's spots**, inside the child's mouth. These look a bit like grains of salt on a red velvet pillow.
- Three to four days later, a red rash appears – usually starting on the head and neck – and spreads to cover the entire body. The spots sometimes join to produce large red blotchy areas.
- The child may have a stomach ache, diarrhoea, vomiting, febrile convulsions and swollen glands.
- After 3 or 4 days, the rash starts to fade and the symptoms subside. The rash disappears within a week in most cases.

See colour section after page 220.

What to do:

- Consult the doctor within 24 hours if you suspect measles.
- To bring the fever down, give the child plenty of fluids and infant paracetamol (suitable for infants over three months old). As it is a viral infection it can't be treated with antibiotics.
- Comfort and reassure the child.
- Darken the room if the light bothers the child's eyes.

General care:

- Let the child choose whether or not to stay in bed. Offer quiet play activities – see page 242.
- Offer plenty of fluids and continue to control the child's fever.
- The doctor may prescribe antibiotics to prevent any secondary bacterial infection.
- Homeopathic remedies are given according to how far the disease has progressed – mainly belladonna and bryonia.

➲ Measles continued

- Traditional Chinese Medicine helps to soothe the symptoms and boost the child's recovery, especially when given together with acupuncture.

Possible complications: Most children recover within a week or ten days and will have lifelong immunity. But some children develop complications such as:
- ear infections, particularly **otitis media** – infection of the middle ear
- chest infections – such as **bronchitis** and **pneumonia**, and
- serious complications such as **encephalitis** (inflammation of the brain) can occur on rare occasions.

Contact your GP straight away if 7 to 10 days after the appearance of the rash, the child gets a headache, becomes drowsy or vomits – it can be a sign of encephalitis.

Further information: Measles is not usually a serious disease; most children recover completely within about 10 days of the onset of symptoms. A single attack of measles should give lifelong immunity.

Mumps

What is it? Mumps is a mild infection that was common among children before the introduction of routine immunisation. It causes a fever and characteristic swelling of one or both of the salivary glands, which are just in front of and below the ears.

Cause: Mumps is caused by a virus and is spread by direct contact with saliva or airborne droplets.
The incubation period is from 15 to 24 days.

Signs and symptoms:
- At first the child may be mildly unwell with a slight fever.
- The child may complain of pain around the ear or being uncomfortable when chewing.
- Swelling then starts under the jaw up by the ear. Swelling often starts on one side, followed (though not always) by the other. The child's face is back to normal size in about a week.
- May complain of headache and a dry mouth, caused by a reduction in saliva.
- The child will be infectious from a few days before becoming unwell until the swelling goes down – about 10 days in all.

See colour section after page 220.

What to do:
- Call the doctor if the child has a severe headache with neck stiffness, a persistent earache or abdominal pain. Also consult the doctor to confirm the diagnosis of mumps.
- Offer baby or junior paracetamol to reduce fever and to ease pain in the swollen glands.
- Give plenty to drink, *but not fruit juices*, as these stimulate the production of saliva, which is affected by the illness.

General care:
- The child may not feel especially ill and may not want to be in bed.
- Offer plenty to drink – apart from fruit juices – and soft foods such as soups and purees.
- Give paracetamol half an hour before a meal to ease the discomfort when eating.

Possible complications:
- Viral meningitis or encephalitis can occur up to 10 days after the first symptoms of mumps. ➲

➲ Mumps continued

- Inflammation of the testes in boys; it is rare for mumps to affect boys' testes. This happens rather more often with adult men with mumps. For both boys and men, the risk of any permanent damage to the testes is very low. Infertility following mumps is extremely rare.
- Deafness in one or both ears, which may be permanent; any deterioration in hearing after an attack of mumps should be checked by a hearing test.
- Pancreatitis (inflammation of the pancreas) is a rare complication, but can lead to diabetes.

Polio (Poliomyelitis)

What is it? Polio is an infection mainly affecting the brain and spinal cord (the central nervous system). It can cause paralysis of the affected muscles.
The incubation period is 5–21 days.

Cause: Polio is caused by a virus.

Signs and symptoms:
- Slight fever and generally feeling suddenly unwell.
- Headache, sore throat, and vomiting.
- Stiff neck and back.
- Loss of movement and paralysis.
- If the muscles used for breathing are affected, there will be difficulty in breathing.

What to do: **Call the doctor immediately**.

General care: The child will be admitted to hospital for treatment and physiotherapy. Treatment is for the problems caused by the polio virus rather than the disease itself.

Possible complications: Permanent paralysis of the affected muscles, usually in the legs.

Further information: The polio vaccine is offered routinely by mouth (as opposed to injection). It is very safe and effective.
Anyone working with children should ensure that their polio immunisation is up to date.
Polio is rarely seen in the UK today, but the odd case does occur.

Roseola infantum (3-day fever)

What is it? Roseola infantum is a mild illness that causes a rash and high fever. It occurs sporadically, but most often during the spring or summer. It is a common infection in early childhood, particularly before the age of three years.

Cause: It is caused by the herpes virus; it is not the same virus that causes sexually transmitted herpes.

Signs and symptoms: Roseola infantum has two distinct stages.
After an incubation period of 5–15 days, the first symptoms appear:
Stage 1:
- Fever of more than 39–40 °C (102–104 °F), typically lasting for 3 to 5 days.
- The child may be irritable and may have one or more **febrile convulsions**. These convulsions tend to appear during the first 24 hours of illness, maybe even before you know that the child is ill, and last for a couple of minutes. (See also page 82.) ➲

➲ Roseola infantum (3–day fever) continued

Some children also have:
- mild diarrhoea
- swollen glands in the neck
- cough
- earache.

After about 4 days, the illness enters its 2nd stage.

Stage 2:
- The fever drops suddenly and the temperature quickly returns to its normal level.
- A 'lacy', pink-red, raised rash of tiny distinct spots appears mainly on the chest, back and abdomen, spreading to the arms, legs and face after the fever drops.
- This rash is not itchy or uncomfortable for the child. It may last anywhere from a few hours to 3 or 4 days.

See colour section after page 220.

What to do:
- Focus on lowering the fever to prevent a febrile convulsion. Give infant paracetamol if the child is at least three months old. Encourage him or her to sip it with a drink of water or well-diluted juice.
- Undress the child to nappy or underpants to reduce the fever while you are waiting for the paracetamol to take effect.
- Give plenty of fluids – water or dilute juice. If breastfed, offer a feed every hour or on demand.

Call the doctor if:
- the fever does not come down with paracetamol and tepid sponging
- the child has a febrile convulsion
- the child appears to have roseola infantum, but the rash worsens or does not go away within a few days.

General care:
- This will probably not need any treatment. By the time the child's fever has dropped and the rash has appeared, the virus has nearly run its course.
- The rash itself does not require treatment and should disappear on its own within a few days.
- Homeopathy can help to ease symptoms. Belladonna, pulsatilla or phytolacca are useful remedies often prescribed by homeopaths.

Possible complications:
- Febrile convulsions – or seizures – occur in about 10 to 15 per cent of roseola infections.
- Other complications are rare.

Further information: There is no way to prevent roseola infantum. However, children who have had the condition usually build immunity to the virus and do not get the condition again.

NOTE: Never give aspirin – even baby aspirin – to a child who may have a viral illness, because its use during viral infections has been linked to Reyes syndrome, a rare but potentially fatal condition.

Rubella (German measles)

What is it? Rubella is a mild viral infection that is most common in children between the ages of four and nine who have not had the rubella immunisation. The *incubation period* is 14–21 days.

Cause: Rubella is caused by a virus. 

➲ Rubella (German measles) continued

Signs and symptoms:

- Often starts like a mild cold.
- There may be a mild fever and the child may feel generally unwell.
- The rash appears in a day or two, first on the face, then spreading to the back, chest and limbs. Features of the rash:
  - Tiny, flat spots; on a light skin they are pale pink.
  - As the rash spreads the spots may merge together, but appear less red and blotchy than the measles rash.
  - A non-irritating rash of tiny spots.

See colour section after page 220.

- Glands in the back of the neck may be swollen.
- May be enlarged lymph nodes in other parts of the body.
- The child won't usually feel too unwell.
- May have some pain in the joints.

What to do:

- Consult the doctor to confirm the diagnosis. Do not take the child to the surgery because of the risk to pregnant women.
- Give plenty to drink and paracetamol for fever or pain.

General care:

- Children usually recover quickly from rubella infection.
- Keep the child away from anybody you know who is up to four months pregnant (or trying to become pregnant).
- If the child was with anyone pregnant before you knew about the illness, let her know. If an unimmunised pregnant woman catches German measles in the first four months of pregnancy, there is a risk of damage to her baby.

NOTE: Any pregnant woman who has had contact with German measles should see her GP. The GP can check whether or not she is immune, and if not, whether there is any sign of her developing the illness.

Possible complications: The main complications from a rubella infection occur in the foetus – or unborn child – of a pregnant woman. These include:

- deafness and blindness
- heart defects
- learning disability.

Further information: The child will be infectious from one week before and at least four days after the rash first appears.

Scarlet fever

What is it? Scarlet fever is a mild bacterial infection which has become less common since the use of antibiotics. The main feature of the illness is a widespread rash, which gives the child a scarlet appearance.

The incubation period is typically 2–4 days.

Cause: Scarlet fever is caused by a particular strain of the streptococcal bacteria, and is spread by airborne droplets – through coughing or sneezing.

Signs and symptoms:

- Sudden fever.
- Headache.
- Vomiting, loss of appetite and tummy ache.
- Swollen glands.
- Sore throat. 

➲ Scarlet fever continued

Within 12 to 24 hours of these early symptoms, a rash develops. The main features of the rash:
- There is a mass of tiny red raised spots.
- It starts on the neck and chest, but does not affect the face.
- It spreads rapidly, but is most dense on the neck, in the armpits and the groin.
- It lasts for up to 6 days, and then the skin peels.

- Cheeks are flushed, but the area around the mouth is pale.
- In the early stages the tongue may have a white coating with raised red spots; 2 or 3 days later this coating peels to reveal a bright red tongue with raised red spots (known as a 'strawberry tongue').

See colour section after page 220.

What to do:
- Consult a doctor within 24 hours to confirm the diagnosis.
- **Call the doctor immediately** if you notice that the child's urine is pink, red or smoky in appearance as this is a sign of glomerulonephritis – see below.

General care:
- The doctor may take a throat swab to confirm the diagnosis and will prescribe a 10-day course of antibiotics.
- Give liquid paracetamol to reduce the fever and relieve the pain.
- Give plenty of fluids.
- Ensure the child completes the prescribed course of antibiotics, and keep the child away from other children until the course is finished.
- The child should feel better within a week of the onset of the symptoms.

Possible complications: With the prompt use of antibiotics the following complications are rare:
- Rheumatic fever – a disorder that can lead to permanent heart damage.
- Glomerulonephritis – a kidney disorder which results in damage to the filtering units in the kidneys (see also page 223).
- Middle ear infection (otitis media).

Tetanus

What is it? Tetanus is an acute illness affecting the central nervous system. It causes severe muscular rigidity and painful contractions. It is now rare in developed countries because of immunisation.

The incubation period is 3–21 days.

Cause: Tetanus is a bacterial infection, usually caused by infected dirt entering a cut or open wound.

Signs and symptoms:
- Inability to open the mouth (lockjaw).
- Stiffness of the neck, jaw and other muscles, often accompanied by a fixed, grinning expression
- Difficulty in swallowing.
- Irritability.
- Uncontrollable spasms of the jaw and neck muscles.
- Painful, involuntary contraction of other muscles, particularly the back, neck, abdomen, arms and legs; these occur over a period of 10–14 days and may cause difficulty in breathing.

In some cases, symptoms will develop in the absence of any cut or wound that you can recall. In addition, you may notice restlessness, lack of appetite and drooling. ➲

➲ Tetanus continued

What to do: **Call an ambulance immediately.** This is a medical emergency.

General care: The child will be admitted to hospital. In mild cases, a light diet and sedative drugs are given. In more severe cases, where breathing is difficult, the child may be put on a life-support machine.

Possible complications: Most children who contract tetanus recover completely with prompt hospital treatment within three weeks, although it is still a rare cause of death.

Further information:
- Routine immunisation against tetanus is offered in early childhood – see page 65.
- If a child has a deep wound, take him or her immediately to the nearest hospital accident and emergency department, even if already immunised. Doctors may operate on the wound to ensure that all foreign bodies are removed, and may give a booster of tetanus vaccine.

Tuberculosis (TB)

What is it? Tuberculosis (TB) is a chronic infection which typically affects the lungs, but may affect other areas of the body, particularly the lymph nodes, the kidneys, bones and joints and the brain.

Cause: TB is caused by bacteria spread from person to person through the contaminated fluid droplets of coughs and sneezes.

Signs and symptoms:
- Persistent cough.
- Tiredness.
- Poor appetite.
- Problems gaining weight (failure to thrive).
- May have a slightly raised temperature.

What to do:
- **Call the doctor** if the child has a persistent cough that does not respond to treatment.
- The child will be admitted to hospital for chest X-ray and other investigations.
- After diagnosis, antibiotics will be given for up to a year to combat the bacteria.

General care:
- After hospital treatment, the child will recover at home, with plenty of rest and a high quality diet.
- The source of the disease will be investigated (by contacting family members and friends) and immunisation offered to those at risk.

Possible complications:
- Tuberculous meningitis

Further information:
- According to World Health Organisation estimates, about one-third of the world's population is infected with TB, although most of these people have not developed the active TB disease.
- Among the minority who do suffer from active TB, there are at least 3 million deaths each year, making TB one of society's most deadly infectious diseases.
- TB is increasing in the UK, partly because UK citizens travel to areas where TB is endemic, and partly because of people travelling to the UK from areas where immunisation is not offered.
- BCG immunisation against TB is offered to all children at secondary school (between the ages of 10 and 14 years) after a **HEAF test** to detect antibodies. ➲

➲ Tuberculosis (TB) continued

- Babies born to parents recently arrived from areas of high incidence of TB – e.g. the Indian subcontinent, parts of Africa and South America – are given a BCG immunisation soon after birth.
- TB contact tracers work within health authorities to find all known contacts of a person who has been confirmed as having TB and to arrange appropriate treatment for them.

Whooping cough (Pertussis)

What is it? Whooping cough is a serious, highly infectious disease which leads to an inflamed respiratory tract. The condition mainly affects children and varies from a slight cough to bouts of coughing, which end in a characteristic whoop.
The incubation period is 7–10 days.

Cause: It is caused by bacteria and spread in airborne droplets coughed out by an infected person.

Signs and symptoms: Whooping cough progresses in two distinct stages:
Stage 1 (lasts 7–10 days):
- After the incubation period, the child will have symptoms similar to those of an ordinary cough or cold:
  - sneezing
  - runny nose
  - sore throat
  - slight fever
  - poor appetite.
- The child may also develop a dry cough that is worse at night and after eating. This is the most infectious stage of the illness.

Stage 2 (lasts 8–12 weeks):
- A week or two later, the coughing will become more persistent and severe, especially at night.
- In most, but not all children, you'll hear the characteristic crowing sound or whoop as the child struggles to breathe in.
  - Younger babies may not whoop as they cough, but may stop breathing for a few seconds before starting to breathe again.
  - Older babies may stop breathing after a coughing fit and may also vomit during a coughing spasm.
- During coughing spasms:
  - the eyes will water and bulge
  - the face may turn red, or even blue
  - the veins on the neck and head will swell
  - saliva pours from the mouth.
- The child may have a convulsion or seizure, caused by the lack of oxygen to the brain.
- When not having a coughing attack, the child will feel well.

NOTE: In very young children or babies, there may be *no* spasms of coughing; the symptoms are similar to a prolonged catarrhal cold.

What to do: **Contact the GP at once if:**
- The child or baby under six months old has a cough so severe it makes them vomit.
- The child or baby under six months old has a cough that lasts for more than a week, or seems unusually ill with it. ➲

➲ Whooping cough (Pertussis) continued

- **Always contact the doctor**, whether or not the child has been immunised, and explain that you suspect whooping cough.
- Stay with the child and comfort and reassure him or her while they are coughing.
- If the child stops breathing, just hold securely and reassure them – they will start again.

General care:

- The GP may prescribe antibiotics for the ill child and any other children in the family. This will help to make the cough less severe, but it will not clear it completely. It will also help to prevent the disease spreading.
- Very young children and babies may need a hospital stay in order to monitor their breathing.
- To help to relieve the cough:
  - Remain calm and comfort and reassure the child – it can be very frightening.
  - Sit the child on your lap and pat the back firmly to help bring up any mucus.
  - Ask a physiotherapist to show you some simple techniques for clearing the lungs.
  - Ensure that no-one smokes in the house – and avoid other irritants, such as cleaning materials and aerosol sprays.
- Avoid changes of temperature which can bring on a coughing attack.
- Provide plenty of drinks and soft food, attractively presented. Do not give crumbly food, which may provoke a coughing attack.
- Allow the child plenty of rest as the coughing attacks can leave them exhausted.
- Try to take caring duties in turns with other carers or family members so that you do not become overtired yourself.

Possible complications:

- The cough can last for 2 to 3 months after the infection has been cleared.
- Children who have had whooping cough tend to cough for the next 12 months or whenever they catch an infection.
- In some children whooping cough can develop into **bronchopneumonia**. This can be treated with antibiotics.
- Hernias – after severe coughing spasms, a hernia in the groin may occur.
- Bleeding into the eye and nose bleeds can occur as a result of strenuous coughing.
- In very young babies, the lack of oxygen during the breathless spells can cause brain damage.

Further information:

- Although most children are immunised for whooping cough, it is not always completely effective and not all children are suitable for the vaccination.
- The infectious period lasts from the first signs of the illness until about six weeks after coughing first starts. If an antibiotic is given, the infectious period is up to five days after beginning the course of treatment.
- Children may need to convalesce for several weeks.
- Chinese and Western herbalism, acupuncture and homeopathy can help to relieve the symptoms of whooping cough.

Revision questions

1 What does the measles rash look like?

2 What are Koplik's spots?

3 Describe the rubella rash. Why is rubella immunisation important?

4 Give two other names for fifth disease. Describe the signs and symptoms.
5 Describe the stages of the rash in chickenpox. Name two common complications of the illness.
6 What is the main complication of roseola infantum?
7 What causes scarlet fever? What is the main complication of this illness?
8 In mumps, which glands are swollen? How would you care for a child with mumps?
9 What causes whooping cough? How is whooping cough spread? What are the signs and symptoms of the illness?
10 Why should you never give aspirin to a child?

Life-threatening conditions

◆ *Childhood cancer* ◆ *HIV infection and AIDS* ◆ *Leukaemia*

What are life-threatening conditions?

Life-threatening conditions are those in which medical intervention may prove successful but which carry a substantial possibility of premature death, or those which make the child more vulnerable. Some of the conditions described earlier in this book can also be life-threatening – for example, **hepatitis**, **Duchenne muscular dystrophy**, **sickle cell anaemia**, **thalassaemia** and **cystic fibrosis**. In this section you will learn about the conditions which occur *without* a genetic cause and which are likely to threaten a child's life.

Childhood cancer

What is cancer? Children's cancers are rare. Only 1 in every 600 children under 15 years of age develops a cancer, and these are quite different from cancers affecting adults. They tend to occur in different parts of the body, they look different under the microscope and they respond differently to treatment. In general, cancer occurs when cells in the body become out of control and multiply. They stop working properly and as their numbers increase they form a lump or **tumour**. When cancer cells break away and spread to other parts of the body they may produce secondary tumours known as **metastases**.

Cause: Nobody knows the cause of cancer, although there are many theories. A great deal of research is currently underway studying a number of possible causes. Sometimes 2 or 3 children develop cancer in the same school or village, causing local concern. These cases are carefully investigated but at present they do seem to arise by chance. Some current theories are that childhood cancer may be caused by:

- *Exposure to radiation* – both the radiation that occurs naturally in the environment and the use of X-rays.
- *Exposure to chemicals* known to be associated with specific cancers in adult life.
- *Exposure to infection*, for example by viruses which cause cells to behave in an unusual way.
- *Exposure to electro-magnetic fields,* for example where the child is living close to power lines or electricity sub-stations. ➲

Childhood cancer continued

Signs and symptoms: The signs and symptoms of cancer in children will vary according to which part of the body is affected. Warning signs include:

- A marked change in bladder or bowel habits.
- An unexplained swelling or lump anywhere on the body.
- Excessive tiredness and lethargy.
- Nausea and vomiting with no apparent cause.
- Weight loss.
- Unexplained pain or persistent crying in a baby or child.
- Generally appearing unwell and lacking energy in spite of a good diet and plenty of sleep.
- Anaemia and easily bruised skin.

What to do: **Consult a doctor** if you suspect there may be a malignancy. Often the doctor will be able to reassure you that it is not cancer, but if a diagnosis is confirmed, treatment will depend upon where the tumour is and whether it has spread to other parts of the body.

Treatments for cancer include:

- **Surgical removal**. If surgery is possible, it may well cure a cancer. This will depend on:
  – whether the cancer can be completely removed
  – whether a border of healthy tissue, free of cancer cells, is removed with the cancer
  – whether the cancer has already spread before the surgery.
  Sometimes removal of a tumour is done for **palliative** reasons – to improve the quality of the child's life, even where there is no hope of recovery.
- **Radiotherapy**. Radiotherapy means the use of 'radiation', usually X-rays, to treat disease. The radiation used is similar to that used for an X-ray, although radiotherapy uses stronger rays than those used for taking X-ray pictures and the radiation beams are very precisely aimed at the child's cancer. As with an ordinary X-ray, the child does not feel anything when having radiotherapy treatment.
  The radiotherapy destroys the cancer cells in the treated area. Although normal cells are also affected, they can repair themselves more effectively than the cancer cells. A course of radiotherapy is usually given over a number of days or weeks. Each treatment is known as a 'fraction'. Fractions are usually given once a day from Monday to Friday with a rest at the weekend to help normal cells recover. The damage to these cells, which is usually temporary, is why radiotherapy sometimes causes side-effects:
  – Tiredness.
  – Nausea and vomiting.
  – Inflammation of the skin around the treatment site.
  – Loss of hair from the treated area.
- **Chemotherapy**. The word 'chemotherapy' comes from two words: 'chemical therapy'. It means 'drug treatment'. Chemotherapy uses anti-cancer ('cytotoxic') drugs to destroy cancer cells. The child may be treated with just one drug or many. The chemotherapy selected depends on many things:
  – The type of cancer.
  – Where in the body it started.
  – What the cancer cells look like under the microscope.
  – Whether the cancer has spread.
  Chemotherapy may be used on its own, with surgery, radiotherapy or both. 

➲ Childhood cancer continued

Because chemotherapy affects cells which are dividing frequently, it can also cause unpleasant side-effects. Cancer cells are dividing in an uncontrolled manner which makes them susceptible to chemotherapy. Some tissues of the body *also* have cells which divide frequently and these tissues can be affected by chemotherapy as well as the cancer. These can cause certain side-effects to:
– the bone marrow, causing anaemia and tiredness and an increased vulnerability to infections
– the lining of the digestive system, causing diarrhoea and vomiting
– hair follicles, causing hair loss from the entire body.
Children react to treatment in different ways so not everyone having chemotherapy has all the side-effects caused by a drug.

General care: It is difficult for parents to understand the benefits of a treatment which causes such unpleasant side-effects when they are grieving and trying to come to terms with the diagnosis. The treatment can seem more distressing than the effects of the illness it is trying to fight.

Support for the child and family:

- Illness as serious as cancer is bound to have an effect on the whole family. Everyone will be worried and therefore under considerable stress. While a child is being treated for cancer it will be best for everyone if life continues as *normally* as possible. Parents are often tempted to spoil their child and relax the usual rules, but this can cause more problems in the long run. The child will feel more secure if discipline is as usual.
- The child should be able to continue with most of his or her usual activities, if they feel able to, as long as parents and carers are aware of some basic precautions. The hospital staff will give guidance on anything connected with the child's treatment and everyday care.
- It is important for the child to continue normal schooling and, for much of the time, there will be no limitation on their activities. The child's head teacher should be kept informed of the child's illness and any side-effects of treatment that they should know about.
- There is still a great fear of death when cancer is mentioned and most parents react to the diagnosis of their child's cancer in similar ways. They first of all have feelings of shock, fear, numbness and disbelief. 'Why has this happened to us?' is a common question to which there is no answer. They often want to deny that such a thing has happened and may take their child from one doctor to another. As well as shock and disbelief, parents may feel guilty. Most parents ask themselves if they could have prevented the cancer from happening. There is no evidence to suggest that this is the case.
- Many centres treating children have parent groups where parents can meet others in the same situation. They may be able to offer support and encouragement. There are also other kinds of support groups, such as for siblings, in some hospitals

In hospital, the child and family are helped and supported by team of professionals:

- Paediatric nurses.
- Doctors.
- Social workers.
- Play therapists and hospital play specialists.
- Counsellors.
- Representatives of different religious faiths.

In the community:

- Primary health care team – the GP, district nurse, health visitor and practice nurse. 

➲ Childhood cancer continued

- Macmillan nurses – trained district nurses who specialise in caring for people with life-threatening conditions.

Possible complications: Complications include the side-effects of the cancer treatments, recurrence of the original tumour or the spread of cancer to other areas of the body.

Further information: Although the total number of children developing cancer has changed little in the last 40 years, the prospects for many have improved dramatically with advances in treatment.
Cure rates for children are much higher than for most adult cancers, and over 60 per cent of all children can now be completely cured.

HIV infection and AIDS

What is HIV infection? HIV, which is short for human immunodeficiency virus, is a tiny virus that attacks the immune system, which is the body's defence against disease. Over time it damages the immune system so badly that it can no longer fight infections and cancers as it would usually do. If a person becomes infected with HIV, it does not mean that they have AIDS. HIV is an unusual virus because a person can be infected with it for many years and yet appear to be perfectly healthy. But the virus gradually multiplies inside the body and eventually destroys the body's ability to fight off illnesses. It is still not certain that everyone with HIV infection will get AIDS. It seems likely that most people with HIV will develop serious problems with their health. But this may be after many years. A person with HIV may not know they are infected but can pass the virus on to other people.

What is AIDS? AIDS is short for Acquired Immune Deficiency Syndrome.
It is a serious condition in which the body's defences against some illnesses are broken down. A person is said to have AIDS when their immune system is so weak that they develop certain serious illnesses. This usually happens some years after becoming infected with HIV.
People with AIDS develop many different kinds of disease which the body would usually fight off quite easily.

Children and HIV infection and AIDS: Most of the children affected by HIV contract the virus from their infected mother either during or around the time of their birth. The risk from contaminated blood products – for example, when blood transfusion is needed in haemophilia – is rare.

Signs and symptoms: Most babies infected before or around the time of birth will have symptoms before the age of two years. However, some children do not develop symptoms until they are over five years old.
There is a wide range of possible symptoms, which typically include:

- Failure to thrive or poor weight gain.
- Frequent infections, such as fungal infections – for example thrush.
- Enlarged lymph nodes.
- Respiratory infections, especially pneumonia.
- Recurrent diarrhoea.
- Developmental delay.

The most common cause of illness and death in infected babies is pneumonia in the first months of life. ➲

➲ HIV infection and AIDS continued

Preventing mother-to-child transmission of HIV infection:

- Most babies born to women infected with HIV will not themselves be infected. About 1 baby in 6 born to an infected mother will have the virus.
- Pregnant women are not automatically tested for HIV. In some antenatal clinics the test is offered and in others women have to ask for it. All pregnant women can have an HIV test, but a woman will never be tested without her consent.
- If a pregnant woman has a positive HIV test result there are now drugs that can reduce the risk of her passing HIV on to her baby in the womb or at birth.
- Delivery by elective caesarean section also reduces the risk of a baby becoming infected.
- It is usually best for babies to be breastfed. However, if a mother has HIV, breastfeeding will increase the risk of her baby becoming infected, so it is recommended that the mother bottle-feeds her baby.

Helping a child who has HIV infection or AIDS:

Children who have been infected with HIV or who have AIDS will need careful medical supervision. Treatment usually involves:

- Anti-viral drugs.
- Regular injections of gamma-globulin, which boosts the child's immunity.
- Antibacterial drugs to fight infections such as pneumonia.

Some of the drugs have side-effects or are difficult to take, so children need to be encouraged to take the prescribed dose.

Children are not infectious to others. The virus cannot be transmitted through everyday social contact, such as sharing crockery or cutlery, or using a toilet. Children should not be excluded from school or other normal social contacts.

The main risk is to the HIV-infected child, who can develop complications after contracting illnesses such as measles, chickenpox or herpes.

Many health districts have specialist services for HIV-infected children and their families. Parents will need counselling and support to help them care for their child.

Leukaemia

What is leukaemia?

Leukaemia is a form of cancer which can occur in people of any age, from young children to the elderly. The main form of leukaemia in children is **acute lymphoblastic leukaemia**. Normally, the body's cells are replaced by dividing in an orderly way, allowing your body to grow and to heal after an injury. Sometimes some cells act in an abnormal way and may grow into a lump which is called a tumour. Tumours can be **benign** (not a cancer) or **malignant** (a cancer). Malignant tumours can spread to other parts of the body forming secondary cancer deposits in other areas of the body. In leukaemia it is the **blood-forming cells** which multiply abnormally and grow out of control. Even though leukaemia may not produce lumps it is still a type of cancer.

Cause: There is no known cause of leukaemia, although there are many theories.

Signs and symptoms:

In children, acute lymphoblastic leukaemia usually develops at around the age of five years; signs and symptoms include:

- Anaemia – causing tiredness, lethargy, breathlessness on exertion and pale skin.
- Bleeding from the gums – due to a reduction in platelet cells needed to stop bleeding.
- Swollen lymph nodes in the neck, armpit and groin. 

➲ Leukaemia continued

- Pain in the limb bones and joints.
- Easily bruised skin.
- Pinkish-purple flat spots on the skin.
- Nose bleeds.
- Chest or throat infections – the immature white cells are unable to resist infection.

What to do: **Consult a doctor immediately** if you suspect that the child may have leukaemia. The diagnosis is based on a **bone marrow biopsy** that confirms an abnormal number of immature white blood cells.

Care of the child with leukaemia: Children with any form of cancer are treated by specialists. Medical professionals who have expertise in diagnosing and treating children with cancer include **paediatric oncologists**, **pathologists**, **haematologists**, **radiotherapists, surgeons, radiographers**, and others, all of whom work closely together, often in dedicated children's cancer centres. Treatment is by:

- Anti-cancer drugs – **chemotherapy**.
- Blood and platelet transfusion.
- Radiotherapy.
- Bone marrow transplant.
- Protective isolation nursing – to prevent the child becoming infected.

Children undergoing treatment for leukaemia will often require repeated blood tests and insertion of needles to enable chemotherapy and other drug treatment to be given. Even though doctors and nurses are very experienced at taking blood and inserting needles it can sometimes hurt and is not a pleasant experience for the child. Many children therefore have a special device called a **central line**, which is used to take samples of blood and to administer chemotherapy and other drugs (such as antibiotics). It can also be used to give blood or platelet transfusions.

Further information:

- After the first period of hospital treatment, children with leukaemia are often in a state of **remission**; this means that a further bone marrow biopsy and special blood tests show that there are no abnormal cells present in the blood. Children still need further treatment to prevent a recurrence of the illness and this often lasts two years.
- Over 60 per cent of children with any form of cancer are completely cured after treatment; acute lymphoblastic leukaemia is the childhood cancer with the highest cure rate.
- There are many voluntary organisations which offer information, help and support for children and their families.

Side-effects of anti-cancer treatment

Some anti-cancer treatments have distressing side-effects:

- □ *Sudden hair loss.* Wigs are provided for children who lose their hair during treatment, but they should not be forced to wear them if it makes them feel uncomfortable.
- □ *Nausea and vomiting.*
- □ *A change in body shape.* Some corticosteroid drugs cause the child to develop a characteristic 'moon face' and the build up of fatty tissue.

Revision questions

1 How may children be infected with HIV?
2 What are the signs and symptoms of AIDS?
3 What measures should you take in an early years setting to ensure the safe disposal of body waste products?
4 What is leukaemia? What are the care needs of children with leukaemia and their families?
5 What support exists for children with cancer and their families?

Muscle, bone and joint disorders

- *Congenital dislocation of the hips (CDH)* ◆ *Cramp* ◆ *Juvenile chronic arthritis*
- *Perthes' disease*

What are muscle, bone and joint disorders?

Children have a high risk of problems with their bones, muscles and joints. This is because they are very active and because their bones and joints are still growing and are immature. Most bones are broken when children are playing or taking part in sports. Children often fall, and it is a natural instinct to throw the hands out in an attempt to stop the fall. Therefore, most fractures occur in the upper extremities: the wrist, the forearm, and above the elbow. Some disorders are caused by genetic abnormalities or birth defects. Many of these can be successfully treated by an **orthopaedic** specialist.

Congenital dislocation of the hips (CDH)

What is it? Congenital dislocation of the hips is one of the most common abnormalities in new-born babies. The hip is made up of a ball, formed by the end of the thigh bone (femur) and socket joint, formed by the pelvis. If the socket is not properly formed, the ball tends to slip out or dislocate, making a slight click when the hip is moved. It is also known as clicky hips.

Cause: The underlying cause is unknown. It is more common in **breech presentation** babies and babies who have been tightly squashed in the uterus due to lack of space. For this reason, it is more common in first-born babies as the uterus tends to be tighter the first time around. CDH is also more common in girls, due to the female hormones which can cause the joint to be more lax. CDH tends to run in families; so if one girl in the family has CDH, the chances are that her sisters will, too.

Signs and symptoms: Congenital dislocation of the hips is usually detected soon after birth. The doctor manipulates a new-born baby's thighs to check for the condition. If a hip is dislocated, the doctor may feel a jerking sensation as the head of the femur moves into the socket. The problem may be detected later, during one of the routine checks during the first year. Occasionally, the disorder may not be detected until the child begins to walk. You may notice that: ➲

➲ Congenital dislocation of the hips (CDH) continued

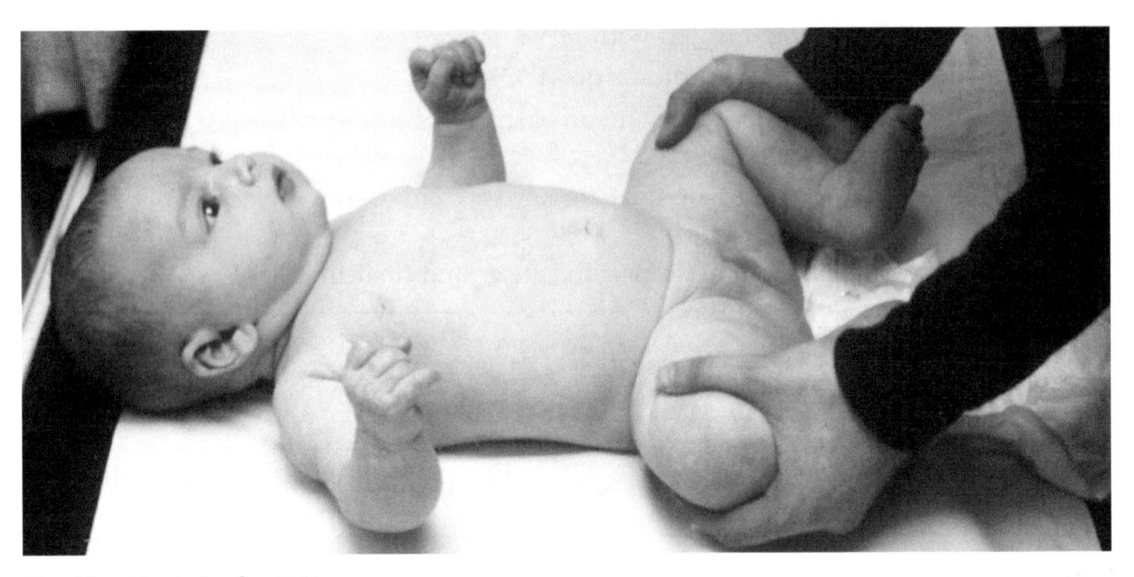

Checking the baby for CDH

- one leg looks slightly longer than the other
- there are extra skin creases on one thigh or buttock
- as you change the child's nappy, one hip may not open as much as the other
- in rare cases, the child may start to walk with a limp or walk on the toes on the affected side.

What to do: The problem often corrects itself soon after birth. If this has not happened by about two weeks of age, a splint may be applied:

- A lightweight splint will be fitted that pushes the baby's legs apart and keeps the hips in position. It will usually be put on within a few days of the diagnosis.
- You may be asked to use double nappies on the child until then, which will act like a temporary splint. The splint is worn under his or her clothes and left on for the duration of the child's treatment – around 6 to 12 weeks.
- You will not be able to bathe the child while the splint or plaster is in place, so you will need to use a sponge or flannel. Also check for any signs of soreness caused by the plaster.
- Buy clothes a couple of sizes too big for the child and always with poppers or velcro.
- A larger than usual pram or buggy is ideal, but the child won't fit into a conventional child car seat. A booster seat may do for a toddler, but a small baby may need to have the seat adapted.

Possible complications:

- When the disorder is detected late, there is a risk of a permanent limp forming.
- Early onset of arthritis in the affected hip.

Further information:

- If the disorder is detected early it can be successfully treated. But if it is only discovered when the child starts to walk with a limp, it is more difficult to treat and may need surgery.
- *Alternative remedies.* Chiropractic can be used to support conventional treatment by helping to improve and monitor the mobility of the child's spine and joints.

Cramp

What is it? Cramp is a strong painful contraction – or spasm – of a muscle. It is sudden and severe but usually only lasts a few minutes. It frequently affects the calf muscle.

Cause: Cramp is caused by the sudden and involuntary contraction of a muscle or group of muscles which then fail to relax. It may be triggered by vigorous exercise, by repetitive movements or by sitting or lying awkwardly. Exercise-related cramp may be partly caused by loss of salt from sweating.

Signs and symptoms:
- Pain around the affected area.
- A lump or swelling may appear in the affected area.

What to do: *Relieve the cramp:*
- Gently massage and stretch the affected muscle.
  - Ask the child to point his toes down as hard as possible and to hold the position.
  - Pull the toes of the affected leg up towards the child's kneecap and hold.
  - Then push the foot back so that the toes point upwards.
  - Hold each position for a few minutes.

  Repeat this process until the cramp passes.
- If pain persists, place a hot water bottle wrapped in a towel to the affected area – or encourage the child to take a hot bath.
- Give the child paracetamol or ibuprofen.
- Reassure the child that the pain is only temporary; stay with the child until the pain has gone.

General care: *To prevent cramp:*
- Make sure that the child does a warm-up routine before taking exercise.
- Ensure the child takes plenty of fluids before, during and after exercise.
- Encourage the child to take a hot bath after exercise to relax the muscles.

If the cramps continue and there is no obvious cause, consult a doctor.

Possible complications: None known.

Juvenile chronic arthritis

What is it? Three types of chronic arthritis – inflammation of the joints – affect children:
1. The most usual type is known as *pauci-articular arthritis*. In this case only one or two of a child's joints are affected, normally a knee or ankle.
2. In other children the arthritis is more widespread, affecting many joints, including the hands and feet; it is called *polyarthritis*.
3. For a few children the small joints are affected and the illness usually begins with high fevers, rashes and enlarged glands; it is called *systemic juvenile arthritis* because it affects the whole body system. (This form of arthritis is sometimes called Still's disease.)

Juvenile chronic arthritis can occur at anytime throughout childhood, but usually starts between the ages of 1 and 4.

Cause: There is no known single cause for childhood arthritis.

Signs and symptoms:
- Joint stiffness and pain in the early mornings, for anything from a few minutes up to three or four hours.
- Redness and swelling of the affected joints, and sometimes a raised temperature. 

➲ Juvenile chronic arthritis continued

- When many joints are affected, the child may have to take a hot bath and do exercises to get mobile before school.
- In systemic arthritis, the following symptoms may appear several weeks before the joints are affected:
  - A temperature above 39 °C (102 °F).
  - Swollen glands throughout the body.
  - A blotchy, non-itchy rash.

What to do:

- Consult a doctor within 24 hours of any of the symptoms.
- The doctor will arrange for blood tests to confirm the diagnosis and to exclude other disorders.

General care:

- The child will need to rest, with the affected limbs supported in light splints.
- Physiotherapy is used to maintain strength, reduce stiffness and increase joint mobility.
- Some children may be given special anti-inflammatory drugs which will require regular visits to the doctor's surgery or the hospital to monitor blood or urine.
- On rare occasions a child may need to spend a short time in hospital for a fuller assessment, for an injection into a joint or even an operation. In these cases it is important that they are welcomed back into their environment as soon as possible.
- **Hydrotherapy** – exercising in water – can help by relieving the pressure on the joints and making them easier and less painful to move.

Possible complications:

- Even though it is a serious illness which can go on for years, the outlook for children affected by arthritis is better than for people who develop it in later life. In most cases the progress of the disease is arrested. The degree of disability or deformity a child is left with depends to some extent on the care received in the early stages.
- Some children may need certain aids and adaptations to help them achieve maximum independence. Special pencils, computers, adapted cutlery, toilet aids, ramps and lifts are just some of the items available. These are usually supplied after recommendations by an **occupational therapist** who will be able to give detailed advice for each child's needs, as these vary widely.

Perthes' disease

What is it? Perthes' disease was originally described as a form of childhood arthritis of the hips. It is usually seen in children 4–8 years of age and is five times more common in boys than girls. Perthes' disease is not really a disease, but a condition characterised by a temporary loss of blood supply to the hip. When the blood supply is diverted, the femoral head in the hip joint dies and intense inflammation and irritation develop.

Cause: The cause of Perthes' disease is unknown.

Signs and symptoms:

- A stumbling, lurching gait or walk.
- A marked limp.
- Pain in the hip or knee.
- Restricted movement in the hip or knee.

What to do:

- Consult a doctor within 24 hours if you notice any of the symptoms listed above.
- The doctor will examine the child and may arrange for hospital assessment, for example X-ray of the hip joint. ➲

➲ Perthes' disease continued

General care: The doctor or specialist nurse may show you some simple exercises to do at home. Hip abduction or hip rotation may be recommended.

Hip abduction:
- The child will lie on his or her back, keeping knees bent and feet flat.
- Place your hands on the child's knees and resist as she pushes out.
- Then resist as the child squeezes the knees together.

Hip rotation:
- With the child on his or her back and with the legs out straight, roll the entire leg inward and outward.

When Perthes' disease is so severe that hip deformity is a real risk, then surgery may be necessary.
- Surgical treatment realigns the bony structures so that the head of the femur is placed deep within the **acetabulum**. Screws and plates are used to fix the bones and will be removed at a later date. In some cases, the socket must also be deepened because the ball actually has enlarged during the healing process and no longer fits snugly within.

Possible complications:
- The risk of arthritis in later life.

Further information:
- After 18 months to 2 years of treatment, the majority of children return to normal activities without major limitations.
- Usually, deformity of the hip joint can be prevented and the joint will then function normally.

Revision questions

1 What is CDH and how is it diagnosed? What are the possible reasons for CDH? What treatment is recommended for CDH in babies?
2 What is cramp? What causes cramp and how could you prevent it? How would you relieve cramp?
3 What is Perthes' disease? What is the complication of Perthes' disease?
4 What is juvenile chronic arthritis?
5 How can hydrotherapy help?

Nervous system disorders

◆ *Cerebral palsy* ◆ *Encephalitis* ◆ *Epilepsy* ◆ *Spina bifida*

Cerebral palsy

What is it? Cerebral palsy is the general term for disorders of movement and posture resulting from injury to a child's developing brain in the later months of pregnancy, during birth, in the neonatal period, or in early childhood. The injury does not damage the child's muscles or the nerves which connect them to the spinal cord – only the brain's ability to control the muscles. (Palsy literally means 'paralysis'.) ➲

➲ Cerebral palsy continued

Types of cerebral palsy: Cerebral palsy jumbles messages between the brain and muscles. There are three main types of cerebral palsy which correspond to the different parts of the brain affected:

1 Spastic cerebral palsy.
2 Athetoid cerebral palsy.
3 Ataxic cerebral palsy.

- Children with **spastic cerebral palsy** find that some muscles become very stiff and weak, especially under effort, which can affect their control of movement. This is the most common type of cerebral palsy, affecting different areas of the body.
- Children with **athetoid cerebral palsy** have some loss of control of their posture, and tend to make involuntary movements. Their speech can be hard to understand, and hearing problems are also common.
- Children with **ataxic cerebral palsy** usually have problems with balance. They may also have shaky hand movements and irregular speech.

Often children will have a mixture of the different types of cerebral palsy.
In some children, cerebral palsy is barely noticeable; others will be more severely affected. No two children will be affected in quite the same way.

Cause: Cerebral palsy is most commonly the result of a failure of part of the brain to develop, either before birth or in early childhood. Occasionally it is due to an inherited disorder. It is sometimes possible to identify the cause of cerebral palsy, but not always. Possible causes include:

- An infection in the mother during the first weeks of a baby's development in the womb (e.g. rubella or a cytomegalovirus).
- A difficult or pre-term birth, perhaps because the baby fails to breathe properly (resulting in cerebral hypoxia).
- Toxic injury, or poisoning, from drugs or alcohol used by the mother during pregnancy.
- Infections of the nervous system, such as meningitis or encephalitis.
- Cerebral bleed (haematoma) which particularly affects pre-term babies.
- Bleeding into cavities inside the brain which may occur in pre-term babies.
- Head trauma resulting from a birth injury, fall, car accident or other causes.
- The baby's brain is formed abnormally, for no apparent reason.
- A genetic disorder which can be inherited even if both parents are completely healthy.

The effects of cerebral palsy: Cerebral palsy may not be recognised until the child is several months old. A child with cerebral palsy may have some or most of the following features, in varying degrees of severity:

- Slow, awkward or jerky movements.
- Stiffness of the arms and legs when being picked up.
- Delayed sitting or walking.
- Feeding difficulties.
- Muscle spasms.
- Floppiness.
- Unwanted (involuntary) movements.

Other areas affected by cerebral palsy:

- **Eyesight**. The most common eye problem is a squint that may need correction with glasses or, in more severe cases, an operation. Some children may have a cortical vision defect, where the part of the brain that is responsible for understanding the images the child sees is not working properly. ➲

➲ Cerebral palsy continued

- **Spatial perception**. Some children with cerebral palsy find it difficult to judge distances or to think spatially (e.g. to visualise a three-dimensional building). This is due to an abnormality in a part of the brain and is *not* related to intelligence.
- **Hearing**. Children with athetoid cerebral palsy are more likely to have severe hearing difficulties than other children, but glue ear (see page 132) is as likely to develop in the child with any type of cerebral palsy as it is in unaffected children.
- **Speech**. Speech depends on the ability to control tiny muscles in the mouth, tongue, palate and voice box. Speech difficulties and problems with chewing and swallowing often occur together in children with cerebral palsy.
- **Epilepsy**. Epilepsy (or abnormal electrical discharge from the brain, causing seizures) affects about one in three children with cerebral palsy.
- **Learning ability**. Some children with cerebral palsy *do* have learning difficulties, but this is by no means always the case. Some have higher than average intelligence and some have average intelligence. Some children have difficulty in learning to do certain tasks (e.g. reading, drawing or arithmetic) because a particular part of the brain is affected; it is then termed a **specific learning difficulty** and should not be confused with the child's general intelligence.
- **Other difficulties**. Some children with cerebral palsy may experience the following difficulties:
  - Tendency to chest infections.
  - Constipation.
  - Difficulty in controlling body temperature.
  - Not putting on much weight.
  - Frustration leading to behavioural difficulties.
  - Sleeping problems.
  - Negative attitudes of others towards them.
  - People sometimes treat children with cerebral palsy as if they are stupid. The term 'spastic' became a taunt used by other children for anyone they felt was inferior in any way. The negative way in which children are treated in society can lead to the child feeling isolated and having poor self-esteem.

Care of children with cerebral palsy: There is no cure for cerebral palsy. It is a non-progressive condition; this means that it does not become more severe as the child gets older, but some difficulties may become more noticeable.

How therapy can help children with cerebral palsy: Physiotherapists, occupational therapists and speech therapists often work very closely together to devise a treatment programme that will meet the needs of both the child and the family. As the nature of cerebral palsy varies immensely, the therapy is adapted to the needs of the individual child. These are some of the things that therapists might do:

- Therapists work at teaching children with cerebral palsy how to inhibit **spasticity** (stiffness) in their muscles in order to promote and produce good patterns of movement. They do this through the use of exercise, structured physical activity and, if necessary, the use of splints.
- **Physiotherapists** and **occupational therapists** will look at the best posture, walking pattern and seating for the child. The occupational therapist may try to develop certain physical and learning skills using special play equipment and advise on equipment to help mobility such as tricycles and trolleys. They will also give advice on equipment and aids that may enable the child to achieve greater success with everyday activities of living. ➲

➲ Cerebral palsy continued

- **Speech and language therapists** may also be involved very early on if a child has feeding, drinking or swallowing problems. If speech is difficult, or if there are any other problems with language, the speech and language therapist will produce programmes to help.
- Some children with cerebral palsy have delayed language because they are unable to play and explore like non-disabled children. Speech and language therapists will work with teachers, occupational therapists and parents to encourage suitable learning activities.
- Speech and language therapists may also provide communication devices, which help a child who is having serious problems with language or speech. The use of sign language, symbol speech or a communication aid will often lessen the frustration that an individual experiences at not being able to communicate their wishes and desires.

Many parents whose children have cerebral palsy seek new ways of improving their progress through education. Three such programmes are:

1. **Conductive education**. This has the backing of the charity for people with cerebral palsy (SCOPE).
2. **Doman-Delacato therapy**. This is based on the theory that the brain, like a muscle, will grow if given regular exercise.
3. **Bobath therapy**. This is specialised physiotherapy for children with cerebral palsy.

CASE STUDY

Callum

Callum has cerebral palsy. When he was about four months old, his parents noticed that he often held his right arm pressed against his body with the fist clenched tightly. He didn't sit unaided until he was thirteen months old and now, at the age of four, Callum is unable to walk without difficulty. He wears splints on his legs that help him to maintain his balance but he tends to walk jerkily.

Callum is a lively, intelligent boy who attends a local play group three mornings a week and gets on well with the other children there. He becomes frustrated when other children are playing football or using the playground equipment and he can't join in.

Questions

1. Find out what is involved in the following therapies:
   - **a** Conductive education.
   - **b** Bobath therapy.
   - **c** Doman-Delacato therapy.
2. Where can parents go to have their child assessed?
3. How can Callum be helped to reach his full potential, both now and when he moves to primary school?
4. In groups, design a poster which explains the different types of cerebral palsy and how each type affects the individual.

SCOPE (formerly The Spastics Society) is the largest charity working with children who have cerebral palsy, their families and their carers. They produce a number of fact sheets on education and therapy for children with cerebral palsy. If you send off for any fact sheets, remember to enclose a s.a.e. Or you can visit their website.

Encephalitis

What is it? Encephalitis is an inflammation of the brain.

Cause: The most common causes of encephalitis are viral infections like chickenpox or mumps.

Signs and symptoms:
- Abnormal drowsiness.
- Fever.
- Severe headache and pain when the neck is stretching.
- Intolerance of bright light.
- Loss of appetite and perhaps vomiting.
- Confusion, and in later stages, convulsions and coma.
- Double vision or an obvious squint.

What to do:
- **Call a doctor immediately** if the child is abnormally drowsy or has a fever plus any two of the symptoms listed above.
- The child will be admitted to hospital for diagnostic tests to determine the severity of the illness. Tests will include a lumbar puncture in which spinal fluid is drawn off under anaesthetic for examination.
- Usually the child is kept in hospital for treatment of symptoms.

General care:
- Once the child is discharged from hospital, keep him or her comfortable and give a nutritious diet.
- If the child has any weakness or stiffness in the muscles, the hospital physiotherapist will show you how to do some exercises to improve muscular control.

Possible complications: Most children recover completely from encephalitis.
In a few cases, there is permanent brain damage, which may cause limb weakness, learning difficulties or behavioural problems.

Further information: A child who has had encephalitis has suffered a serious illness which has possibly required a considerable amount of time in hospital and convalescence at home before returning to school. In particular, on return to school, the child may:
- tire more easily in such activities as PE and games, as well as from general lessons
- have problems with co-ordination and balance
- (rarely) suffer from **epilepsy** following encephalitis. The child may be taking anti-convulsant drugs which can in turn have side-effects such as drowsiness
- find it harder to concentrate, think and remember.

Epilepsy

What is it? Epilepsy is a condition of the nervous system affecting about 1 in 200 people. It is not a mental illness and cannot be 'caught'. A person with epilepsy experiences convulsions, usually called seizures or fits. The seizure is caused by a temporary 'electrical storm' in the brain.

Cause: In most cases of epilepsy there is no known cause, but sometimes a structural abnormality of the brain may be found. In some children, individual attacks may be brought on by a trigger, for example a flashing light; in others, the attacks have no trigger.

Signs and symptoms: What happens during a seizure depends upon the type of epilepsy. There are three main types of seizure:
1 Partial seizure: complex and simple.
2 Petit mal seizure or generalised absence.
3 Grand mal seizure or generalised tonic clonic. ➲

➲ Epilepsy continued

Partial

These seizures affect only part of the brain. There are two types:

Complex:

- Seizures may start with an 'aura' or warning, such as a funny taste in the mouth, flashing lights or a peculiar sound that the child hears.
- There is no seizure *as such*, but the child may be unaware of his or her surroundings and start to make odd, lip-smacking noises or pluck at their clothes.

Simple:

- Seizures may involve some twitching of the body and the child may complain of 'feeling strange'.
- There is no loss of consciousness.

Petit mal (or generalised absence)

This type of seizure affects the whole brain. There may be:

- Sudden 'switching off' in which the child appears to be in a trance.
- Slight twitching movements of lips, eyelids or head.
- Strange 'automatic' movements such as chewing, making odd noises, fiddling with clothing.

Grand mal (or generalised tonic clonic)

This type of seizure usually follows a pattern:

- The child suddenly falls unconscious, often with a cry (caused by a tightening of the voice muscles).
- He or she goes rigid, arching the back (**tonic phase**).
- Breathing may stop and the lips go blue.
- Convulsive movements begin (**clonic phase**). The child's limbs make rhythmic jerks, the jaw may be clenched and the breathing noisy.
- Saliva may appear at the mouth.
- Bladder or bowel control may be lost.
- Muscles relax and breathing becomes normal.
- Consciousness is usually regained in a few minutes; the child may feel dazed or fall into a deep sleep.

What to do: **Send for an ambulance only if:**

- It is a child's first seizure and you don't know why it happened.
- It follows a blow to the head.
- The child is injured during the seizure.
- The seizure is continuous and shows no sign of stopping – a rare condition called status epilepticus.

Caring for a child during a seizure: **During a 'grand mal' seizure:**

1. Protect the child from injury by moving any furniture or other solid objects out of his or her way during a seizure.
2. Make space around the child and keep other children away.
3. Loosen the clothing around the child's neck and chest and protect the child's head.
4. Stay with the child until the seizure has finished.
5. **Don't** try to restrain the child in any way and **don't** try to hold the child's teeth apart if they are clenched. **Don't try to put anything in the child's mouth** – any injury to the tongue will occur at the beginning of the attack, so there is nothing you can do until the attack is over.
6. When the seizures have stopped, place the child in **the recovery position** – see colour section after page 236 – and stay with the child until they have recovered. ➲

➲ Epilepsy continued

During a 'petit mal' seizure:
1 Sit the child down in a quiet spot.
2 Stay with the child until he or she is fully recovered and alert.
3 Talk calmly and reassuringly to the child – never try to shake or slap the child in an attempt to stop the seizure.

General care:
- Try to minimise embarrassment for the child. If the child has been incontinent during the attack, deal with it discreetly.
- Inform the parents. Observe the child closely and write down exactly what happened, as this will help the doctor to make a diagnosis.
- Supervise children with epilepsy during activities such as cycling or swimming.

Possible complications: Most grand mal seizures can be controlled by drugs. Children who have the petit mal type of seizure generally grow out of it by the time they reach adolescence.

Further information: Teachers and nursery managers need to know how to cope with a child's epilepsy. Parents can provide useful information such as:
- What kind of seizure the child usually has and how long it lasts.
- Any known triggers – for example flashing lights, stress, etc.
- If the child has to take medication at school.
- Any restrictions on activities suggested by the GP.
- If anyone needs to be contacted after a seizure.
- If extra precautions are needed – for example protective headgear.

Epilepsy does not affect intelligence and 80 per cent of children attend mainstream schools.

Spina bifida

What is it? Spina bifida is a defect in the formation of the spinal cord which occurs 14–25 days into pregnancy. The condition occurs due to a split in the neural tube which forms the spine and spinal cord.

Cause: Although the exact cause of spina bifida is not known, diet plays a vital role. Folic acid is effective in preventing spina bifida developing and it is advisable that all women trying to become pregnant take a supplement of folic acid for the first three months of pregnancy.

Signs and symptoms:
- A blood test at 16–18 weeks of pregnancy will indicate if there is an abnormality such as spina bifida.
- An ultrasound at 16–20 weeks will also reveal whether the child has the condition.
- At birth, the baby may have either a small dimple or tuft of hair in the small of the back. If the spinal cord is damaged, there may be a large blister-like lump over the base of the spine.

The size of the split in the neural tube determines the severity of spina bifida. In the mildest of cases where there is a fault in only one vertebrae, the nerves will not be damaged. However, if the nerves and spinal cord are affected, this usually leads to some paralysis and loss of sensation. Symptoms include:
- Weakness or paralysis of the legs.
- Urinary and/or faecal incontinence.
- Hydrocephalus (a condition in which excessive fluid accumulates in the brain); 9 out of 10 babies with spina bifida also have hydrocephalus, which shows as an excessively large head.
- In some cases, there are learning difficulties. 

➲ Spina bifida continued

What is the treatment?
- There is no cure for spina bifida and any defects in the spinal cord cannot be corrected.
- The degree and extent of paralysis is assessed as soon as possible by a paediatrician, and a brain scan will be carried out to see if there is excessive fluid on the brain.
- Surgery can repair the skin defect and prevent infection, but this will not restore function to the spinal cord.
- If hydrocephalus is present, a drainage tube is inserted into the brain to drain off fluid.

Possible complications:
- A child with a mild defect may have no symptoms at all except for the skin markings and require no treatment.
- Children with severe defects may require physiotherapy and rehabilitation.

Further information: If there is a family history of spina bifida, it is important to carry out screening procedures during pregnancy. These include:
- Ultrasound scanning.
- Measurement of alphafetoprotein in the mother's blood.
- Analysis of the amniotic fluid.

Revision questions

1. What is epilepsy? Describe the two most common types of epileptic seizure.
2. What is encephalitis? What are the most common causes of encephalitis? What are the signs and symptoms?
3. What is cerebral palsy? What difficulties might a child with cerebral palsy experience? What therapies are available?
4. What is spina bifida? What is hydrocephalus?
5. What treatments and therapies are available for children with spina bifida?

Respiratory tract disorders

◆ *Allergies* ◆ *Asthma* ◆ *Bronchitis* ◆ *Common cold* ◆ *Enlarged adenoids* ◆ *Epiglottitis* ◆ *Hay fever (Allergic rhinitis)* ◆ *Influenza* ◆ *Pneumonia* ◆ *Sinusitis* ◆ *Tonsillitis*

What are respiratory tract disorders?

Babies and young children are particularly susceptible to respiratory tract infections – most commonly infections of the upper respiratory tract. Children attending playgroup, nursery or school for the first time are suddenly exposed to a variety of viruses and bacteria to which they are not yet immune. Most of these infections are caused by droplet infection, so it is vital that child care workers follow safe hygiene routines to try to limit the spread of infection.

Allergies

What are they? An allergy is a negative physical reaction, which occurs within the body, to a particular substance. This substance might not necessarily be harmful to an individual but can cause miserable symptoms.

Cause: The word **allergen** is used to describe the substance(s) to which an individual is allergic. The most common allergens are:

- pets
- eggs
- pollen
- cats
- peanuts
- house dust mites
- milk
- grass
- dogs

Signs and symptoms: Symptoms range from very mild to extremely serious – for example **anaphylaxis** (see below).

The most common symptoms of an allergic reaction are:

- Skin rashes.
- Coughing and sneezing.
- A runny nose.
- Itchy eyes and ears.
- Wheezing.
- Vomiting and diarrhoea.
- Shortness of breath.

Many of these symptoms are experienced by a child with **hay fever** – see below.
In severe cases 2 per cent of the population experience a life-threatening whole body allergic reaction, which is called **anaphylaxis.** (See also page 202.)

What to do: Consult the doctor if you think the child has an allergy.
There are skin and blood tests that can determine the cause of the allergy.

General care: Once the allergens have been identified, it's a matter of avoiding them or treating the symptoms with medication.

Further information: Some people self-diagnose their negative reaction to a particular substance as an allergy, when it really it should be termed an **insensitivity** or an **intolerance**. For example, some people are intolerant or sensitive to certain foods – the most common being shellfish or fruit. They will feel sick, and often will actually *be* sick, within half an hour of eating the offending food. If it were an allergy, the reaction would be much more extreme and produce more of the general 'allergic' symptoms listed above.

- **Sensitivity** is used to describe a reaction to a substance, which is an exaggeration of a *normal* side-effect produced by that substance.
- **Intolerance** happens when unpleasant symptoms occur after eating a substance, which your body cannot handle because the digestive system does not produce sufficient quantities of a particular enzyme/ chemical, which is needed to break down the food and aid digestion.

Asthma

What is it? Asthma is a condition that affects the airways – the small tubes that carry air in and out of the lungs. People with asthma have airways that are almost always red and sensitive (inflamed). When a person has asthma their airways react to a **trigger** by ➲

Asthma continued

becoming narrower, as the muscle surrounding the airway tightens and inflammation inside the airway leads to swelling and a build up of mucus. This causes a cough, wheezing or breathlessness.

Cause: It is difficult to predict who is going to develop asthma. Like eczema and hay fever, it often runs in families and may be inherited. It can develop at any age.

Triggers in childhood asthma: A trigger is anything that irritates your airways and causes the symptoms of asthma to develop. Most children who develop asthma will have several triggers and these vary from one child to another. Triggers include the following:

- **Allergens**. House dust, feathers, animal fur, grass pollens, some foods.
- **Emotional factors**. Crying, excitement or disappointment – both pleasant and unpleasant – can provoke attacks.
- **Drugs**. A few drugs, notably betablockers, can worsen asthma in susceptible children.
- **Exercise**. Some children will suffer an attack during moderate or strenuous exercise and will require treatment before sports activities.
- **Infection**. Colds and other upper respiratory infections.
- **Environmental factors**. House dust mite present in all household dust, air pollution from fumes or pollens.
- **Weather**. Rapid changes of temperature can provoke an attack; some children are worse in damp weather – others suffer in dry conditions when there is an increase in grass pollens.

It is important to try and identify possible triggers, so that they can be avoided. 

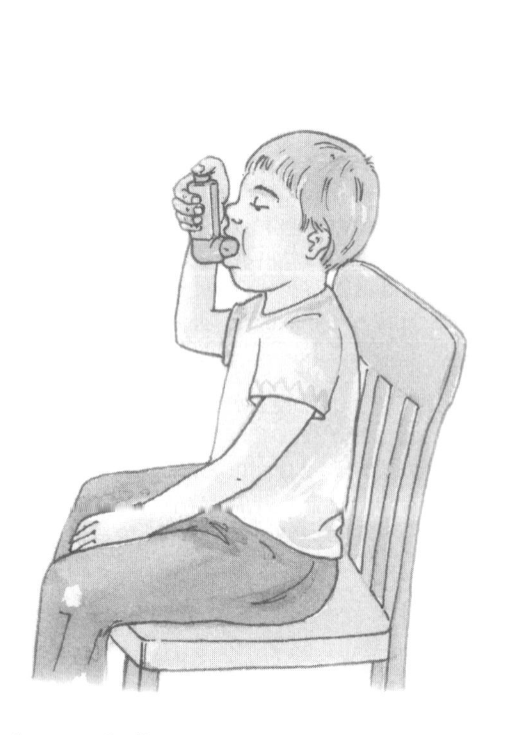

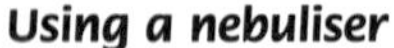

Using a nebuliser

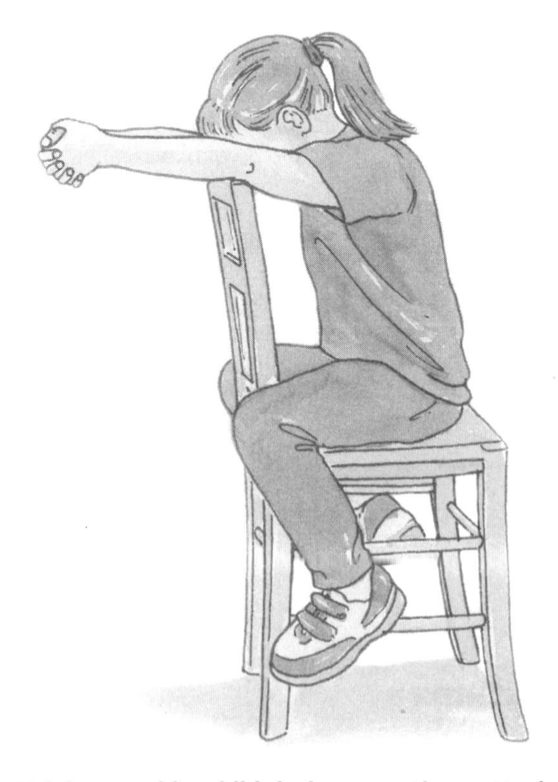

Helping an older child during an asthma attack

➲ Asthma continued

Signs and symptoms: When a child is having an asthma attack, they are often very frightened. You will notice:
- Wheezing. The difficulty is in breathing out rather than in catching one's breath.
- Dry persistent cough (often the first sign of asthma is a night-time cough).
- Difficulty in breathing.
- Rapid breathing.
- Sweating.
- The child may be very anxious or panic as they feel they are suffocating.
- The child becomes pale (a darker-skinned child may appear drained of colour, particularly around the mouth).

What to do immediately:
- If the asthma attack is the child's first, then **call a doctor** and the **child's parents**.
- If the symptoms are severe, **send for an ambulance**.

How to manage an asthma attack:
- Never leave the child alone during an attack.
- Stay calm and reassure the child, who may be very frightened; try not to ask too many questions that require answers – the child needs all available energy to help with breathing.
- Encourage the child to sit up to increase lung capacity; small children are often comforted by sitting on the carer's lap. An older child can sit upright, straddling a chair, with his or her arms over the chair back and their head resting on their arms. Pillows and cushions can give extra support.
- If the child has a **reliever** inhaler or **nebuliser**, then supervise them while using the inhaler.
- Try not to let other children crowd around.

If these measures do not stop the wheezing and the exhaustion caused by the attack, **call a doctor.** He or she will either give an injection of a drug to expand the child's airways or arrange admission to hospital.

When to call an ambulance:
- If the attack is the child's first.
- If the steps above have been taken and the child shows no improvement after 5–10 minutes.
- If the child becomes increasingly distressed and is unable to talk because of the difficulty in breathing.
- If the child shows signs of **cyanosis** – that is, the lips and tongue become tinged blue because of lack of oxygen.

General care after the attack:
- Continue to comfort and reassure the child.
- Offer a warm drink to relieve dryness of the mouth.
- Inform the parent or carer when the child is collected. If the child is distressed by the attack, then contact the parents immediately.
- Once the child has recovered, let him or her take part in normal quiet activities, but be observant for any further symptoms.

Treatment for asthma: Most asthma medication is delivered using an inhaler. This makes sure that very small amounts of medication are delivered directly into the lungs. There are three types of medication to treat asthma – **relievers**, **preventers** and **protectors**.
- **Relievers**. Reliever inhalers are usually blue. They act by opening up the airways by causing the muscles to relax and so allowing you to breathe more easily. The reliever should only be used when the symptoms of asthma appear or, *if recommended,* ➲

➲ Asthma continued

before exercise. Relievers are literally a lifeline during an asthma attack. Their effect is instant but they don't reduce the long-term swelling or inflammation in the airways.

NOTE: If the child needs to use the reliever three times a week or more this could mean that there is inflammation in the airways and preventer treatment may be needed.

- **Preventers**. Preventer inhalers are usually brown or orange. They work by reducing the swelling and inflammation in the airways and can take between 10 and 14 days to build up the preventative effect. They must be used every day, even when the child is feeling perfectly well.
  Most preventers are **steroids**, but because they are *inhaled*, only low doses need to be used. (It is important to understand that these steroids are NOT the same as anabolic steroids used by athletes to improve their performance.)
- **Protectors**. Protectors are long-acting medicines which reduce asthma symptoms and work by keeping the airways open and relaxed. This makes it easier for air to get in and out of the lungs, and so helps to ease asthma symptoms. They are available as inhalers or tablets.
  A protector would usually be taken with a preventer. Like preventers, it is important that protectors are taken every day.

Managing asthma: Asthma symptoms can happen at any time. It is important to understand what to do if you feel that the child's asthma is getting worse. Once the child is about 5 or 6 years old, he or she can be taught how to use a peak flow meter.

- A **peak flow meter** measures the performance of the lungs. The meter has a marker that slides up and down as the child blows into it. The marker stops at a point where they blow hardest. Each time the child uses the meter (usually morning and evening) you mark the result on a chart. Used over time, it gives a very clear idea of the asthma being controlled. Some peak flow meters are fitted with a ➲

Guidelines for early years settings

The **National Asthma Campaign** recommends that all schools should draw up an asthma policy. Schools should:

- □ Welcome all children with asthma, recognising it as an important condition affecting many students.
- □ Ensure that children with asthma participate *fully* in all aspects of school life, including physical education (PE).
- □ Recognise that *immediate* access to reliever inhalers is crucial.
- □ Keep records of children with asthma and their medication.
- □ Ensure that the school environment is favourable to children with asthma by removing *triggers* such as furry and feathery animals, strong fumes and tobacco smoke.
- □ Ensure that other children understand asthma.
- □ Ensure that all staff who come into contact with children with asthma know what to do in the event of an asthma attack.
- □ Work in partnership with all interested parties, including all school staff, parents, governors, doctors and nurses, and children, to ensure that they fully support an asthma policy so that it is implemented and maintained successfully.

➲ Asthma continued

'windmill trainer' for very young children to use. It has sails that are turned as the air is forced out of the lungs. Many asthma attacks can be predicted by regularly measuring the peak flow – the level of air expelled often falls a few days before an asthma attack.

- **Nebulisers and spacer devices**. Very young children sometimes use a nebuliser to inhale the medication. Nebulisers are electrical machines which turn liquid medication into a fine spray. This is then inhaled through a face mask. Spacer devices are large plastic bubbles which fit onto an aerosol inhaler and make it easier for young children to use and ensures that more of the medication gets into the airways.
- **House dust mites.** If the trigger for the child's asthma is house dust mites, take the following precautions:
  – Vacuum carpets and soft furnishings when the child is out of the house.
  – Damp dust regularly.
  – Avoid feather pillows and duvets.
  – Ensure that all rooms are well ventilated.
  – Cover the child's mattress with a plastic cover.
- **Sport and physical exercise**. Regular exercise is important for general health and well-being. Make sure that a child with asthma has *immediate* access to a reliever inhaler at all times; some children are advised to use their reliever inhaler immediately *before* taking part in any vigorous exercise, such as swimming or running.

Further information: One in seven children has asthma in the UK and this number is growing. Most classrooms will have an average of 4 or 5 children with asthma, making it the most common long-term medical condition in schools today.
For additional information contact:
The National Asthma Campaign
www.asthma.org.uk

ACTIVITY

In small groups, design and produce a colourful poster for use in a nursery or primary school to raise awareness of asthma; include the following information:

- A brief description of what asthma is.
- The main factors known to trigger an asthma attack.
- What to do when a child has an asthma attack.

Bronchitis

What is it? Bronchitis is infection of the air passages in the lungs called the bronchi.

Cause: Bronchitis is usually caused by a virus, following a common cold or flu, but occasionally is caused by bacteria.

Signs and symptoms: The child may have a runny nose for a few days before bronchitis develops. Symptoms are:

- Constant, persistent cough – starting off dry, then producing green or yellow phlegm.
- Shortness of breath.
- Rapid breathing even when resting.
- Wheezing.
- Sometimes a slight fever. ➲

➲ Bronchitis continued

What to do:
- **Call the doctor** if:
  - – the child has difficulty breathing
  - – the temperature rises to over 39 °C
  - – there is coloured phlegm.
- Antibiotics or a bronchodilator drug may be prescribed.
- Encourage the child to rest in an upright position as this helps breathing and coughing.
- If the child has a fever and is not vomiting, give children's paracetamol.
- Do not give cough medicine, unless prescribed by the doctor.
- Keep the air moist and humid: you can do this by using a humidifier or by hanging damp towels or sheets over a hot radiator.
- Offer warm soothing drinks.

General care:
- Continue to allow the child to rest and make sure they have plenty of fluids.
- During a coughing attack, sit the child forward on your lap and gently rub his or her back.
- Avoid overheating the house as this can cause a dry atmosphere which will irritate the cough.

Possible complications: Children usually recover from an attack of bronchitis within a week. Children who regularly have bronchitis infections generally grow out of it by about the age of five years.

Common cold

What is it? The common cold is a minor contagious illness that occurs frequently in children, especially in children attending nursery or school. It usually lasts less than two weeks. The common cold causes irritation and drainage in any or all of the airways including the nose, sinuses, throat, voice box, and often the bronchial tubes.

Cause: Many different viruses can cause the common cold. Each virus may have a slightly different pattern of symptoms and severity. Immunity gained as a result of infection with one virus does not protect the child from another cold virus. The cold virus is spread in droplets that are sneezed or coughed out and inhaled by others; it can also spread by direct contact with an infected child or object.

Signs and symptoms: Colds usually begin abruptly.
- A tickly feeling in the throat is often first, followed by some or all of the following:
- Sneezing.
- A runny nose.
- A blocked nose, which may make feeding difficult for babies.
- Babies and young children may have a fever.
- Watering eyes.
- Aching muscles.
- A cough and a sore throat.

What to do: Consult a doctor if:
- a baby refuses feeds for more than 24 hours, has a fever over 39 °C (102 °F) or seems very unwell ➲

➲ Common cold continued

- the child has symptoms of a chest infection, ear infection or a cough that persists for more than five days. The doctor can prescribe antibiotics for any bacterial infection.

General care:

- Make sure the child drinks plenty of fluids.
- Keep the child's room warm – but not too hot.
- Increase the moisture in the atmosphere by humidifying the air (see page 98).
- Sometimes babies who are snuffly can't breathe easily when feeding or asleep. Raising the head of the mattress slightly by putting a blanket underneath may help.
- The doctor may prescribe nose drops, which can help. Nose drops should not be used for more than a few days, otherwise they may make the situation worse. Or you could try gently tickling the baby's nostrils – a sneeze might help to clear your baby's nose.
- A menthol rub or capsules containing a decongestant liquid, which you can put on to clothes, or a cloth, may help the child breathe more freely, especially at night. You can buy them from most pharmacists. **NOTE:** Don't use menthol products for babies under three months without asking the doctor, and be careful not to let the baby swallow a menthol capsule.
- Give paracetamol liquid to reduce a high temperature or to relieve the pain of a sore throat.
- Apply vaseline to any soreness around the nostrils.

Possible complications:

- If the cold virus spreads to the lungs, it is commonly referred to as a 'chest cold':
  - Mucus becomes thick.
  - Coughing, if present, can last 2 to 3 weeks.
  - Green or yellow sputum or nasal secretions suggest a secondary bacterial bronchitis or sinusitis.
- Bacteria that live in the nose and throat can gain a foothold and cause secondary infection such as ear infections, pneumonia or bronchitis. ➲

Managing a cough

Although it is distressing to hear a child cough, in fact coughing serves a purpose. When there is phlegm on the chest, or mucus from the nose runs down the back of the throat, coughing clears it away. If the child is feeding, eating and breathing normally and there is no wheezing, a cough is not usually anything to worry about.

Consult a doctor if:

- ◆ a cough continues for a long time, especially if it is more troublesome at night or is brought on by the child running about – it might be a sign of asthma. Some children with asthma also have a wheeze or some breathlessness.
- ◆ the child seems to be having trouble breathing – call the doctor immediately – even in the middle of the night.

Most doctors believe cough mixtures do not work and are a waste of money. To ease the child's cough, give him or her plenty of warm, clear fluids to drink.

If your child is over the age of one, try a warm drink of lemon and honey. There is no need to try to stop the cough completely.

➲ Common cold continued

- Children with asthma may trigger an asthmatic attack after 'catching' a cold.

Further information:
- It is normal for a child to have a cold eight or more times a year. This is because there are hundreds of different viruses and young children are meeting each one of them for the first time. Gradually they build up immunity and get fewer colds.
- Colds are caused by viruses, not bacteria, so antibiotics do not help.

Enlarged adenoids

What are they? There are four areas of tissue at the back of the throat which are concerned with the development of **defences against infection** in early infancy. These are the right and left **tonsils**, the base of the tongue and the **adenoids**.
The adenoids are located above the tonsils, at the back of the nose. They get larger between birth and four years of age and then become progressively smaller. By adulthood they have disappeared altogether. When a child's adenoids are enlarged following repeated infections, they block the back of the nose, causing breathing difficulties.

Cause: Enlarged adenoids are caused by viral infections and allergies, for example to house dust mites, pollen, animal fur, etc.

Signs and symptoms:
- **Nasal obstruction**. This causes the child to:
  - breathe through his or her mouth, causing a dry mouth and throat and unpleasant-smelling breath (halitosis)
  - snore when sleeping
  - eat with the mouth open
  - wake often because of difficulty in breathing
  - have difficulty in pronouncing sounds, such as 'm' and 'n'
  - talk with a nasal voice.
- **Glue ear**. In some cases large adenoids are associated with the development of fluid in the middle ear ('glue ear').
- Recurrent ear infections, particularly otitis media, because of blockage of the Eustachian tubes.

What to do:
- In most cases large adenoids can be left alone as they will become smaller as the child gets older. Symptoms caused by enlarged adenoids decrease when the child is about seven years old, due to natural shrinkage of the adenoids.
- Humidify the air in the child's bedroom to help breathing and the problems of a dry mouth and throat.
- Encourage the child to sleep on their side or front to prevent snoring.

General care:
- If the cause of enlarged adenoids is found to be an allergy, then attempts should be made to remove the allergen from the child's environment as far as possible.
- When enlarged adenoids are associated with 'glue ear', recurrent ear infections or sleep apnoea, surgical removal is recommended. Removal of the adenoids is carried out by specialist ear, nose and throat doctors. It is a simple procedure which only takes a few minutes to perform.

Possible complications:
- Sometimes large tonsils and adenoids are associated with a condition called sleep apnoea syndrome, in which the child stops breathing during sleep.
- Glue ear and hearing problems.
- Speech delay.

Further information: There is no evidence that removing children's adenoids causes any problems. This is because they are necessary in babies, but have no function in older children.

Epiglottitis

What is it? A disorder caused by inflammation of the epiglottis. (The epiglottis is a piece of cartilage by the base of the tongue; it prevents food from entering the trachea – or windpipe.) Epiglottitis is most common in children between 2 and 6 years old.

Cause: Epiglottitis is usually caused by the bacterium *haemophilus influenzae*, although it may be caused by other bacteria or viruses. It results in the rapid swelling of the epiglottis and can obstruct breathing.

Signs and symptoms: **Epiglottitis is a life-threatening disease** and comes on suddenly. The main symptoms are:

- A high fever and very sore throat.
- Difficulty in breathing as the epiglottis swells; breathing is noisy and rasping.
- Severe difficulty in swallowing – the child will dribble as a result of being unable to swallow.
- A barking cough – as in **croup**.
- A bluish tinge to the lips and tongue.
- Exhaustion.

What to do: **This is a medical emergency**.

- **Get the child to hospital as quickly as possible, by car or by ambulance.**
- Comfort and reassure the child.
- Help the child to breathe by sitting them up, leaning forward slightly.
- **Do not attempt to look down the child's throat;** this is because if the child starts to cry, the extra mucus can cause the throat to go into spasm and to block the airway further.
- The child will be admitted to hospital where treatment includes:
  - Intubation: a tube is passed through the nose or mouth into the trachea (the airway to the lungs).
  - Humidified oxygen.
  - Intravenous fluids are given to increase hydration.
  - Antibiotics are used to treat the infection and corticosteroids may be used to decrease the swelling. ➲

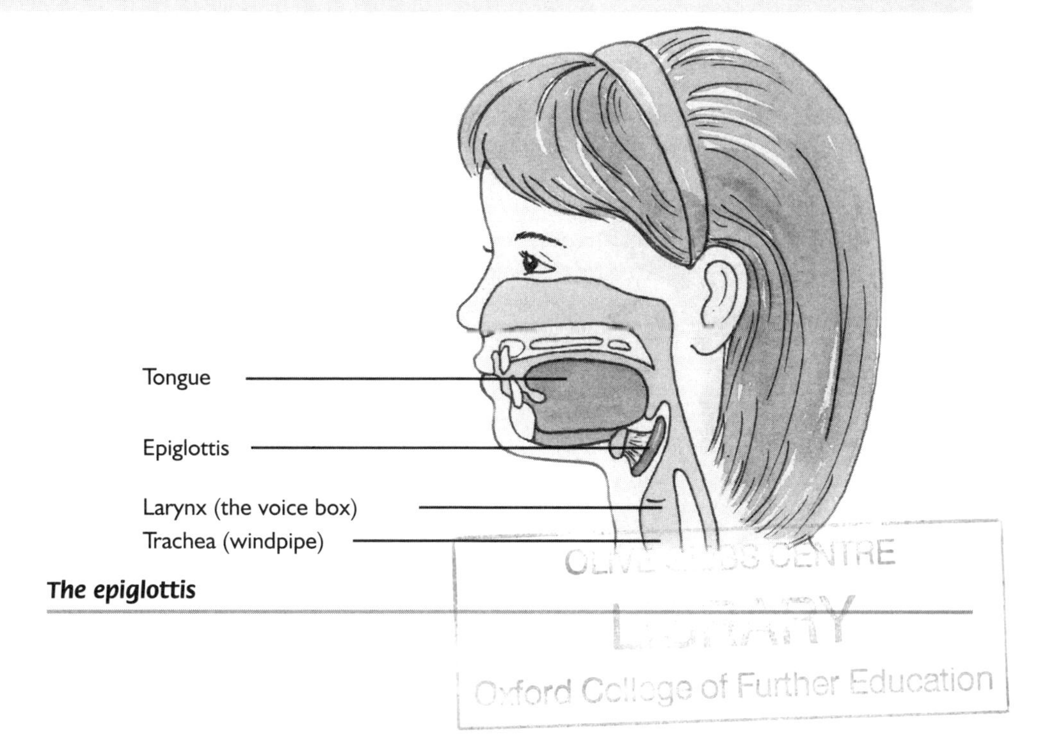

The epiglottis

➲ Epiglottitis continued

General care: • Most children recover completely within a week and should become immune to the condition.

Possible complications: • Complete obstruction of the airway which can result in death.

Further information: The incidence of epiglottitis has been decreasing since the inclusion of Hib (Haemophilus influenzae group B vaccine) as a routine childhood immunisation.

Hay fever (Allergic rhinitis)

What is it? Hay fever (or **allergic rhinitis)** is an allergic reaction to tree pollen or grass which causes a runny nose, sneezing, itchy and watery eyes. Hay fever commonly affects people who suffer from allergy-related disorders whose immune systems over-react to harmless substances and produce antibodies against them. This leads to a release of inflammatory chemicals that cause hay fever symptoms. Children under the age of five rarely get hay fever, but it is a condition that probably affects 1 in every 6 children by the time they become teenagers.

Cause: In spring, hay fever is caused by tree pollen and in the summer it is caused by grass.

Signs and symptoms: The child develops:
- an itchy nose, mouth and throat, and a stuffy nose every spring or summer
- itchy, watery eyes
- a sneezy cold.

What to do: • Check that the child does not have a raised temperature. If the child *does* have a fever, he or she is more likely to have a cold or an infection.
– To ease symptoms, the doctor can prescribe eye drops and nasal sprays.

General care:
- To ease the itching lay a damp face cloth over the child's eyes. Smear vaseline around the nose as this will prevent it from becoming sore.
- Keep bedroom windows closed at night as this will limit the child's exposure to pollen.
- When pollen counts are high keep the child away from grassy areas.
- Oral antihistamines often help to relieve severe symptoms of hay fever.

Further information: The British Allergy Foundation advise:
✓ checking the pollen count each day (local radio, newspapers and TV); and *if it is high*:
✓ staying indoors
✓ sleeping with the windows closed
✓ wearing sunglasses to stop pollen entering eyes
✓ staying away from grassy areas
✓ treating symptoms with treatment from your pharmacist or doctor.
Another form of allergic rhinitis affects people throughout the year; this differs from hay fever which affects people only in the spring and summer months. This perennial form of allergic rhinitis is usually caused by house dust mites or animal **dander** and cannot be relieved by taking antihistamines.

Influenza

What is it? Commonly called flu, influenza is an acute viral infection of the upper respiratory tract, which affects all age groups. It is highly contagious and occurs in epidemics, usually in the winter. ➲

➲ Influenza continued

Cause: Influenza is caused by the influenza virus and spread by coughing and sneezing and by direct contact. There are different strains of the flu virus; this means that while a child may be immune to one particular strain, he or she will succumb to a new one.

Signs and symptoms: The symptoms of flu usually come on rapidly, 1 to 3 days after infection, and may include:

- A high fever – often above 40 °C.
- Chills.
- Headache.
- Muscle aches.
- A dry cough.
- Stuffy nose.
- Tiredness and weakness.
- Sometimes a sore throat and nausea.

In most cases, the acute symptoms usually last for 4 or 5 days and clears up completely within 10 days.

What to do:

- Call the doctor if :
  - the child is under two years of age.
  - the temperature rises above 40 °C.
  - the child is breathing abnormally fast or is excessively drowsy.
  - there is no improvement within 48 hours.
- Give paracetamol to control the fever and to ease aches and pains.

General care:

- Care for the child in bed in a warm – but not too hot – well-ventilated, humidified room until the temperature returns to normal.
- Offer warm, soothing drinks at frequent intervals.

Possible complications:

- Pneumonia
- Bronchitis
- Sinusitis
- Otitis media
- Febrile convulsions in babies.

Further information: An annual influenza vaccine is advisable for children with chronic medical conditions, such as asthma, diabetes, heart disease, renal failure and those with a depressed immune system.

Pneumonia

What is it? Pneumonia is an inflammation of the lungs. It ranges in severity from a mild illness to a severe infection and can develop as a result of inhaling food or drink into the lungs, or even an object such as a toy or coin. Pneumonia may start with symptoms of a common cold, such as a runny nose and sneezing, and over a period of a few days, the child quickly becomes very unwell.

Cause: Most cases are caused by the respiratory syncitial virus (RSV), an infection which affects young babies in particular. Bacterial pneumonia is less common. Sometimes, the condition can be caused by both viruses and bacteria. Children with cystic fibrosis are very vulnerable to pneumonia. ➲

➲ Pneumonia continued

Signs and symptoms:
- Loss of appetite and may feel generally very unwell.
- Rapid, difficult breathing – 40 or more breaths per minute even when resting.
- Coughing, which can be severe and may produce green, yellowish or blood-flecked **phlegm**.
- Fever – often very high temperature (40 °C or 104 °F).
- Headache.
- In severe cases, drowsiness, blueness of the lips and tongue (cyanosis).

What to do:
- Contact the doctor immediately; if the child has breathing difficulties while resting, or signs of cyanosis – **call an ambulance**.
- Keep the child warm and offer drinks.
- The doctor will listen to the child's lungs and will prescribe antibiotics if the child has a mild case of bacterial pneumonia. Parents should keep the child at home until they have recovered.
- If the child is very young or has breathing difficulties, they may be admitted into hospital where extra oxygen will be given. Tests may be carried out to discover the cause of the pneumonia.

General care:
- Prop the child upright as this may help them to breathe more easily.
- If the child has a fever, is over the age of three months and is not vomiting, give children's paracetamol. Do not give cough medicine.
- Keep the air moist and humid: you can do this by using a humidifier or by hanging damp towels or sheets over a hot radiator.
- Offer warm drinks.
- Avoid vigorous exercise for about two weeks after the infection is first noticed.

Possible complications:
- Sometimes a cough persists for a further two weeks when the child has otherwise recovered.
- Bronchopneumonia may result after whooping cough or measles.
- Pneumonia does not cause any long-lasting damage to the lungs.

Further information:
- Pneumonia can affect one or both lungs – or even just one lobe of a lung (lobar pneumonia). The temperature can be very high – for example 40 °C.

Sinusitis

What is it? This is inflammation of the lining of the sinuses (air-filled cavities in the bones which surround the nose).

Cause: Sinusitis is usually caused by a bacterial infection following a cold as the drainage holes that lead from the sinuses into the back of the nose become blocked.

Signs and symptoms:
- Initially the child has a cold with a blocked or runny nose with a thick white or yellow-green discharge.
- Pain around the nose, eyes or forehead.
- Fever.
- Recurrent attacks of sinusitis.
- Coughing during the night.
- Sometimes severe pain in the upper back teeth.

What to do:
- Contact the doctor if the child has a high temperature and give the child children's paracetamol. The doctor may prescribe antibiotics and nose drops to help reduce the inflammation and allow the sinuses to drain. ➲

➲ Sinusitis continued

General care:
- If the child is in pain, wring out a face cloth in hot – but not too hot – water and lay it over the affected area.
- Use either a vaporiser or prepare a bowl of warm water and encourage the child to breathe in the steam.
- Encourage the child to drink plenty of fluids.

Possible complications: Although this condition may require antibiotics, it rarely leads to complications.

Tonsillitis

What is it? Tonsillitis is inflammation of the tonsils. The tonsils are the two glandular swellings at either side of the throat that help to trap and destroy viruses and bacteria. The tonsils respond to viruses and bacteria by swelling as they produce antibodies to fight off the infection. Tonsillitis develops when the tonsils become overwhelmed by the viruses and bacteria, causing the tonsils to become chronically swollen. The condition usually clears up within ten days.

Cause: Tonsillitis is caused by viruses and streptococcal bacteria.

Signs and symptoms:
- Fever.
- Inflamed sore throat – the tonsils look fiery red and swollen, sometimes with white patches.
- The child feels unwell.
- Loss of appetite and pain when swallowing.
- Stomach ache and vomiting.
- Swollen and tender glands in the neck.
- The child may have bad breath (halitosis). ➲

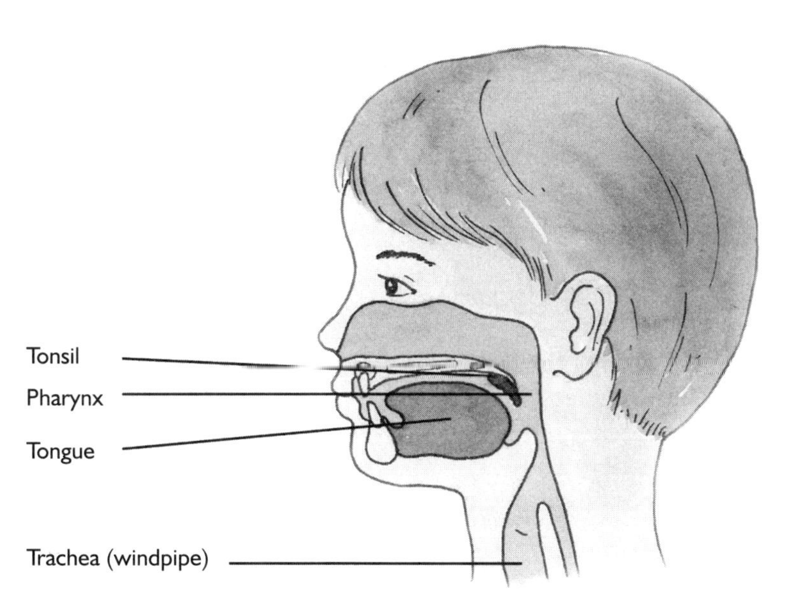

The tonsils

➲ Tonsillitis continued

What to do:	• Contact the doctor if the child is very unwell or has repeated attacks of tonsillitis. Antibiotics may be prescribed if the cause is bacterial. • Give children's paracetamol to reduce the fever. • Offer the child chilled drinks.
General care:	• Keep the child at home and away from other children; a child with a sore throat is infectious for about three days after the symptoms appear. • Offer soft foods such as yoghurt, ice cream, fruit mousses, etc. Ice lollies help to ease a sore throat. • In most cases, the symptoms disappear within three days. • The tonsils can be removed if the child has repeated infections of the throat, although this treatment is rare nowadays.
Possible complications:	• Quinsy. This is where an abscess forms around a tonsil and causes severe pain, a high fever and extreme difficulty in breathing. It may need to be surgically drained in hospital.
Further information:	Surgical removal of the tonsils is usually only done if the child has frequent infections or if a quinsy develops.

Revision questions

1 What are the signs and symptoms of influenza? How can you tell the difference between a common cold and influenza?

2 Why is coughing an important reflex? How would you help a child who is coughing?

3 What is epiglottitis, and what should you do if a child has difficulty in breathing?

4 Why are tonsils and adenoids important in childhood?

5 What are the possible complications of (**a**) enlarged adenoids, and (**b**) recurrent tonsillitis?

6 What is sinusitis? How can you help to relieve the pain of sinusitis?

7 What is asthma?

8 What are the possible trigger factors in asthma?

9 List five ways in which you could reduce the presence of house mites in the family home.

10 Asthma management: What is

a a peak flow meter
b a reliever inhaler
c a preventer inhaler
d a nebuliser?

Skin disorders

◆ *Alopecia* ◆ *Athlete's foot* ◆ *Cold sores* ◆ *Eczema* ◆ *Impetigo* ◆ *Infestations: Fleas – Head lice – Scabies* ◆ *Molluscum contagiosum* ◆ *Psoriasis* ◆ *Ringworm* ◆ *Verrucas* ◆ *Warts*

What are skin disorders?

Skin disorders are common in childhood, as young skin is very sensitive. Some common skin rashes in children are those associated with infectious diseases such as chickenpox and measles. Other skin disorders may be the result of local bacterial infection, allergies, insect bites, sunburn, or irritation (for example, by chemicals in detergents). Most skin disorders are minor and usually clear up rapidly. The first steps in dealing with a skin disorder are to find out what has caused it and to seek the appropriate treatment.

Alopecia

What is it? Alopecia means baldness. Patchy hair loss in children, often sudden in onset, is known as **alopecia areata**.

Cause: There may be several reasons for hair loss in children:

- A baby may lose hair by rubbing their scalp against the mattress; babies sometimes develop bald patches on the back of their heads as they are laid to sleep on their backs.
- It can be caused by hair pulling; children who pull their own hair – often subconsciously – may be anxious or distressed.
- Tight braiding and using rollers or hot curlers can damage and break hair, and running hair picks through tight curls can scar hair follicles and cause bald patches.
- The causes of alopecia areata – resulting in patchy hair loss – are unknown, although it can be caused by a simple illness or emotional upset.
- Ringworm can also cause hair loss.
- Chemotherapy (drug treatment) used to treat children with cancer usually results in severe hair loss.

Signs and symptoms:

- Hair loss.
- Bald patches on the scalp.
- Hair coming out in handfuls when washing or brushing the hair.

What to do:

- Consult the doctor if you suspect **ringworm** (see page 220) or if there is no obvious cause.
- Remove any braids or hair accessories that may be causing the problem.

General care:

- Reassure the child – who will be very anxious – that their hair will grow back.
- Discourage children from pulling at their hair.
- Try to find out what has caused the problem and deal sympathetically with any anxieties or emotional upsets.

In most cases of alopecia the hair grows back, although it may be very fine and possibly white before the normal colour and thickness return.

Possible complications: Loss of confidence because of teasing and bullying about their appearance can lead to deep-rooted psychological problems.

Athlete's foot

What is it? Athlete's foot is a fungal infection between the toes, which is common in children in the summer months, especially if they wear trainers all the time.

Cause: Athlete's foot is caused by the same fungus which causes ringworm. The fungi thrive in closed, warm, moist environments and feed on keratin, a protein found in hair, nails and skin. Athlete's foot is mildly contagious; it can be spread through direct contact with the infection and by skin particles left on towels, shoes, floors of shower cubicles and around swimming pools.

Signs and symptoms:

- Very itchy areas between the toes, particularly the webs between the fourth and fifth toes.
- Sore, cracked skin between the toes.
- Toenails may become thick and brittle.

What to do:

- Treat athlete's foot at the first sign of itchy feet or redness between the child's toes.
- Most cases of athlete's foot can be cured with over-the-counter anti-fungal powder and basic good hygiene.

General care:

- Wash and dry the feet thoroughly morning and evening.
- Change socks daily, and don't wear the same shoes day after day.
- Sprinkle anti-fungal powder on the feet and in the shoes daily.
- Make sure the feet get plenty of air. If the child can't go barefoot or wear sandals, use cotton socks and shoes made of a natural, porous material such as leather or fabric, not water-resistant synthetics.
- As an alternative to anti-fungal treatment, try the following remedy:
  - Soak the infected feet in warm, salted water (1 tsp salt per cup) for 5 to 10 minutes every day.
  - Dry the feet thoroughly, then apply a baking soda paste between the toes, or dab on an aluminium chloride solution, available from the local pharmacy.
- As long as the area is not blistered or cracked, remove flakes of dead skin with a soft brush before using a topical powder or ointment. Do not tear off flaking skin; you may break nearby healthy skin and spread the infection.
- Keep the child's toenails short, and clean out debris under and around nails to prevent spread of the infection.
- Make sure that the child's shoes fit properly. Small shoes make it more likely that the infection will spread to nearby nails.

Possible complications: If not treated properly and promptly, the infection can be very hard to get rid of. Even when treated with anti-fungal drugs, the infection may take several weeks to disappear.

Further information:

- Although walking barefoot in the shower at the gym or around the pool may increase the chance of contracting athlete's foot, you are more likely to develop the infection from not changing sweaty socks and shoes.
- The risk of developing athlete's foot can also depend on your susceptibility. For example, people who have diabetes are at greater risk.

Cold sores

What are they? Cold sores are small painful blisters that develop on and around the lips. They are very common in nursery-age children.

Cause: Cold sores are caused by a member of the herpes simplex virus. They are caught by kissing or close contact with someone who has the infection and cold sores. The ➲

➲ Cold sores continued

virus passes through the skin, travels up a nerve, and hides in the nerve root until it is reactivated by a stressful event. Cold sores can also be triggered by:
- illness, e.g. colds and flu
- emotional upset
- fatigue
- bright sunlight
- cold winds.

Signs and symptoms:
- A tingling sensation is usually felt around the lips and mouth a few hours before the blister appears.
- Small blisters, which may be itchy or sore, surrounded by an inflamed area.
- The blisters burst within a few days to form a yellow crust.
- The sores heal on their own within two weeks.

What to do:
- If the sore is bothering the child, consult the doctor who will probably prescribe an anti-viral cream; these creams are much less effective once the sore has developed – they are best applied when the first tingling sensation is felt.
- Offer cold drinks and ice lollies to soothe the pain.
- Apply a lip balm which contains a sunblocking agent.

General care:
- Keep the child's hands clean and discourage him or her from touching the sore.
- Never let the child put their fingers near their eyes.
- Until the sore has healed up, make sure the child does not kiss anyone.
- Try to prevent further cold sores by:
  - ✓ avoiding sunlight/cold winds
  - ✓ avoiding triggers if possible
  - ✓ applying a lip balm daily – containing UV protection
  - ✓ reducing stress
  - ✓ eating a diet rich in vitamins A, C, and E, zinc, and iron
  - ✓ taking garlic – fresh or supplements
  - ✓ applying melissa herb.

Possible complications:
- The virus can be spread to other parts of the body by transfer from the cold sore site.

Further information: Once the child has contracted the virus it is there for life and children may have frequent recurrences throughout life.
Despite what people might say, you cannot catch cold sores from cups, flannels, or towels.

Eczema

What is it? Eczema (also know as atopic eczema) is a skin condition characterised by excessive dryness and itching. The condition often flares up, resulting in the appearance of red, scaly, bumpy, rough patches on the body. It is common to see eczema in children who have allergies, hay fever, asthma, or close family members with eczema. The term eczema comes from the ancient Greek and literally means 'to boil over'.

Cause: It is almost impossible to pinpoint the exact cause of eczema, but it is thought to be triggered by the same allergens as asthma, such as:
- house dust mite droppings
- dairy products
- pollen, etc. ➲

➲ Eczema continued

Signs and symptoms: Atopic eczema usually appears between 18 months and 2 years, but can occur for the first time – or reappear after an earlier episode – between the ages of 4 and 10 years.

- The skin becomes itchy, dry, flaky, and often red and painful. Eczema can appear anywhere on the body but most commonly it is found in the skin creases of the elbows and wrists, and behind the knees. For babies it commonly affects their face, in particular the cheeks.
- The skin may be cracked with patches of redness and scaling; in dark-skinned people, there may be changes in skin colour.
- Sometimes the pimples appear as blisters that may ooze fluid.
- Lack of sleep due to the intense itching.

NOTE: When eczema appears on fair-skinned people, the affected areas typically turn a brownish-grey colour; on people with dark skin, it usually alters their natural pigmentation, making the affected area either lighter or darker.
See colour section after page 220.

What to do:

- **Consult the doctor** if a child has a sore, itchy rash.
- In severe cases of eczema, the doctor will prescribe steroid treatment.
- Observe the child closely to try to discover possible triggers of the condition – for example, hot atmospheres, house dust mites, etc.

General care: There is no cure for eczema but there are a few things you can do to alleviate the symptoms.

- Dress the child in cotton clothes and use cotton bedding to prevent skin irritation.
- Avoid over-warm rooms, especially at night, as heat can irritate the condition.
- Don't let the child become too cold or hot as both can aggravate the symptoms.
- Keep the child's fingernails clean and short and use cotton scratch mitts on a young child to prevent scratching.
- Avoid drying or perfumed toiletries, such as soap and bubble bath or baby lotion which can irritate the skin.
- Use an emollient (or skin-softening) cream or bath oil, such as E45 to keep skin soft and supple and to prevent the dryness which can cause itching and inflammation. (Emollients are also available on prescription.)
- A bath or shower with lukewarm water will soothe the skin. Bathing should be limited to once per day, or every other day when the eczema has flared-up. Frequent bathing (more than once per day) can actually cause the skin to become *more* dry.
- Many soaps irritate the skin of a child with eczema. Use minimal amounts of soap to cleanse the skin and choose one that is super-fatted.
- Wash the child's clothes in a non-biological washing powder to prevent further skin irritation, and do not use fabric conditioners.
- Wet wrapping involves using stretchy wet and dry bandages to seal in moisturisers next to the skin. Many parents and carers find that, although time consuming, wet wrapping keeps the eczema under control and prevents the need for long-term steroid use; it also improves sleep.

Using prescribed and over-the-counter drugs.

- An **antihistamine** (anti-itch) medication, such as Benadryl, is sometimes needed to give the child relief. Benadryl is available without a prescription. It can be given every six hours to relieve itching. Consult the doctor before giving Benadryl to a child under two years old or if you are unsure of the correct dosage. The most common side-effect of Benadryl is drowsiness. ➲

➲ Eczema continued

- Hydrocortisone cream 1% is most commonly used during a flare up of eczema. Hydrocortisone cream is a steroid cream and should be applied to the skin *sparingly.* It does not need to be slathered on to be effective. In fact, overuse of steroid creams can cause serious problems. The steroid cream is usually applied to the rash two times per day.

NOTE: Always wear gloves when applying steroid cream to prevent the medication being absorbed into *your* skin and to minimise the risk of infection.

- Antibiotics may be prescribed to treat skin infections, which occur because of the scratching; they may be given by mouth as a medicine or applied to affected areas as a cream or lotion.

Possible complications:

- Recent studies have shown that bacteria called **staphylococcus aureus** that lives normally on the skin can be responsible for a flare up or worsening of eczema. Scratching causes breaks in the skin allowing the bacteria to get in and upset the skin.
- **Impetigo** can occur as a result of scratching the spots (see page 212).

Always consult a doctor if you notice any of the following signs and symptoms:

- Signs of skin infection appear: increasing redness, swelling, tenderness, pus oozing from the spots, red streaks on the skin, or fever in association with these other signs.
- The rash becomes worse, changes in its appearance or if new symptoms develop along with the rash.
- If there is no improvement after one week of treatment.

Further information:

- 50 per cent of children with eczema tend to be clear of the condition by the age of two and 90 per cent by the age of 15.
- In more than 70 per cent of people with atopic eczema there is a family history of eczema, asthma or hay fever.
- Eczema is often associated with asthma, so children with that disorder may be at greater risk of skin problems. ➲

ACTIVITY

Design a leaflet for use in a nursery or infant school to outline the support and coping strategies available for children with eczema. Areas to include are:

- ☐ Communicating with the parents and carers of the child with eczema to find out the individual child's particular needs; for example, you could devise a questionnaire for parents.
- ☐ Use of play materials such as dough, paints, sand, clay and water (e.g. when on a swimming trip). How could the use of such materials be adapted for a child with eczema?
- ☐ Use of pencils, brushes and cutlery. How can this be made easier for children with sore hands and fingers?
- ☐ The effects of heat in the setting – including direct sunlight. How can the problem of overheating be avoided?
- ☐ Personal hygiene. Consider the setting's arrangements for toileting and hand washing and how these could be adapted for a child with eczema.
- ☐ Self-esteem and confidence. How could staff ensure the development of the child's self-esteem and confidence while in the setting?

➲ Eczema continued

- Children with visible skin rashes can be teased and bullied by other children at school. You should always deal with this promptly to discourage such behaviour.
- Overheating, dry air and cold weather, teething, colds and other infections can all make eczema worse.

Impetigo

What is it? Impetigo is a highly contagious skin infection. It can appear anywhere on the body but usually attacks exposed areas. Children tend to get it on the face, especially around the nose and mouth, and sometimes on the arms or legs.

Cause: It is caused by bacteria – usually streptococcal or staphylococcal – that live on the skin, entering the skin through a cut, graze, cold sore or even a patch of eczema. While it is rarely serious, it is highly contagious. Children spread it by touching the scabs and transferring the bacteria via their toys, clothes or towels.

Signs and symptoms: A small patch of impetigo near the mouth can be mistaken for a cold sore, but impetigo can be recognised by the following signs and symptoms:

- There are tiny blisters, particularly around the nose and mouth.
- The blisters burst easily, exposing a wet, weepy patch that oozes a cloudy yellow liquid that dries to a thick honey-coloured crust.
- Sometimes the blisters join up to form clusters.
- The affected area may spread at the edges, or a new patch may develop close by.
- In severe cases, the child's glands may swell and there may be a raised temperature.

See colour section after page 220.

What to do:

- See the doctor immediately.
- Although it is not usually serious, impetigo should be treated quickly to prevent it spreading and making the child ill. The doctor will prescribe some antibiotic cream which should be applied as directed – usually several times a day.
- Contact the child's parents immediately if away from home and keep him or her away from other children.

General care:

- Gently wash off any loose crusts with soap and water, then dab the area dry. Wear gloves when treating the affected areas.
- Apply the antibiotic cream as directed – always wear gloves.
- To prevent the skin from getting too dry, use emollient bath oils, such as Oilatum, available over the counter and on prescription.
- Don't use talcum powder or bubble bath. Ask the GP to prescribe an emollient cream if child eczema.
- Keep the child's nails short to avoid picking at the scabs. Cut your own fingernails short and wash your hands after treating the child.
- Keep the child's towels, flannels and bedding separate from the rest of the family's. To stop the sores from spreading, use a clean towel every time the affected areas are washed. Remember to pat rather than rub the skin dry.

Contact the GP if:

- the child's condition does not improve after three days of treatment
- the child becomes ill and has a raised temperature (above 37.5 °C/99.5 °F). 

➲ Impetigo continued

Possible complications:
- The most serious potential complication of impetigo is **glomerulonephritis**, a severe kidney disease that occurs in about 1 per cent of cases, mainly in children. Look for changes in the appearance of the child's urine, headache, nausea and puffiness of the face and limbs (see page 223).
- Small, very itchy, pus-filled ulcers form, with a dark brown crust. This indicates an ulcerated form of impetigo that penetrates deep into the skin. If left untreated, it may cause scarring and permanent changes in pigmentation.

Further information:
- Anyone in a household who develops impetigo should use a clean towel every time they wash.
- All clothing, towels and bedding used for the child must also be laundered separately.

Infestations

Fleas

What are they? Fleas are small wingless insects that are able to bite through skin and suck blood. The human flea is virtually extinct in the UK.

Cause: Children may be bitten by fleas which usually infest cats (and sometimes dogs). The increased number of pets being kept and the tendency for their beds to be neglected during cleaning has provided an environment favourable to fleas. Wall-to-wall carpeting also provides a relatively undisturbed area for flea larvae to develop. Fleas can live for several hours without contact with the host animal and will bite humans instead.

Signs and symptoms:
- Adult fleas are normally 1.08 mm long, brownish in colour, with no wings but muscular legs adapted for jumping. The potential life span of a female flea is two years during which she can lay up to 1000 eggs.
- Although small, fleas can be seen clearly with the naked eye.
- Bites may be painful and extremely itchy.
- Severe cases can result in painful lumps and swellings.

What to do:
- Wash the bite with unperfumed soap and water.
- Apply calamine lotion or antihistamine cream to soothe the itching.
- If the problem persists, consult the doctor who may prescribe antihistamine medicine or antibiotics for infected bites.

General care:
- Treat the host animal first by applying an approved insecticide. Flea collars are not always an effective method of preventing fleas.
- Treat the animal's bedding, carpets and soft furnishings with insecticide.
- Place insect powder into your vacuum bag before vacuuming the floor and soft furnishings. This will kill any fleas vacuumed.
- The treatment may take a few weeks to be entirely successful, as new adult fleas will hatch from eggs left in carpets, etc.

Possible complications:
- Allergic reaction to the flea bites.
- Impetigo if bacteria enters through the site of the flea bite.
- Fleas carry many other germs which can be transmitted to humans, for example typhus and anthrax.

Head lice

What are they? Head lice are small wingless insects which infest the scalp and suck blood. They are a common affliction. Anybody can get them but they are particularly prevalent among children.

The features of head lice:

- They are tiny insects with six legs.
- They are between 1 and 4 mm in size – slightly larger than a pin head.

See colour section after page 220.

- They only live on human beings; they cannot be caught from animals.
- They live on, or very close to, the scalp, and they don't wander down the hair shafts for very long.
- They have mouths like small needles which they stick into the scalp and drink the blood.
- They are unable to fly, jump or hop.
- They do not discriminate between clean and dirty hair, but tend to live more on smooth, straight hair.
- They are not the same as nits. Nits are the egg cases laid by lice. Nits may be found 'glued' onto the hair shafts; they are smaller than a pinhead and pearly white.

Cause: Head lice are caught just by coming into contact with someone who is infested. When heads touch, the lice simply walk from one head to the other.

Signs and symptoms:

- The first sign of head lice infestation is usually intense itching of the head and neck; children will scratch their head repeatedly.
- Sometimes you can see the nits or egg cases, which may look like dandruff, but which, unlike dandruff, cannot be brushed out of the hair.
- You may be able to see the lice moving when using a fine-toothed comb.
- Children who have had the infestation for some time will feel literally 'lousy', with a lack of energy because of interrupted sleep.

What to do: *How to detect head lice:*

You will need a plastic detection comb (from the chemist), good lighting and an ordinary comb. Lice are most easily detected by fine tooth-combing wet hair. Some parents find that using a hair conditioner helps to lubricate the hair and ease the combing process. Others report that such lubricants make it more difficult to see the eggs.

- Wash the hair well, and then dry it with a towel. The hair should be damp, not dripping.
- Make sure there is good light; daylight is best.
- Comb the hair with an ordinary comb.
- Start with the teeth of the detection comb touching the scalp at the top of the head. Draw the comb carefully towards the edge of the hair.
- Look carefully at the teeth of the comb in good light.
- Do this repeatedly, from the top of the head to the edge of the hair in all directions, working around the head.
- Do this for several minutes. It takes 10–15 minutes to do it properly for each head.
- If there are head lice, you will find one or more grey or brownish lice on the teeth of the comb.
- Use the comb over a pale surface, such as a paper towel or over a basin of water to aid detection.
- Clean the comb under the tap; a nail brush helps to do this. 

➲ *Head lice* continued

Preventing infestation by head lice:
The best way to stop infection is for families to learn how to check their own heads. This way they can find any lice before they have a chance to breed. They can then treat them and stop them being passed around the family. If a living, moving louse is found on one of the family's heads, the others should be checked carefully. Then any of them who have living lice should be treated at the same time.
NOTE: Contrary to popular belief, head lice are not easily damaged by ordinary combing. However, regular combing may help to detect lice early and so help to control them.
Treatment
Treatment should only be used if you are sure you have found a living, moving louse. Anyone who has a moving, living louse should be treated at the same time. There are two main methods of treatment for head lice:

1 Insecticide lotions

Lotions and rinses that are specifically formulated to kill lice and their eggs are available from chemists and from some child health clinics. Your school nurse, health visitor or pharmacist will advise you which lotion to use, or you can ask your GP for a prescription. The lotion is changed frequently, as the lice become resistant to it and it no longer works. Follow the instructions on the product carefully. Some general guidelines are:

- ✓ Put the lotion onto dry hair.
- ✓ Use the lotion in a well-ventilated room or in the open air.
- ✓ Part the hair near the top of the head, put a few drops on to the scalp and gently rub it in. Part the hair a little further down and repeat the process. Do this over and over again until the whole scalp is wet.
- ✓ You do not need to put lotion down long hair any further than where you would put a pony tail band.
- ✓ Use enough lotion – at least one small bottle for each head, more if the hair is thick. Use all the lotion up.
- ✓ Keep the lotion out of the eyes and off the face. One way is to get the child to hold a cloth over the face.
- ✓ Do not use a hair dryer. Let the lotion dry on the hair naturally. Some lotions are flammable, so keep well away from flames, cigarettes, stoves and other sources of heat.
- ✓ Treat all of them again seven days later in the same way, using the same brand of lotion.
- ✓ Check all the heads a day or two after the second treatment. If you find living, moving lice, ask your local chemist, health visitor, school nurse or GP for advice.

See colour section after page 220.

2 Herbal/Aromatherapy lotions

Aromatherapy lotions have been found to be very effective by parents in treating head lice. However, they have not been tested in large, controlled trials. The Tisserand Institute of Aromatherapy has been advocating a specifically formulated blend of essential oils for treatment of head lice:

Eucalyptus, 10 drops
Tea-tree oil, 10 drops
Geranium, 5 drops
Rosemary, 5 drops
Mix with 30 ml of vegetable oil. ➲

➲ *Head lice* continued

Treatment guidelines are:

✓ Apply the mixture liberally to dry hair.
✓ Cover with shower cap for half an hour and then shampoo.
✓ Use detection comb on dry hair and not when the blend is in.
✓ Two applications are enough, either on subsequent or consecutive days.

Essential oils can be bought from health food shops, chemists and from the Tisserand Institute.

Bug Busting method

The Bug Busting method launched by Community Hygiene, a charity, has the backing of the Department of Health. It is a two-week programme that is safe and works when shampoos of all varieties fail. The method is:

- Wash the child's hair and towel dry.
- Put on a lot of conditioner, maybe three times what you would normally use.
- Comb through with an ordinary comb.
- You then take a fine-toothed comb and go through the hair absolutely scrupulously, backwards and forwards and from side to side, covering every bit, even those tiny hairs at the back of the neck and beside the ears, wiping the comb every time.
- Rinse hair but do not blow-dry.
- Repeat every three days (following the life cycle of the head louse).

The Bug Busting kit includes detailed instructions, a cape and a fine-tooth comb specially designed to hook the lice off close to the scalp.

General care:

- Once the infection is treated there is no need to repeat the treatment unless you find a living, moving louse.
- Regular combing of children's hair can help to prevent head lice by aiding early detection.
- Never use insecticide lotions 'just in case' or as a preventative measure, since the lotions may be harmful to young children when used repeatedly.
- Wash all combs and brushes in hot, soapy water after use.
- Inspect the child's hair regularly for early signs of infection.

Possible complications:

- Although head lice are very unpleasant, they rarely do any harm other than causing an itchy scalp.
- If children really do keep on having head lice, this is most likely to be due to not doing the treatment properly and not treating those close contacts who have also been found to have head lice.

Further information: Parents and carers should remember that just one infected child can infect an entire nursery or school, so it is important to treat the family members as soon as the problem is detected.

General information for early years settings:

- It is important to remember that head louse infection is not primarily a problem of early years settings, but of the wider community. Most head lice are caught within the family and in the local community, not in the early years setting. The popular perception is that there is a serious 'outbreak' in the setting, with many of the children infected. This is rarely the case; at any one time, most schools will have a few children who have active infection with head lice. This is often between 0 per cent and 5 per cent, rarely more.
- The age-old stigma which linked head lice with poor hygiene and general neglect is gradually disappearing, but there is still often an atmosphere of agitation and alarm which aggravates the problem. ➲

➲ *Head lice* continued

- Some parents believe that school nurses should resurrect the old practice of doing regular head checks on children in schools – the 'Nitty Nora' method. Such checks are ineffective against the problem, but the school nurse can advise and support parents to check their own families.

Recommended procedure for early years settings

DOs

✓ *DO* have a written protocol on the management of the head louse problem. If possible, write a protocol for your area in consultation with the local education authority, the local consultant in communicable disease control, infection control nurses, the school nurses, and, if appropriate, colleagues in other schools.

✓ *DO* make sure that your school nurse is informed in confidence of cases of head louse infection. The school nurse will assess the individual report and may decide to make confidential contact with the parents to offer information, advice and support.

✓ *DO* keep individual reports confidential, and encourage all staff to do likewise.

✓ *DO* collaborate with the school nurse in providing educational information to parents and children about head lice, but do not wait until there is a perceived 'outbreak'. Send out information on a regular basis, preferably as part of a package dealing with other issues.

✓ *DO* consider asking the school nurse to arrange a talk to parents at the school if they are very concerned.

✓ *DO* ensure, with the school nurse, that parents are given regular, reliable information, including instructions on proper diagnosis by detection combing and effective treatment guidelines.

✓ *DO* advise concerned parents to seek the professional advice of the school nurse, the family practice or the local pharmacist.

DO NOTs

✗ *DO NOT* send out an 'alert' letter to other parents.

✗ *DO NOT* exclude children who have, or are thought to have, head lice.

✗ *DO NOT* recommend or support any mass action, including wet combing campaigns.

✗ *DO NOT* agree with parents that routine head inspection should be reintroduced; they were never effective.

✗ *DO NOT* refer parents directly to the consultant in communicable disease control. The appropriate clinical advisors are the school nurse, the local pharmacist, the health visitor and the general practitioner.

✗ *DO NOT* take, or support, actions simply 'to be seen to be doing something' (such as sending out alert letters).

ACTIVITY

Prepare an information sheet for parents about head lice. Using the information on pages 214–217, answer the following questions:

- ☐ What are head lice?
- ☐ How do children get head lice?
- ☐ How can you recognise the condition?
- ☐ How should you treat head lice?
- ☐ Where could parents go for further information?

NOTE: Remember to reassure parents that head lice are not a result of poor hygiene or neglect.

You could also design a poster to be put on the nursery or school parents' notice board.

Scabies

What is it? Scabies is an extremely itchy, contagious condition due to infestation of the skin by parasitic scabies mites

Cause: Scabies is caused by a mite which is very difficult to detect (it's only just visible to the human eye at less than half a millimetre in diameter). It can cause a fierce itch, enough to keep the child awake at night, which is due to an allergic reaction to the mite and its products. The mite burrows under the skin, laying eggs and secreting substances which cause the itch. The eggs develop into larvae which travel to the skin surface and develop into adult mites in what look like red spots on the skin.

Signs and symptoms: It can take some weeks for an infection to get established, and you may not notice anything for up to a month. Symptoms then include:

- A rash of tiny little red pimples which usually begin in the folds and crevices of the body, especially between the fingers, on the elbows or wrists, buttocks or belt line. The mites also tend to hide under rings, bracelets or watchbands, or under the nails.
- Itching, particularly at night (this may be generalised around the body, not just in the area of the rash, as it is an allergic reaction).
- Children with scabies may be very tired and irritable because of loss of sleep from scratching.
- In more advanced cases, the spots may be seen to form red lines, along the burrow of the mite, and the skin may be crusty or scaly.

What to do:

- Call the doctor within 24 hours.
- The doctor may take scrapings of the child's skin to check for the mite.
- Pesticide treatments must be applied to the whole body (including palms and soles – there must be no possible hiding place left for the mite) and left on for up to 12 hours (the best way is overnight).
- Everyone in the family should be treated, even if they are not yet showing any signs of the condition.

General care:

- It may be necessary to repeat the treatment a week later.
- It may then take as long as four weeks for the skin to heal fully.
- All clothing, bed linen and towels will also have to be washed after treatment.
- Itchiness caused by the allergic reaction can be treated with an antihistamine cream. ➲

➲ Scabies continued

Possible complications: Spots may become very inflamed if a secondary infection with bacteria occurs, for example impetigo.

Further information: Ensure that any other people that the child has been in close contact with know about the infection so that they can be examined and also treated if necessary.

Molluscum contagiosum

What is it? Molluscum contagiosum is a very common skin infection among children, especially nursery-age children.

Cause: It is caused by a virus and, without treatment, will probably sort itself out and disappear within a few weeks. It is easily spread, either by direct contact or indirectly, for example in a public swimming pool or by touching infected clothing or towels.

Signs and symptoms:
- Lots of tiny pimply spots form on the skin, usually on the exposed surfaces – that is, the hands, arms, face, neck and also often the chest and tummy.
- The spots are about 2–6 mm across, and are raised from the surface of the skin in a pale pearly dome shape, with a central dimple or pit.
- They usually form in little clusters, although there may be single ones dotted about. After a while each spot crusts over and heals.

Apart from the rash, children rarely have any other symptoms – they usually feel quite well and as lively as usual, and there is no fever.
See colour section after page 220.

What to do:
- **Consult a doctor**.
- Although caused by a virus, molluscum contagiosum *can* be treated, especially if it just affects a small area of the body. The usual treatment consists of:
  - Pricking each spot with a sharp instrument dipped in a chemical called podophyllin. This causes the contents of the pimple (a white cheesy fluid) to burst out and the spot to heal.
  - In severe cases, other reatments which freeze or burn off the pimply spots may be needed.

The chemical (podophyllin) used is very powerful and the treatment can be a little uncomfortable, so it **must be done by a doctor**.

General care:
- Although it doesn't cause any more than a superficial problem, molluscum contagiousum is highly infectious and this is why children with it are sent home from nursery or school until they are better.
- If untreated, the condition will probably disappear within a few weeks to a few months.

Possible complications: There are no complications, although parents and carers are always concerned about the unsightly appearance of the spots

Psoriasis

What is it? Psoriasis (pronounced *so-rye-ah-sis*) is a recurrent inflammatory skin condition which is most common in children over the age of 10 years, but it can occur in younger children with a family history of the disease.

Cause: The cause of psoriasis is unknown, but it tends to run in families and may be inherited. However scientists have identified many of the triggers of the condition, which include physical and emotional stress, certain drugs, throat infection and injury. ➲

➲ Psoriasis continued

Signs and symptoms: In children, the psoriasis rash is often preceded by an upper respiratory tract infection caused by streptococcal bacteria. The signs and symptoms of the psoriasis rash are:

- It can be in a small area or become very widespread. It is not contagious and contrary to popular belief cannot be transferred from one part of the body to another.
- It is usually found on the elbows, knees or scalp.
- Raised patches on the skin, redness, and often there is white scaling and 'crustiness'. This scaling is due to the greatly increased replacement of surface skin cells which normally takes 28 days, but in psoriasis happens in 3 to 4 days. This results in a thick layer of scales, which flakes off in abundance.
- Mild to severe itchiness – or discomfort and a feeling of tightness. The rash may crack and become very sore.
- Pitting, discolouring and thickening of the fingernails and toenails. If psoriasis develops on the nails, they may separate from underlying skin.

What to do: Consult a doctor, who will probably refer the child to a dermatologist (skin specialist).

General care:

- The doctor will probably prescribe corticosteroid creams or lotions, or coal tar preparations.
- Use emollient creams to help to keep the skin soft and supple.
- Light therapy is often used and may be prescribed by the specialist; moderate exposure to sunlight can help, but care should be take to avoid sunburn.

Possible complications:

- Red, scaly, cracked skin on the palms of the hands with tiny pustules can signal **palmar psoriasis**; on the soles of the feet the same condition is **plantar psoriasis**. These forms of psoriasis affect only those areas; the condition can become very inflamed and ooze fluid, making movement very painful.
- It can 'flare up', making the child's skin so inflamed that they need urgent admission to hospital for treatment to replace fluids and to prevent hypothermia. Fortunately this is very rare.
- Around 5 per cent of people with the condition develop a form of arthritis called psoriatic arthritis. This happens because the small joints of the hands and feet become inflamed.
- The condition can make a child feel embarrassed about the way they look; they may avoid situations where affected parts of the body are exposed to the gaze of others.

Further information: Psoriasis is a chronic relapsing condition – that is, it can come and go – and the possibility of it recurring remains with people all their lives.
Early years workers should support a child with psoriasis and be especially alert to the problems caused by teasing and social isolation from their peers.

Ringworm

What is it? Ringworm is a common infection among schoolchildren. It affects the scalp or the skin of the body or face. It is called ringworm because the rash is ring-shaped.

Cause: Ringworm is caused by a fungus usually caught by direct contact with infected children, animals (particularly cats), or soil. What usually happens is that a person has some break in the normal immune defences which allows the fungal spores to enter and start to grow. In skin infections this is often a tiny cut or scratch which breaks the ➲

Visible signs of some common childhood illnesses

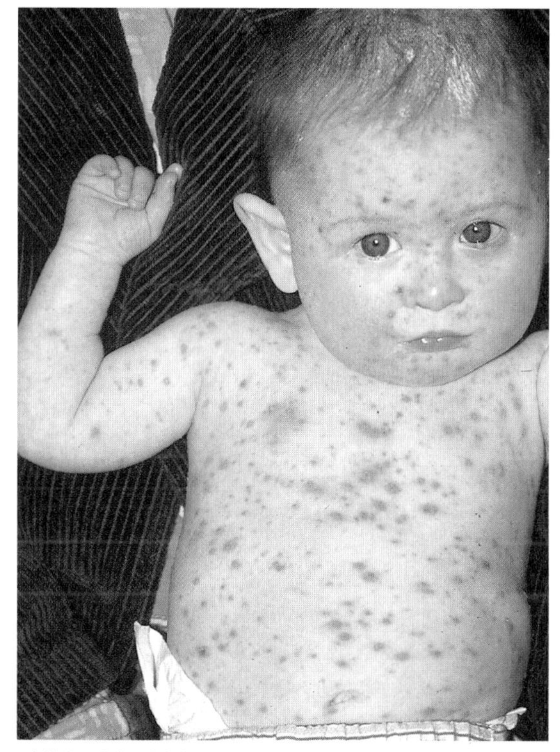

Child with chickenpox rash

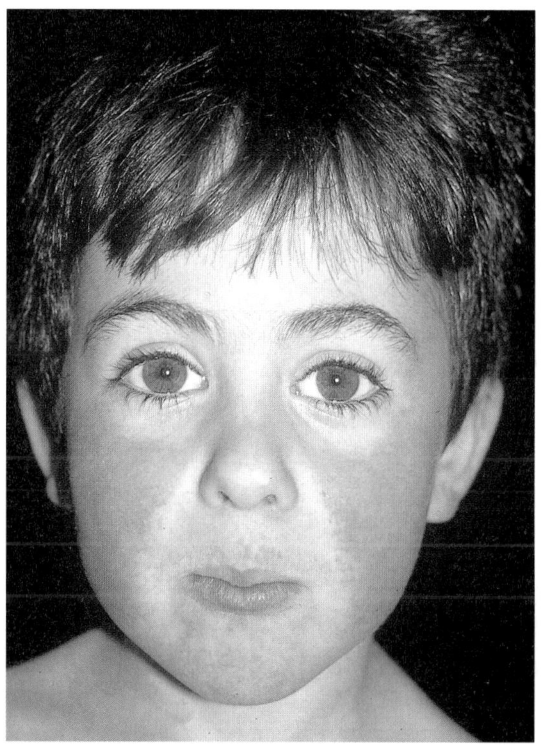

Fifth disease (slapped cheek syndrome)

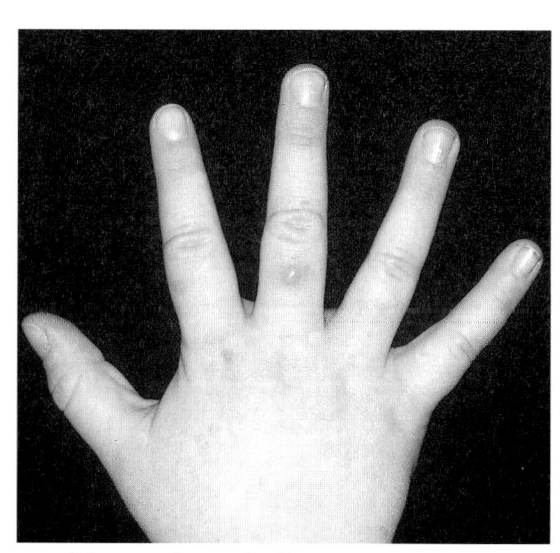

Hand foot and mouth disease

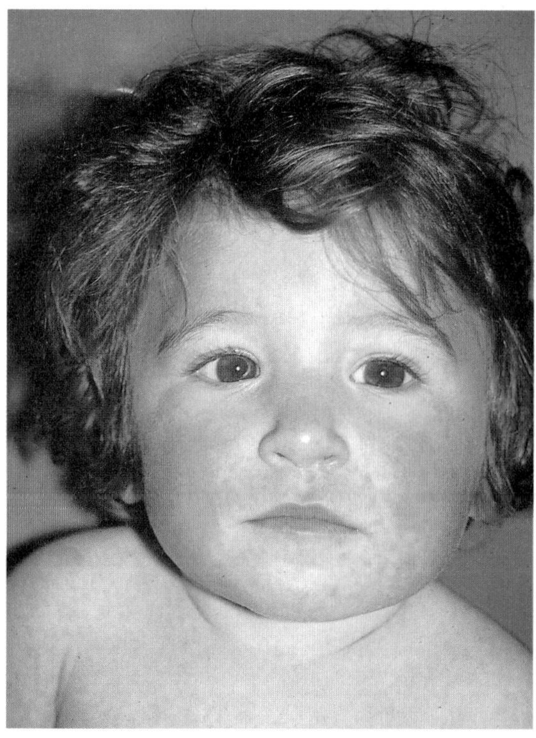

Child with measles rash

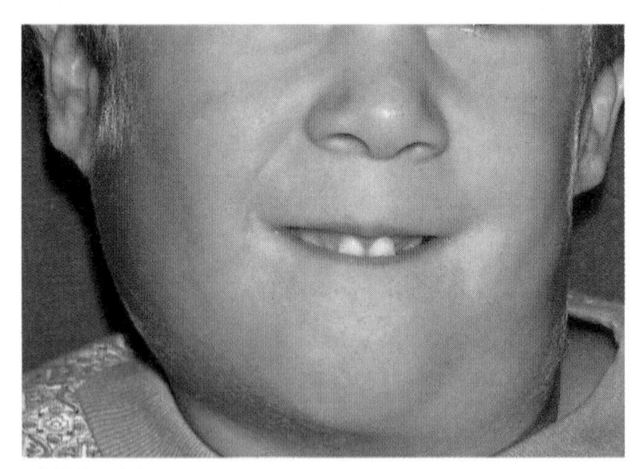

Child with *mumps*

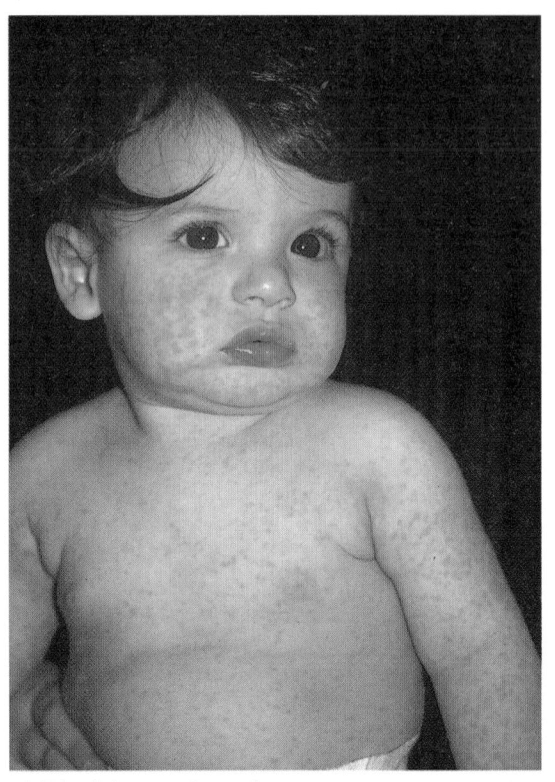

Child with *roseola rash*

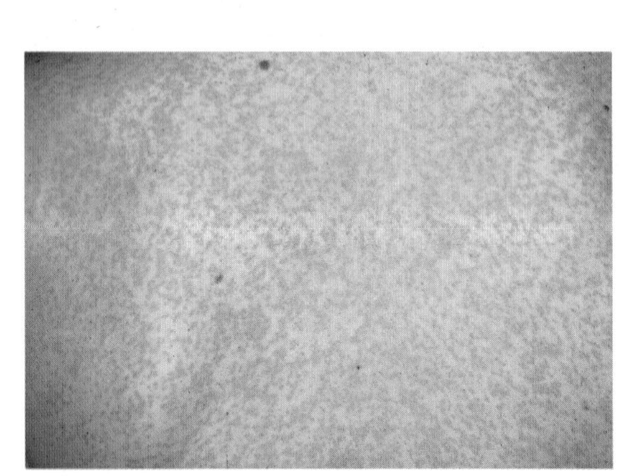

Child with *rubella rash*

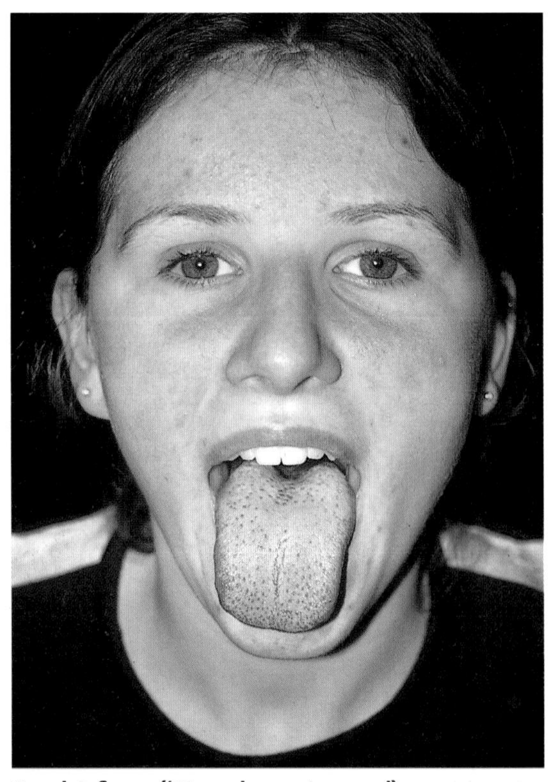

Scarlet fever ('Strawberry tongue')

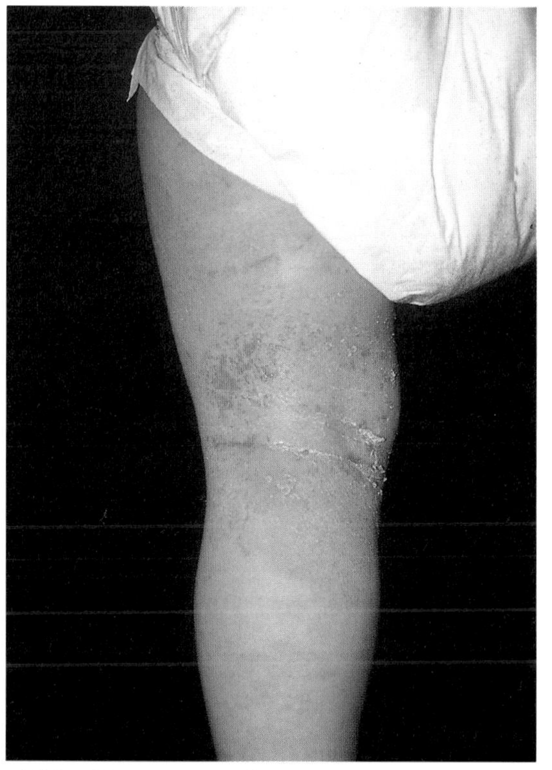

Child with eczema rash

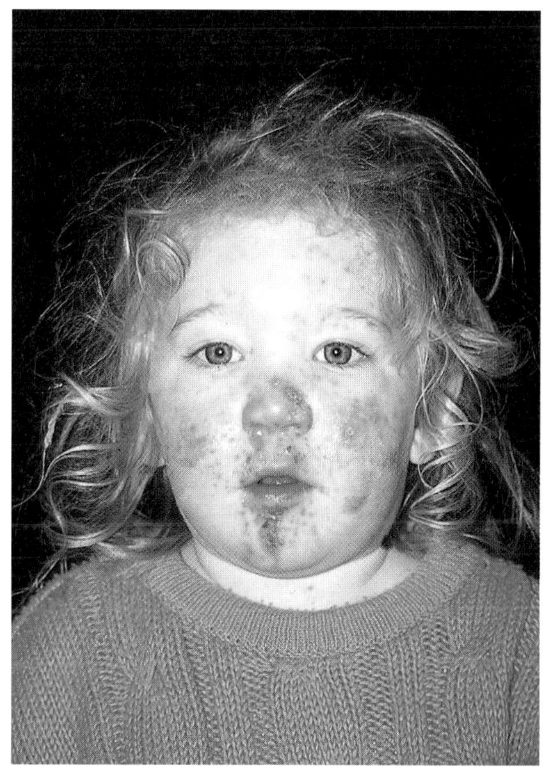

Child with impetigo

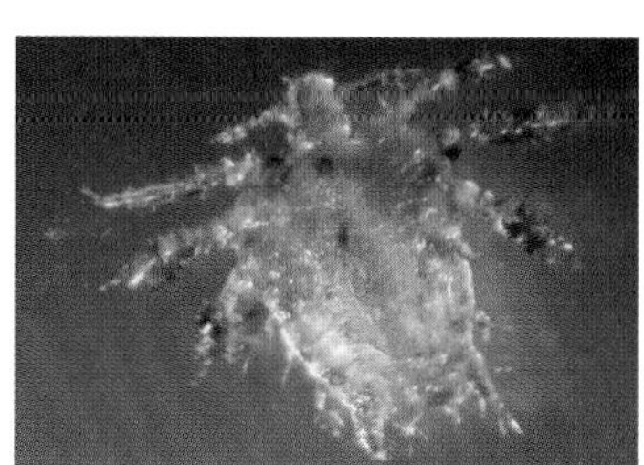

A head louse

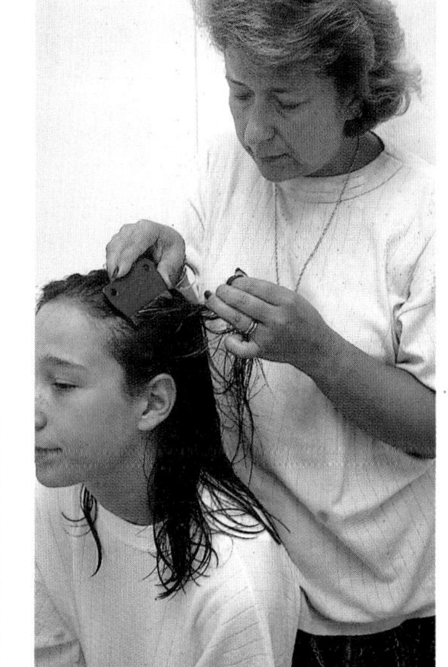

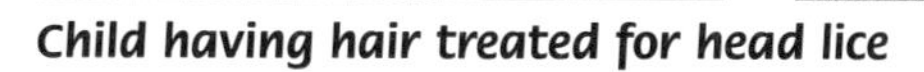

Child having hair treated for head lice

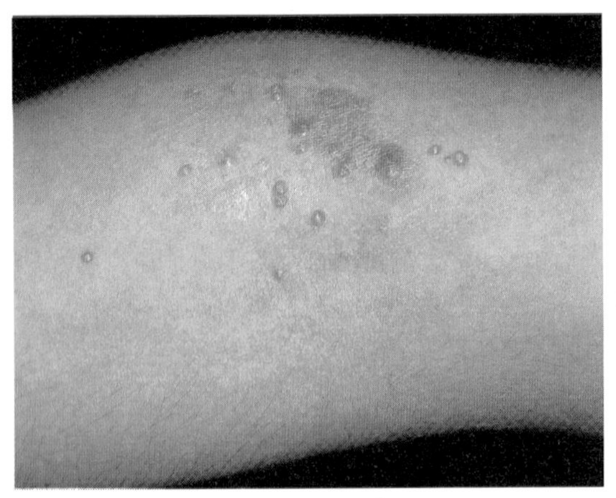

Child with mulluscum contagiosum

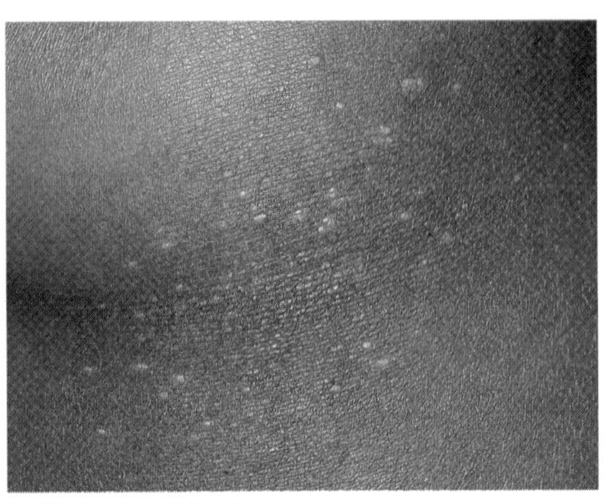

Mulluscum contagiosum on a black skin

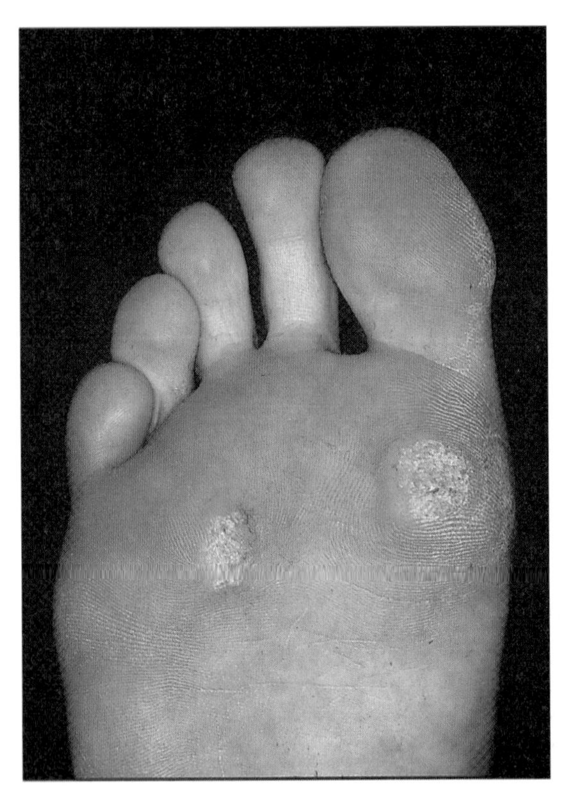

Child with a verruca

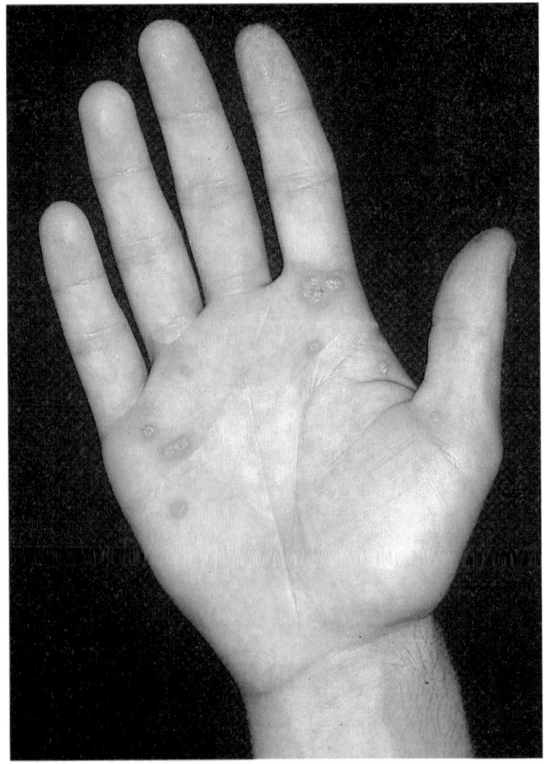

Child with common warts

➲ Ringworm continued

barrier of the skin. This may be so small that the person does not even realise it has happened.

Signs and symptoms: In children, the most common ringworm infections affect the skin on the face or body or the scalp.
On the skin, signs and symptoms include:
- A ring-shaped rash with red or silvery itchy scales which tend to clear in the centre as the ring expands. The edge of the ring may be slightly raised.
- Severe itching.

On the scalp:
- Circular patches of hair loss.
- Large flakes of skin in the hair.
- Severe itching.

What to do: Consult the doctor, who will prescribe a course of anti-fungal cream. In very severe cases or infections of the hair and nails, anti-fungal tablets may also be needed.

General care:
- If the cause is an infected animal, treatment of the animal should be given by a vet.
- Keep the child's towels and flannels separate.
- Keep combs and other personal belongings away from other children.
- Wash hands regularly.

Possible complications:
- Occasionally an inflamed pus-filled blister develops; this is called a kerion and will need to be treated with antibiotics.

Verrucas

What are they? Verrucas (or verrucae) are warts that appear on the sole of the foot. They are also known as plantar warts.

Cause: Verrucas are caused by a virus. They are usually caught from public changing rooms and swimming pools. Catching verrucas has nothing to do with poor hygiene.

Signs and symptoms:
- They appear as small hard growths on the sole of the foot; the surface of the wart is usually specked with black spots (tiny blood clots).
- They can spread quite quickly to other areas of the sole of the foot appearing as 'crops of verrucas'.
- The weight of the body can flatten the verruca and force it into the skin; when this happens the verruca can be very painful and stops the child from walking properly.

See colour section after page 220.

What to do:
- Eventually verrucas will disappear on their own without treatment. However, this can take months so most people choose to have them treated.
- Consult a doctor or chiropodist (foot specialist).
- The usual treatment is to freeze the verrucas with liquid nitrogen; this speeds up the healing process by partly killing the virus and partly destroying the skin that the virus is living in. Many GPs will do this for people in their surgery. It feels cold during treatment, like putting an ice cube on your skin, and sometimes feels a little sore afterwards.

General care:
- A wart paint or gel containing salicylic acid used every day helps to remove the hardened skin. The verruca should be soaked in water for a few minutes then dried before applying treatment. ➲

➲ Verrucas continued

- Hardened skin can be safely removed using a pumice stone or emery board – always remember not to be over vigorous.
- Complementary therapies can work well. The following remedies are tried and tested:
  - Tea-tree oil and tincture of thuja are well known for treating verrucas and warts on other parts the body.
  - Apply the inside of a banana skin to the verruca. Rub the inner skin against the verruca for a few minutes two or three times a day or cut out a piece of banana skin large enough to cover the verruca, tape it over the verruca to hold it in place, and leave it overnight.
- Never be tempted to try to dig or cut the verrucas out because this will do more harm then good.

Possible complications:
- Verrucas can recur, even after treatment; they may require several treatments before they finally disappear.

Having verrucas should not stop children from going swimming. Prevent the spread of verrucas by ensuring that the child wears verruca socks, which are available in different sizes from the pharmacist.

Warts

What are they? Warts are harmless small hard growths on the skin which occur individually or in clusters. They are common in children, usually appearing on the hands, feet, knees or face.

Cause: Warts are caused by a virus, which enters the skin through a *cut* or *scratch* and causes cells to multiply rapidly. Warts are slightly contagious, and you can spread them to other parts of your body by touching them. Usually, warts spread through direct contact, but it is possible to pick up the virus in moist environments, such as showers and locker rooms.

Signs and symptoms: There are three main types of warts:

1. *Common warts* are small, hard, rough lumps that are round and elevated; they usually appear on hands and fingers and may be flesh-coloured, white, pink or bumpy. They are not usually painful.
2. *Plane warts* are slightly raised and have smooth, flat, or rounded tops. They often appear in groups on the face, neck, hands, wrists or forearms; they may be slightly itchy.
3. *Plantar warts* or verrucas – see page 221.

See colour section after page 220.

What to do:
- Nearly every doctor says that the best treatment for warts is no treatment at all.
- Check for other warts – if there is only one and it is not itchy or painful, it is probably best to wait for it to disappear by itself.

General care: If the wart doesn't disappear, or if it's unsightly or uncomfortable, you can try self-treatment.

- An over-the-counter medication in liquid, gel, pad or ointment form. Most of these contain salicylic acid, the main constituent of aspirin, which softens abnormal skin cells and dissolves them. Follow the instructions that come with the treatment pack.
  - First, soak the wart in warm water for five minutes to help the medication penetrate the skin.
  - Then very gently rub off dead skin cells with a flannel or pumice stone. ➲

➲ Warts continued

– Before applying the medicine, coat the area around the wart with vaseline to keep the medicine away from healthy or sensitive skin.

If over-the-counter treatment fails, your doctor can remove a wart by:
- Freezing it with liquid nitrogen.
- Burning it off with electricity or a laser.
- Excising it (a minor surgical procedure).

Possible complications:
- Skin infections.
- Burns to healthy surrounding skin if treatments are not used correctly.

Further information: Most people develop an immune response that causes warts to go away by themselves. One-fifth of all warts disappear within six months, and two-thirds are gone within two years.

Consult the doctor if warts multiply and spread, causing embarrassment or discomfort.

Revision questions

1 Why are children particularly susceptible to skin infections?
2 What is molluscum contagiosum?
3 How would you recognise psoriasis? What treatment is used for this condition?
4 Where on the body does impetigo usually occur and what is the treatment?
5 How is athlete's foot treated and how can it be prevented?

Urinary tract disorders

◆ *Enuresis (Bedwetting) see page 144* ◆ *Glomerulonephritis* ◆ *Urinary tract infections*

What are urinary tract disorders?

Infections of the urinary tract are fairly common in childhood. These are more common in girls than in boys because of the closer position of the female urethra in relation to the anus. Most of these infections clear up quickly without treatment. Sometimes a throat or skin infection by particular streptococcal bacteria can cause a kidney infection called glomerulonephritis. Rarely, there may be a structural defect of the urinary tract present from birth. The majority of urinary tract defects and infections are treatable.

Glomerulonephritis

What is it? Glomerulonephritis is an inflammation of the kidneys – particularly of the glomeruli, which are the filtering units in the kidneys. The inflamed glomeruli are not able to process wastes efficiently, resulting in decreased urine production and loss of blood and protein in the urine.

Cause: Glomerulonephritis is usually caused by an immune reaction following a streptococcal throat infection, such as **tonsillitis.** Boys are affected more often than girls. ➲

➲ Glomerulonephritis continued

Signs and symptoms:
- Reddish-brown or smoky-looking urine– due to the presence of blood. (**NOTE:** Urine can also be discoloured after a child has eaten beetroot.)
- Slight swelling of the face, ankles and abdomen (known as **oedema**).
- Headache.

What to do:
- **Consult the doctor immediately.**
- The doctor will test the child's urine, take the blood pressure (which may be raised) and take a blood sample for analysis.
- The child will probably be admitted to hospital for treatment, usually bed rest at first and a special diet to reduce salt, fluid and protein levels. This diet prevents the build-up of fluids and alleviates any strain on the kidneys.
- If the streptococcal infection is still present, the doctors will prescribe antibiotics and the child will be sent home to convalesce once the urine has returned to normal.

General care:
- Always consult a doctor when a child has a severe throat infection or any other bacterial infection, such as impetigo.
- With treatment, glomerulonephritis usually clears up within one to two weeks.

CASE STUDY

Judith is a six-year-old girl who always seemed to catch any infection that is going around. Within the last year, she had been off school for a total of more than three weeks because of recurrent ear infections. During the last week, two children in her class had been away from school with suspected tonsillitis. Now the Whitsun holiday had arrived and Judith's parents, Judith and her younger sister, Kate, travelled more than 200 miles to visit relatives. Whilst there, Judith started to complain of a sore throat and her mother noticed that she had a high temperature. Judith's parents managed to bring the temperature down by giving children's paracetamol and by tepid sponging, but Judith still complained that it hurt to swallow and she was very reluctant to drink anything as her throat hurt even more.

By the Bank Holiday Monday, Judith seemed very listless and still complained of pain, but now she had a headache and her face and ankles looked puffy. When she went to the toilet she passed dark red urine and was very frightened. The family decided to go straight home and to call their own doctor. Judith's GP immediately diagnosed glomerulonephritis and Judith was admitted to hospital for tests and treatment. Fortunately, she made a complete recovery and is now back to her normal self.

Questions

1 What signs and symptoms did Judith show that would make you suspect glomerulonephritis?
2 Was there anything else that could have been done to help Judith whilst away from home?

Possible complications:
- Very rarely, glomerulonephritis may be followed by **nephrotic syndrome** – a chronic disorder of the kidneys that may require prolonged treatment.

Urinary tract infections

What are they? Urinary tract infections are infections of any part of the urinary tract – the kidneys, the bladder and the urethra (the tube leading from the bladder to the outside). In most cases, the part infected is the bladder; this condition is called **cystitis**. ➲

➲ Urinary tract infections continued

Cause: Urinary tract infections are usually caused by bacteria from the rectum that enter the urethra. Girls tend to be more prone to urinary infections because the female urethra is shorter, so making it easier for bacteria to reach the bladder. If a young girl wipes her bottom from back to front, this may bring faecal matter near the urethral opening , which could cause infection. Rarely, a minor structural abnormality of the urinary tract is the cause.

Signs and symptoms: Children under the age of two years show signs of a more general infection:

- Fever.
- Diarrhoea.
- Vomiting.
- Strong-smelling urine.

In older children, symptoms are usually more specific, and may include:

- A burning sensation when passing urine.
- Wanting to urinate frequently but being able to pass only a dribble.
- Frequent urination, which can lead to bedwetting in a child who was previously dry at night.
- Low back pain and/or low abdominal pain.
- Unpleasant-smelling – and often cloudy – urine.
- Fever.

What to do:

- Consult the doctor if the child complains of pain when passing urine, or if a younger child shows the symptoms listed above.
- The doctor will examine the child and take a urine sample to identify the organism causing the infection; if infection is confirmed, the doctor will prescribe antibiotics.
- The child may be referred to a specialist to be tested for scarring of the kidneys or congenital abnormalities of the urinary tract.

General care:

- Encourage the child to drink plenty of fluids.

To prevent recurrences of urinary tract infection, the child should*:*

- Drink plenty of fluids.
- Pass urine at regular intervals – at least every 4 hours or before each meal, and before going to bed.
- Empty the bladder completely – after passing urine, tell the child to count to 20 and to try again to get out the last drops.
- Always wipe the bottom from front to back.
- Avoid constipation.
- Bath or shower every day, using non-scented soap.
- Wear cotton underwear.

Possible complications:

- Recurrences of urinary tract infections are fairly common, but prompt treatment should prevent permanent damage to the kidneys.

Revision questions

1 Why are girls more prone to urinary tract infections than boys?
2 How can you help to prevent recurrent urinary infections in children?
3 What is glomerulonephritis? What is the cause of glomerulonephritis?
4 What are the signs and symptoms and possible complications?
5 What is oedema? Why is it important to observe a child for signs of oedema?

Chapter 7: Accident prevention and first aid

◆ *Preventing accidents: at home and in early years settings* ◆ *Safety when babysitting and child sitting* ◆ *Your role in keeping children safe* ◆ *Reporting and recording accidents in an early years setting* ◆ *First aid*

Preventing accidents: at home and in the early years setting

Accidents are the main cause of death and serious injury in children. Every child is likely to go to hospital three times before the age of 15 as a result of an accident. Accidents to children happen every day – some of them serious ones – but that doesn't mean they have to be just a part of growing up. Many serious and fatal accidents can be prevented, and injuries caused by accidents can be reduced.

Children need to explore and to learn about the things around them. The safer you make the child's home and nursery, the less likely it is that their exploration will end in an accident. There are dangers outside the home – in the car, on the roads and just being outdoors. Use the list below to help you think about preventing accidents and teaching the children in your care how to be safer. It is impossible to list *all* the dangers, but thinking about some of these should start you thinking about others.

Preventing accidents

From birth to 3 months

Although babies aren't yet mobile, falls from a pram or from a raised surface such as a bed can pose a threat.

- □ Never leave babies alone on the changing table or bed, even for a second. They are safer on the floor.
- □ **Never leave babies alone in the bath**. If you must answer the door or the phone, again place them on the floor or take them with you.
- □ Don't leave babies to sleep with a bottle propped in their mouth – this could cause choking.
- □ Don't leave a baby unattended in a pram.
- □ Use the safety harness on a baby in a pram.

From 3–6 months

Babies may be able to roll now, so what used to be safe may no longer be – for example putting them down in the upstairs hall. They can also use their hands more, so you'll need to watch what they pick up.

- □ Don't leave babies with the cot side down.
- □ Keep plastic bags well out of their reach.
- □ Make sure they can't pick up small objects which could be a choking hazard.
- □ Keep swing doors propped open to prevent babies catching their fingers.
- □ Ensure trailing flexes are safely tucked away.
- □ Cover hot radiators with towels, or turn the heating down

From 6–9 months

A crawling baby can move fast. Once a baby becomes really mobile, and can use her hands well, keep any dangerous objects well out of reach.

- □ Ensure low-standing cupboards don't contain dangerous items such as knives, bleach, scissors, or medicines.
- □ Fit safety locks on cupboards and drawers – though some babies work out how to open them all the same!
- □ Keep a baby away from anything else she might reach up and pull at, such as tablecloths, ironing board, and oven.
- □ Fit safety covers to electric sockets.
- □ Fit stair gates to the top *and* bottom of stairs.
- □ Keep a fireguard in front of the fire.
- □ Don't leave babies with buckets or other containers of water – it is possible to drown in as little as two inches of water. Fence off or fill in garden ponds.

From 9–12 months

Be extra vigilant about what is within a baby's reach – they can now pull themselves to standing, have started 'cruising' around furniture and may be able to climb.

- □ Remove lightweight furniture which a standing baby could pull down on top of herself.
- □ Ensure large doors and windows are fitted with safety glass.
- □ Have safety locks on all windows.
- □ Remove breakable ornaments to a higher shelf.
- □ Fit a cooker guard or keep all cooking to back burners.
- □ Never leave a child unattended with boiling pans on the stove.
- □ Don't leave hot or alcoholic drinks, matches or lighters lying around.
- □ Keep doors locked to hazard areas such as cellar, garage or garden.

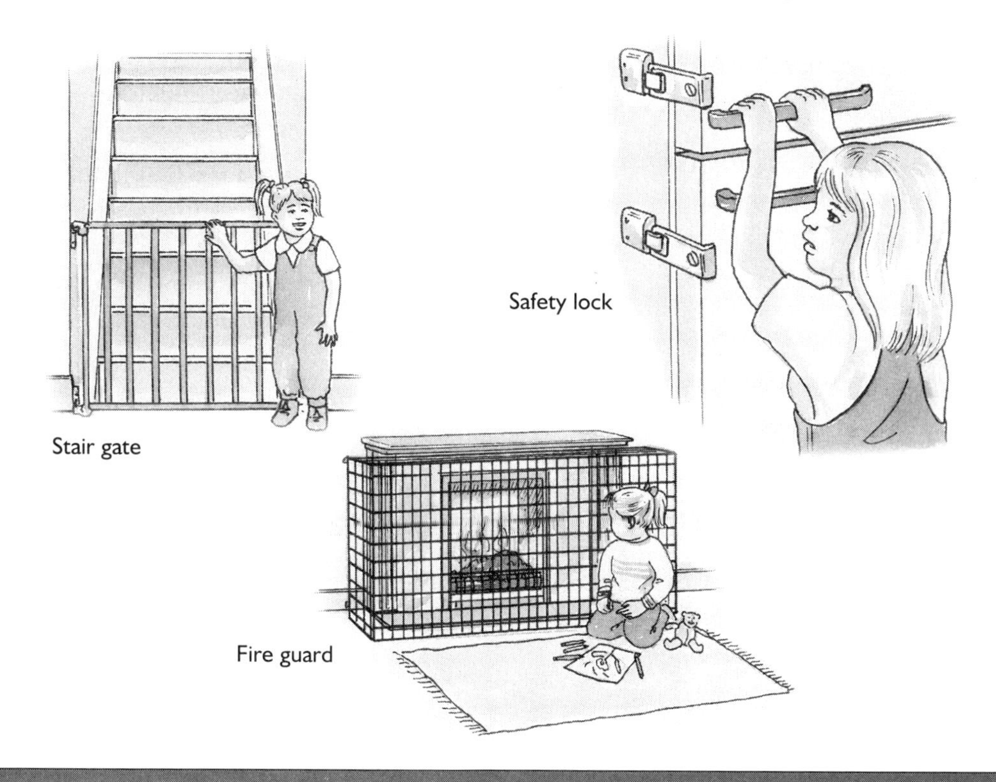

Safety from 1 year onwards

Many toddlers are seriously injured in accidents around the home. These can include falling down stairs, banging their heads, pulling objects on top of themselves, getting seriously scalded or burnt or even falling out of windows that have not been properly shut or locked. Follow these safety guidelines when identifying possible safety hazards in the home and the early years setting:

Choking and suffocation

- ☐ Store small objects away from babies and small children; choose toys suitable for the child's age and stage of development.
- ☐ Keep toys for older children away from younger brothers or sisters to prevent them from choking on small parts.
- ☐ Don't use pillows in babies under 1 year.
- ☐ Remove ribbons and strings that might get wound around a child's neck.
- ☐ Store polythene bags out of children's reach.
- ☐ Make sure that any toys used conform to safety standards. Look for safety symbols, such as the Lion mark and the age-appropriate advice on packaging.
- ☐ Do not give young children peanuts to eat.
- ☐ Always supervise children when eating finger food, especially pieces of banana which can cause choking.

Fires, burns and scalds

- ☐ Fit a smoke detector: check the smoke detector battery weekly.
- ☐ Work out how to get out of your house, nursery or school in case of a fire.
- ☐ Shorten the flexes on kettles and other electrical appliances.
- ☐ Put up a fireguard and fix it to the wall around any open fires or hot stoves.
- ☐ Always use the back rings on the cooker and turn pan handles away from the front of the cooker or fit a cooker hob guard.
- ☐ Keep children at a safe distance while you cook.
- ☐ Make sure children can't reach your hot coffee or tea and keep tea and coffee pots out of reach.
- ☐ Don't leave tablecloths on the table: children can pull hot drinks and food down with them.
- ☐ Always run the cold tap first in the bath and check the temperature before a child gets in.
- ☐ Turn the hot water thermostat to 54 °C or 130 °F to avoid scalds.
- ☐ Only attend well-supervised bonfire and fireworks events.

▶

Falls

- Always put bouncing chairs on the floor – **never** on a table or worktop.
- Encourage children not to play on stairs or in the main walkways in group settings.
- Make sure there are properly fixed stair gates or barriers both at the top and bottom of any stairs.
- Do not use a baby walker; these encourage children to reach areas that are potentially dangerous.
- Check the rails round landings and balconies to make sure children can't fall through, crawl under or climb over them.
- If you have safety catches or locks on upstairs windows to stop a child falling out, make sure you won't be locked in if there is a fire.
- If windows are not locked, put stoppers on them so they can't be opened by more than 10 cm. The best place to put them is at the top of the window so that children can't reach them.
- Move furniture away from windows, so children can't climb up in the first place.
- Use safety harnesses when children are sitting in high chairs and push chairs.
- Supervise play on climbing frames and swings.

Cuts

- Low-level glass in doors and windows is dangerous, especially when the child starts to move about. Fit safety film or safety glass.
- Keep all sharp objects somewhere safe – out of reach of children.
- Make sure children never walk around holding anything made of glass or with anything like a pencil or lollipop in their mouths.
- Low corners on tables and chairs that could poke a child in the eye are especially dangerous. The best way to make them safe is to put plastic corners on them, or foam rubber secured with a rubber band.
- Use a wedge or hook on doors to hold them permanently open so that a child can't get their fingers trapped.
- Only use children's safety scissors when cutting paper and card.

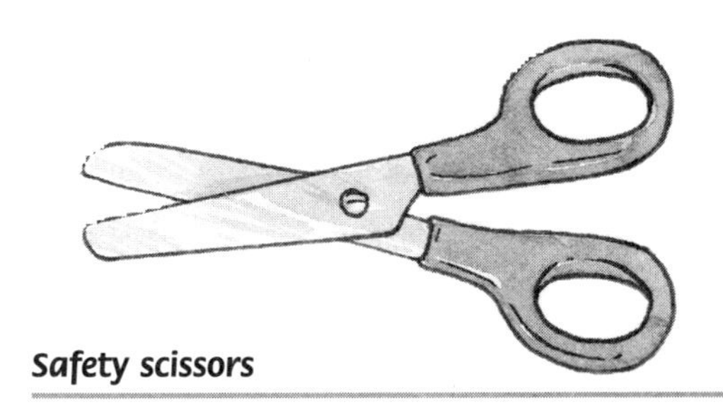

Safety scissors

Electricity

- Cover electric sockets with heavy furniture or safety covers when not in use.
- Repair all worn flexes.
- Do not plug too many appliances into one socket.
- Electric wiring should be checked regularly for safety by a qualified electrician.
- Prevent children from pulling at electric cords by installing a cord holder which will make the cord too short to reach over the edge of the table or work surface.
- Find out if there is a safety relay or circuit breaker in the house and if there isn't, have one installed.

Poisoning

- Lock all alcohol and medicines away or store them high up, out of sight where the child can't climb.
- Put all medicines in child-resistant containers and be alert in other peoples' houses for tablets in drawers and handbags.
- Store all household and garden chemicals in a safe place, high up and locked away – make sure you replace any child resistant caps properly after use. Dish washing agents, cleansing agents, detergent, turpentine, flammable liquids and fertilisers are all toxic if swallowed. Dish washing powder is also dangerous if it comes into contact with skin, e.g. if a child spills a packet over themselves.
- Don't put any dangerous liquids in drinks bottles.
- Teach children not to eat any plants, fungi, berries or seeds.
- If surma is used on child's eyes, make sure it is one of the safe, lead-free brands. Check with a pharmacist.

Drowning

- If a small child's face goes underwater, they will automatically breathe in so that they can scream and this will fill their lungs with water. Children also lose their sense of direction underwater, so they can't react by pulling their head out or standing up as an adult would do.
- Never leave a baby or child under four alone in the bath – even for a moment.
- Cover or fence off any garden ponds or water butts. Never leave a child alone near water.
- Teach children to swim. Children who can swim are safer but it is still no guarantee – always keep a close watch on them when they are near water.

Road safety

- Never let a child on or near roads alone. Young children don't understand the danger of traffic.
- Hold a child's hand when you are near roads. Walking reins are useful for toddlers.
- Teach children to cross roads by always crossing safely yourself and explaining what you are doing. Don't expect a child under the age of eight to cross a road alone.

Sun safety

- Keep children out of the sun between 11 a.m. and 3 p.m. when the sun is highest and most dangerous.
- Keep babies under the age of six months out of the sun altogether.
- Don't let children run around all day in a swimsuit or without any clothes on.
- Cover children in loose baggy cotton clothes such as an oversized T-shirt with sleeves.
- In particular, protect a child's shoulders and back of neck when playing, as these are the most common areas for sunburn: let a child wear a 'legionnaire's hat' or a floppy hat with a wide brim that shades the face and neck.
- Cover exposed parts of the child's skin with a sunscreen, even on cloudy or overcast days. Use one with a minimum sun protection factor (SPF) of 15 and reapply often.
- Use waterproof sunblock if the child is swimming.

Strangers

Parents are often worried about their child being abducted or murdered by a stranger. In fact, this is rare compared, for example, with the risk of a traffic accident. However it makes sense to teach children the following:

- Never go with anyone (even someone they know well) without telling the grown up who is looking after them.
- If someone they don't know tries to take them away, it's OK to scream and kick.
- Tell children always to tell you if they have been approached by someone they don't know.
- Make sure that children know what to do if they are lost.

If they are in a crowded place, tell them to stand still and wait to be found.

Otherwise, teach them to:

- tell a police officer
- go into a shop and tell someone behind the counter
- tell someone who has other children with them
- and as soon as they are old enough, teach a child his or her address and phone number or the phone number of another responsible person.

Safety when travelling in cars

Children in a car who are not fastened with a seatbelt or who are not placed in a child seat may be seriously injured or even die in a car accident. The relatively large weight of their heads as they are thrown forward makes them particularly vulnerable.

- The front seat must be moved as far back as possible. A distance of at least 20 cm (10") must be left between the dashboard and the child seat, in order not to hurt the child in a head-on collision.
- The advice from the Child Accident Prevention Trust (CAPT) and paediatricians is that babies should travel *rearward facing* in a special child safety seat at least until they are able to sit on the floor, unaided, for at least half an hour.
- If you have air bags fitted to your car, make sure the baby always travels in a special fitted baby seat on the back seat.

Recommended safety measures for children aged 3 to 6 years old:

- Children in this age group (weighing 15 to 25 kg) should be carried in the back seat in approved child seats which must be fastened with the car's three-point seat belt.
- Bigger children should use a booster cushion to use with an adult safety belt.
- Make sure you always get children out of the car on the pavement side.

ACTIVITY

A friend is adopting an 18-month-old child soon. She has asked you for advice on making her flat as safe as possible for him. Prepare a fact sheet which includes the following information:

- The expected stage of development and behaviour of the child.
- How to check for safety in the living room, bathroom, bedroom and kitchen.
- Reasons for the advice given.

What to do in an emergency

If a child is ill or has an accident and you need help quickly:

- Phone the GP. You can call at any time of the day or night. If you haven't been given a special number for calls outside surgery hours, phone the usual number and wait for an answer.
- If the GP doesn't answer or can't get there quickly enough, take the child to the accident and emergency department of the nearest hospital with a children's unit. Find out in advance where this is. The health visitor will be able to help you.
- If you think the child's life is in danger, call an ambulance. Dial 999 and ask for the ambulance service. Say it's for a baby or a child. You don't need a coin or phonecard to dial 999 from a public phone box.

If you don't have a phone

Keep a couple of coins and/or a phone card always ready in a special place.

Find out in advance whether neighbours have a phone you could use in an emergency.

Safety when babysitting and child sitting

Many early years workers gain valuable experience about children and child care by taking on babysitting or child sitting jobs. When accepting a new job looking after someone else's children, follow these guidelines to ensure your safety and that of the children entrusted to your care:

- Know who is employing you; only accept jobs from people you know or for whom you have personal, reliable references.
- Make sure that your parent (or someone you live with) knows where you are babysitting. Leave them the name, address and telephone number of the people you are sitting for, and let them know what time to expect you home.
- **Compile a checklist**, photocopy the list to take with you to any new jobs, and make sure you always fill it in before the parents leave you in charge:

Babysitting checklist

1 Address of the house ....

2 Phone number at the house ....

3 Name and phone number of the GP ....

4 Nearest hospital and phone number ....

5 Where the parents will be ....

6 Phone number where the parents can be reached ....

7 What time the parents are expected home ....

8 Name and phone number of neighbours ....

9 Other contacts, e.g. grandparents or other relatives ....

10 Any allergies or special medical information for children ....

Keep this checklist by the phone while you are in sole charge

Additional safety guidelines

- If the house has an electronic security system, learn how to use it.
- Don't open the door to strangers.
- Don't let anyone at the door or on the phone know that you are there alone. If asked, respond that you are visiting, the children's parents cannot come to the door (or phone) and that you'll deliver a message.
- If you plan to take the children out, make sure that you have a key to lock and unlock doors; don't forget window locks.
- When you get back to the house, don't go inside if anything seems unusual – broken window, door open, etc. Go to a neighbour and call the police.
- Make sure that you have an escort home if babysitting at night.

In an emergency

- If there is a fire, get the children and yourself OUT! Go to a neighbour's and call the fire department – dial 999. If you can, call the parents and let them know where you and the children are, and what is happening.
- Try not to panic during an emergency. It will not only prevent you from thinking clearly – it will also frighten the children.
- If you suspect that a child has swallowed a poison, dial 999 immediately. Be able to identify the poison and the amount taken.

Your role in keeping children safe

You should be able to identify potential hazards in the child's environment and should be a good role model for children. This means that you should:

- set a **good example** to children and to others. Children unconsciously imitate the adults they are with. If you show a real concern for safety issues, then children will pick up on this and behave as you do.
- be **vigilant** at all times. When supervising children in a group setting, you need to be aware of their moods and to anticipate any problems.
- follow **safety procedures**: for example, you should learn the **Green Cross Code** and make sure that you *always* adhere to the rules when you are out with children.
- keep the environment as **safe** and **hygienic** as possible: mop up spills straightaway, clear up after activities with children, etc.

Reporting and recording accidents in an early years setting

Reporting to parents

Any accident, injury or illness which happens to children in a group setting must be reported to the child's parents or primary carers. If the injury is minor, such as a graze or a bruise, the nursery or school staff will inform parents when the child is collected at the end of the session. If someone other than the child's parent collects the child, a notification slip will be sent home. Parents are notified about:

- The nature of the injury or illness.
- Any treatment or action taken.
- The name of the person who carried out the treatment.

In the case of a major accident or illness then the child's parents must be notified as quickly as possible.

Accident Report Book

Every early years setting is required by law to have an Accident Report Book and to maintain a record of accidents. Information recorded includes:

Name of person injured ....

Date and time of injury ....

Where the accident happened ....

What exactly happened (e.g. Matthew fell in the outdoor play area and grazed his right knee) ....

What injuries occurred (e.g. a graze) ....

What treatment was given (e.g. graze was bathed and an adhesive dressing applied) ....

Name and signature of person dealing with the accident ....

Signature of witness to the report ....

Signature of parent or guardian ....

First aid

How to get emergency help

1. **Assess the situation**: stay calm and don't panic.
2. **Minimise any danger** to yourself and to others, e.g. make sure someone takes charge of other children at the scene.
3. **Send for help**. Notify a doctor, hospital and parents, etc. as appropriate. If in any doubt.

Call an ambulance: Dial 999

Be ready to assist the emergency services by answering some simple questions.

- ☐ Your **name** and the **telephone number** you are calling from.
- ☐ The **location** of the accident. Try to give as much information as possible, for example familiar landmarks such as churches or pubs nearby.
- ☐ Explain briefly **what has happened**: this helps the paramedics to act speedily when they arrive.
- ☐ Tell them **what you have done** so far to treat the casualty.

Revision questions

1 List the observations and records you should make when a child suddenly becomes unwell in an early years setting.
2 What information must be included in an Accident Report Book?
3 Describe the ABC procedure for resuscitation in:
   a A baby under one year.
   b A four-year-old child.
4 What is the recovery position? When would you place a child in the recovery position?
5 What is the first-aid treatment for a burn or scald?
6 How would you treat a child who is choking?
7 What is a sprain? What is the first-aid treatment for a sprain?
8 How should you treat a child with a grazed knee?
9 What is the Sun Safety Code?
10 Describe how you would call for an ambulance in an emergency.

ACTIVITY

Using a First Aid book, find out what to do in the following scenarios:

- ☐ A three-year-old girl has fallen from a climbing frame and is lying perfectly still on the ground. You suspect that she has a head injury.
- ☐ A six-year-old boy complains of pain just above his elbow. When you examine the arm, you see that it is very swollen and bruised and tender to the touch. You suspect that he has a fracture of the upper arm.
- ☐ A four-year-old complains of feeling sick. You notice that there are berries in and around his mouth. You suspect that he has eaten some berries from a yew tree and may have acute poisoning.

A guide to basic first aid for children

First aid is an important skill. By performing simple procedures and following certain guidelines, it may be possible to save lives by giving basic treatment until professional medical help arrives. Also remember that practice makes perfect. In an emergency there is no time to read instructions. If you've memorised some of the most basic procedures, you will be able to react quickly and efficiently. All those who work with children should take a recognised first-aid course, such as those run by the **St John's Ambulance Association** or the **British Red Cross Society**, and should periodically take refresher courses so that they feel competent to deal with any medical emergency.

The colour section on the following pages explains the major first-aid techniques for babies and children. They should **not** be used as a substitute for attending a first-aid course with a trained instructor. The photographs also show ways of dealing with the more minor accidents which you are likely to encounter in the child's home, nursery or school.

The first-aid techniques included here are:

- Resuscitating a baby (mouth-to-mouth-and-nose ventilation and chest compressions)
- Resuscitating a child (mouth-to-mouth ventilation and chest compressions)
- Recovery position
- Choking
- Bleeding: cuts and grazes; nosebleeds
- Burns and scalds
- Sprains and strains.

ABC of resuscitation: babies up to 1 year old

If a baby appears unconscious and is not responding:

A Open the airway

- □ Place the baby on a firm surface
- □ Remove any obstruction from the mouth – using your finger.
- □ Put one hand on the forehead and one finger under the chin, and gently tilt the head backwards VERY SLIGHTLY – if you tilt the head too far back, it will close the airway again.

If there is no pulse, or the pulse is slower than 60 per minute, and the baby is not breathing, start **chest compressions**:

1. Find a position one finger's width below the line joining the baby's nipples, in the centre of the breastbone.
2. Place the tips of two fingers on this point and press to a depth of about 2 cm ($\frac{3}{4}$ inch) at a rate of 100 times per minute.

B Breathing – check for breathing

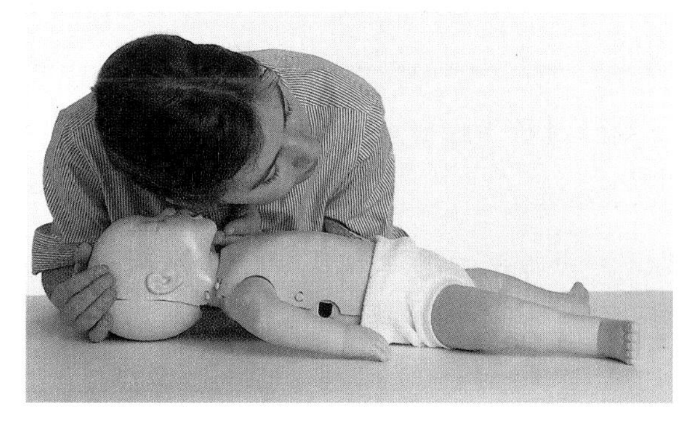

- □ Put your ear close to the baby's mouth.
- □ Look to see if the chest is rising or falling.
- □ Listen and feel for the baby's breath on your cheek.
- □ Do this for five seconds.

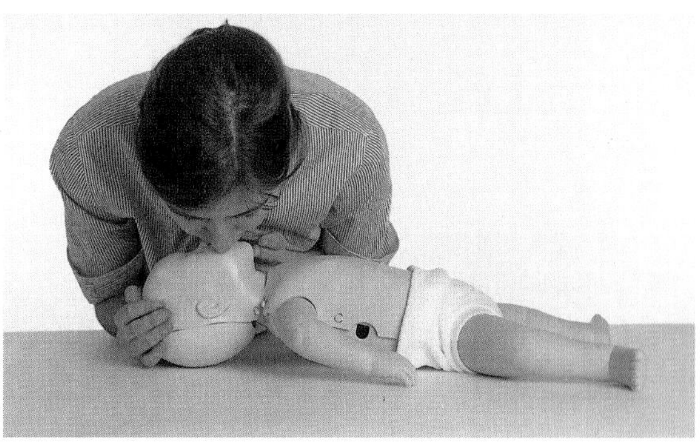

If the baby is *not* breathing:

1. Start **mouth-to-mouth-and-nose resuscitation**:
   - □ Seal your lips around the baby's mouth and nose.
   - □ Blow *gently* into the baby's mouth and nose.
   - □ Remove your mouth and allow the chest to fall.
2. Repeat 5 times at the rate of one breath every 3 seconds.
3. Check the pulse.
4. After 5 chest compressions, blow gently into the lungs once.
5. Continue the cycle for one minute.
6. Carry the baby to a phone and dial 999 for an ambulance.
7. Continue resuscitation, checking the pulse every minute until help arrives.

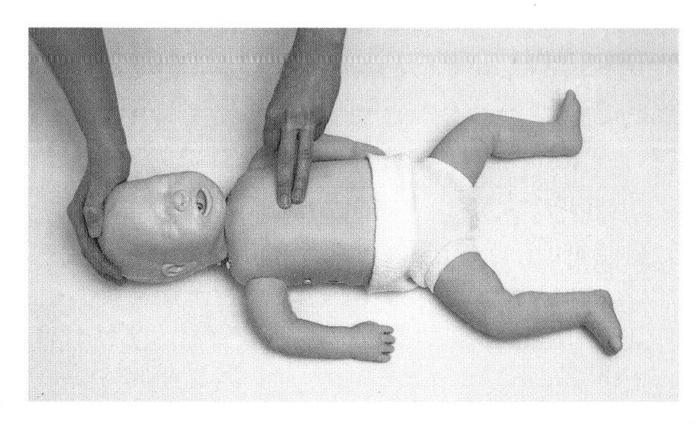

If the baby is *not* breathing but *does* have a pulse:

1 Start **mouth-to-mouth-and-nose resuscitation**, at the rate of 1 breath every 3 seconds.

2 Continue for one minute, then carry the baby to a phone and dial 999 for an ambulance.

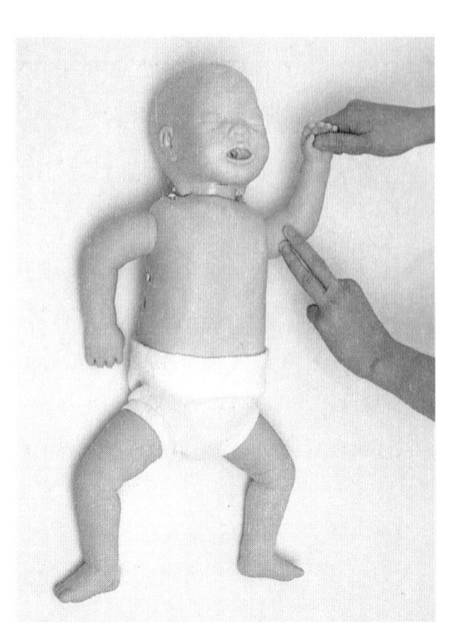

C Circulation – check the pulse

Lightly press your fingers towards the bone on the inside of the upper arm and hold them there 5 seconds.

If the baby *does* have a pulse and is breathing:

1 Lay the baby on its side, supported by a cushion, pillow, rolled-up blanket or something similar.

2 Dial 999 for an ambulance.

3 Check breathing and pulse every minute and be prepared to carry out resuscitation.

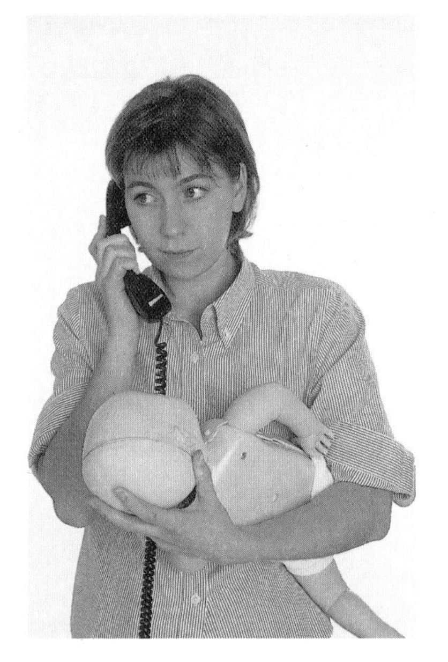

ABC of resuscitation: children aged 1 to 10 years old

A Airway – open the airway

- Lay the child flat on their back.
- Remove clothing from around the neck.
- Remove any obstruction from the mouth.
- Lift the chin and tilt the head back slightly to open the airway.

If the child is *not* breathing and *does not* have a pulse:

1 Begin a cycle of 5 chest compressions (see below) and one breath (see mouth-to-mouth resuscitation). Continue for 1 minute.

2 Dial 999 for an ambulance.

3 Continue at the rate of one breath to 5 compressions until help arrives.

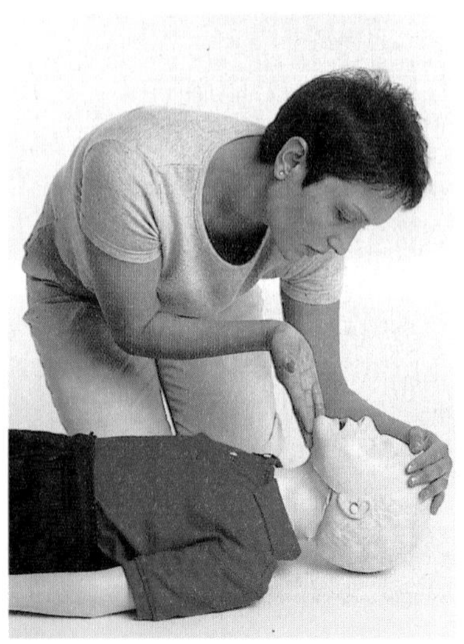

If the child is *not* breathing but *does* have a pulse:

1 Give 20 breaths (see mouth-to-mouth resuscitation) in 1 minute.

2 Dial 999 for an ambulance

3 Continue mouth-to-mouth resuscitation, re-checking the pulse and breathing after each set of 20 breaths, until help arrives or until the child starts breathing again. When breathing returns, place the child in the **recovery position**.

B *Breathing – check for breathing*

- □ Keep the airway open and place your cheek close to the child's mouth.
- □ Look to see if their chest is rising and falling.
- □ Listen and feel for their breath against your cheek.
- □ Do this for 5 seconds.
- □ If the child is not breathing, give 5 breaths (see below), then check the pulse.

Mouth-to-mouth resuscitation

1. Open the airway by lifting the chin and tilting back the head. Check the mouth is clear of obstructions.
2. Close the child's nose by pinching the nostrils.
3. Take a deep breath and seal your mouth over the child's mouth.
4. Blow firmly into the mouth for about 2 seconds, watching the chest rise.
5. Remove your mouth and allow the child's chest to fall.
6. Repeat until help arrives.

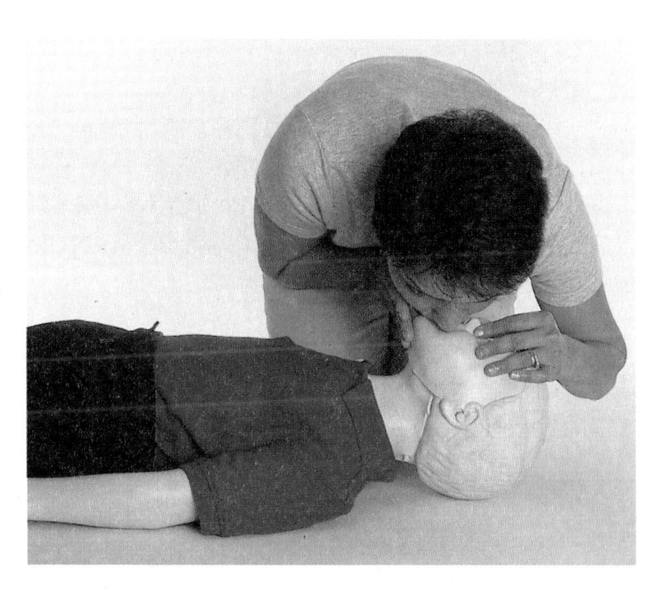

C *Circulation – check the pulse*

- □ Find the carotid pulse by placing your fingers in the groove between the Adam's apple and the large muscle running from the side of the neck.
- □ Do this for 5 seconds.

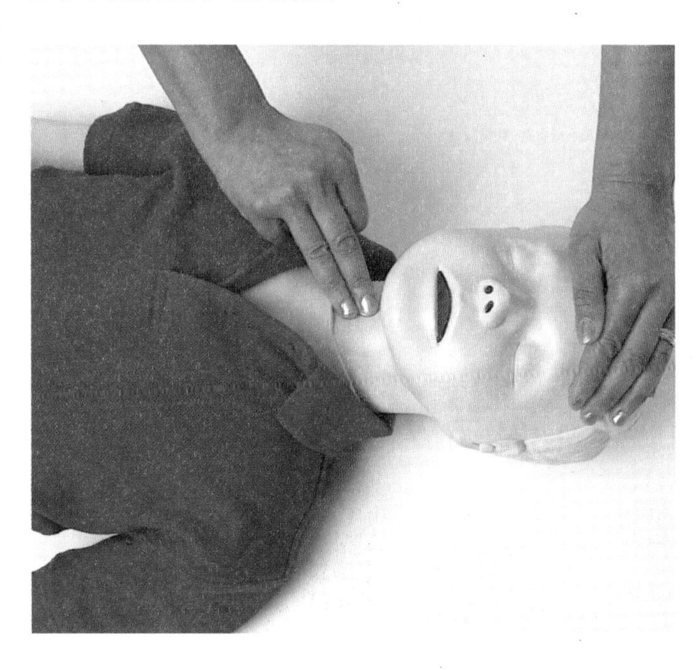

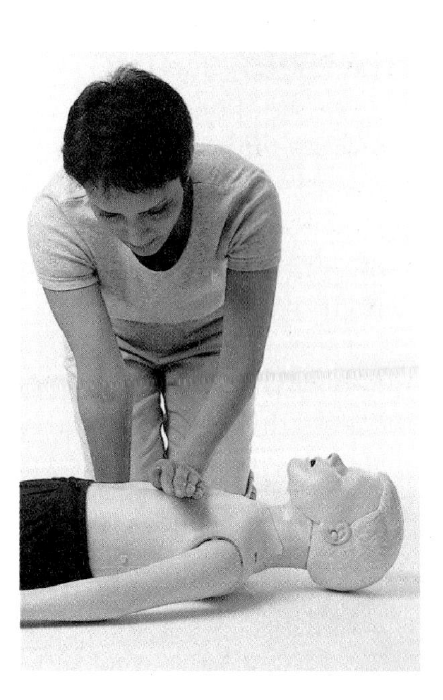

Chest compressions

1 Make sure the child is lying on their back on a firm surface, preferably the ground.
2 Find the spot where the bottom of the ribcage joins on to the end of the breastbone and measure one finger's width up from this point.
3 Using one hand only, press down sharply at a rate of 100 times a minute, to a depth of about 3 cm ($1\frac{1}{4}$ inches). Counting aloud will help you to keep at the right speed.
4 Continue until help arrives.

Recovery position

Any child who is breathing and who has a pulse should be placed in the recovery position while you wait for an ambulance or other medical assistance. This safe position allows fluids to drain out of the child's mouth so that they are not inhaled into the lungs.

An unconscious baby should be held securely, with the head tilted back slightly to keep the airway open.

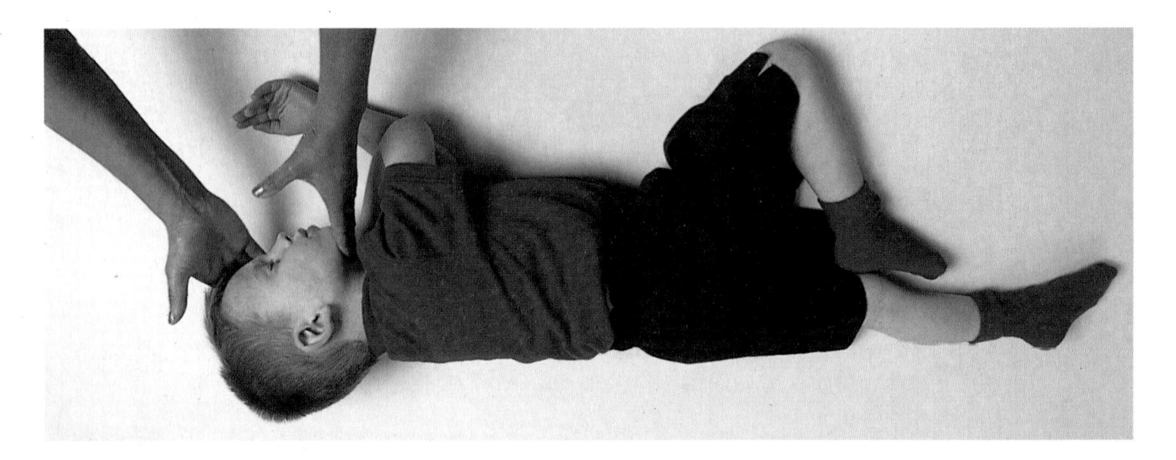

For an unconscious child:

1 Roll child onto side. Grasp the thigh furthest away from you and roll the child over by pulling the bent leg towards you. As you roll, keep the child's head held against his or her cheek.
2 Bend the top leg at a right angle and adjust the position of the bottom arm to prevent the child from rolling forwards. Tilt the head back to keep the airways open.

Make sure that someone stays with the child until the ambulance arrives and check both breathing and pulse frequently.

NOTE: If the child has a spinal injury, only put them in the recovery position if their breathing is obstructed. You should aim to keep the child's head, neck and spine aligned at all times.

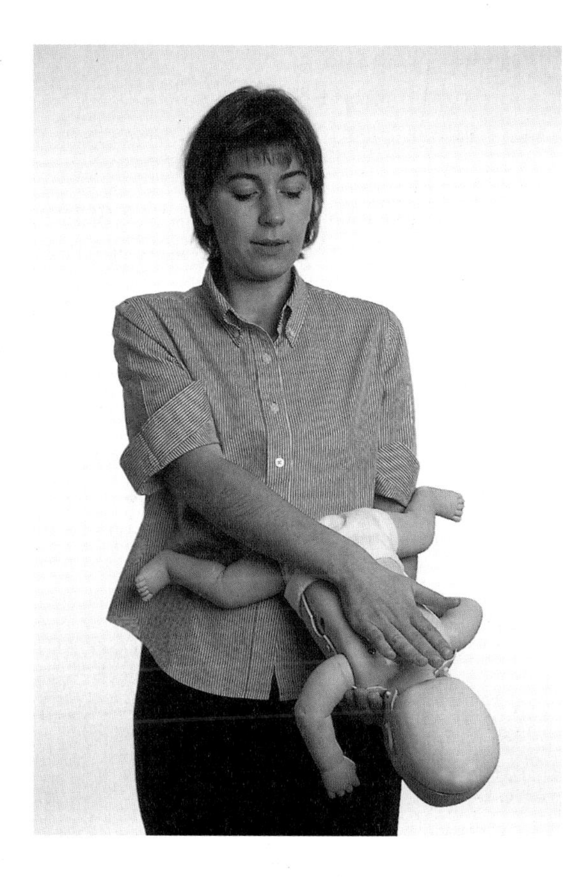

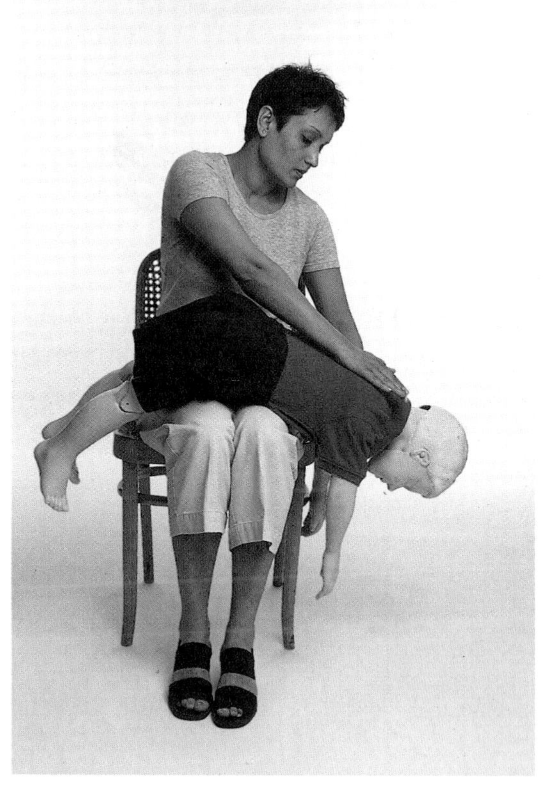

Choking

First check inside the child's mouth. If the obstruction is visible, try to hook it out with your finger, but don't risk pushing it further down. If this doesn't work:

1 **For a baby:** Lay the baby down along your forearm, supporting her head and neck with your hand. The baby's head should be lower than her bottom.

For an older baby or toddler: Sit down and put the child face down across your knees with head and arms hanging down. Keep the child's head lower than the chest.

2 Give five brisk slaps between the shoulder blades.

3 Turn the child over, check the mouth again and remove any visible obstruction.

4 Check for breathing.

5 If the child is not breathing, give five breaths (see **ABC of resuscitation**).

6 If the airway is still obstructed, give five chest compressions.

7 If the child is still not breathing, repeat the cycle of back slaps, mouth-to-mouth-and-nose breathing and chest compressions.

8 After 2 cycles, if the child is not breathing, **dial 999 for an ambulance**.

Never hold a baby upside down by the ankles and slap its back – you could break its neck.

Bleeding, cuts and grazes; nosebleeds

For minor cuts and grazes:

1 Sit or lie the child down and reassure them.
2 Clean the injured area with cold water, using cotton wool or gauze.
3 Apply a dressing if necessary.
4 Do not attempt to pick out pieces of gravel or grit from a graze; just clean gently and cover with a light dressing.
5 Record the injury and treatment in the **Accident Report Book** and make sure the parents/carers of the child are informed.

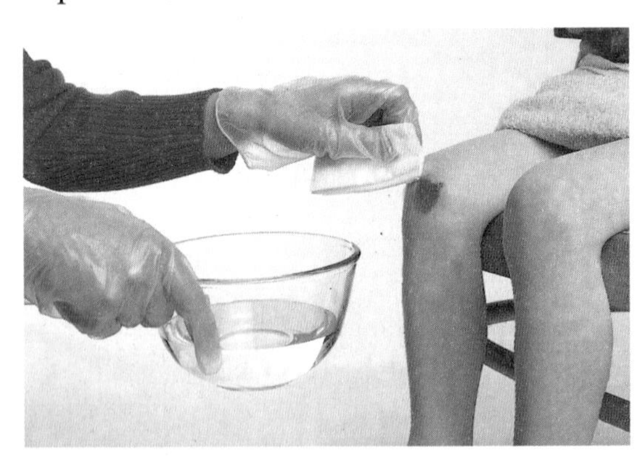

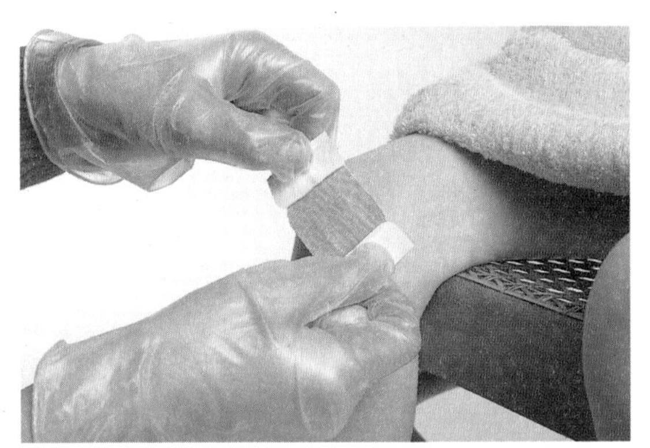

For severe bleeding:

1 Summon medical help – Dial 999 or call a doctor.
2 Try to stop the bleeding:
   - Apply direct pressure to the wound. Wear gloves and use a dressing or a non-fluffy material, such as a clean tea-towel.
   - Elevate the affected part if possible.

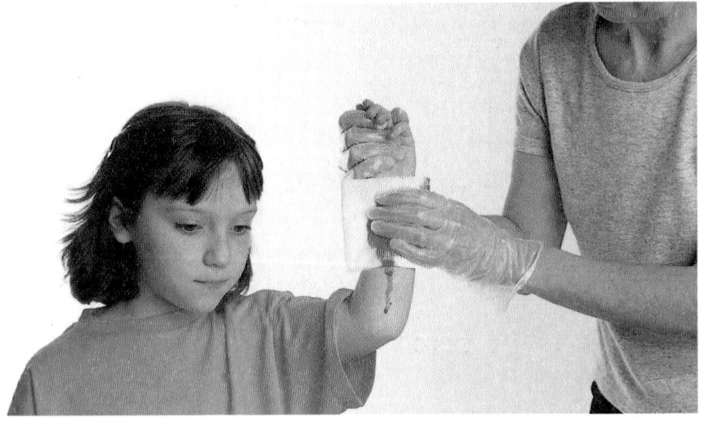

3 Apply a dressing. If the blood soaks through, DO NOT remove the dressing, apply another on top and so on.
   ✓ Keep the child warm and reassure them.
   ✓ DO NOT give anything to eat or drink.
   ✓ Contact the child's parents or carers.
   ✓ If the child loses consciousness, follow the ABC procedure for resuscitation.

NB Always record the incident and the treatment given in the **Accident Report Book**. ***Always wear disposable gloves if in an early years setting to prevent cross infection.***

Nosebleeds

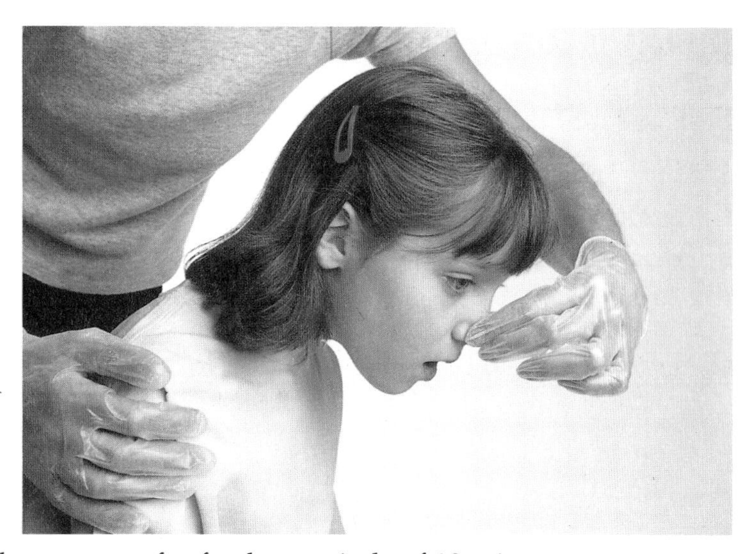

1 Sit the child down with her head well forward.
2 Ask her to breathe through her mouth.
3 Pinch the fleshy part of her nose, just below the bridge.
4 Reassure her and tell her not to try to speak, cough or sniff as this may disturb blood clots.
5 After 10 minutes, release the pressure. If the nose is still bleeding, reapply the pressure for further periods of 10 minutes.
6 If the nosebleed persists beyond 30 minutes, seek medical aid.

Minor burns and scalds

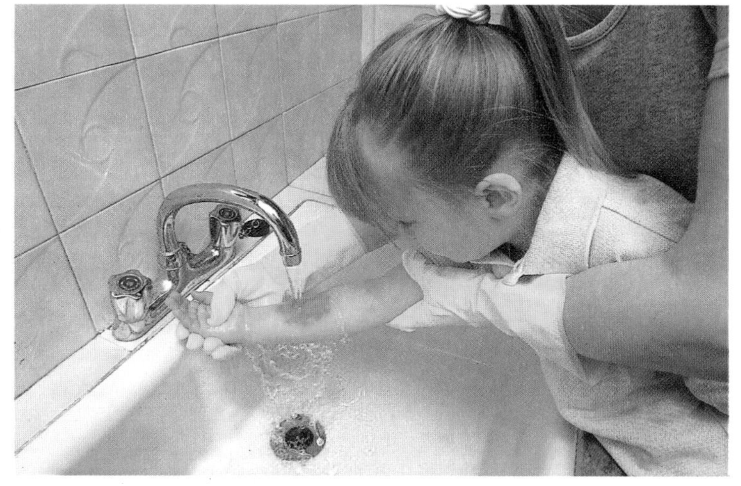

1 Place the injured part under slowly running cold water, or soak in cold water for 10 minutes.
2 Gently remove any constricting articles from the injured area before it begins to swell.
3 Dress with clean, sterile non-fluffy material.

DO NOT use adhesive dressings.

DO NOT apply lotions, ointments or grease to burn or scald.

DO NOT break blisters or otherwise interfere.

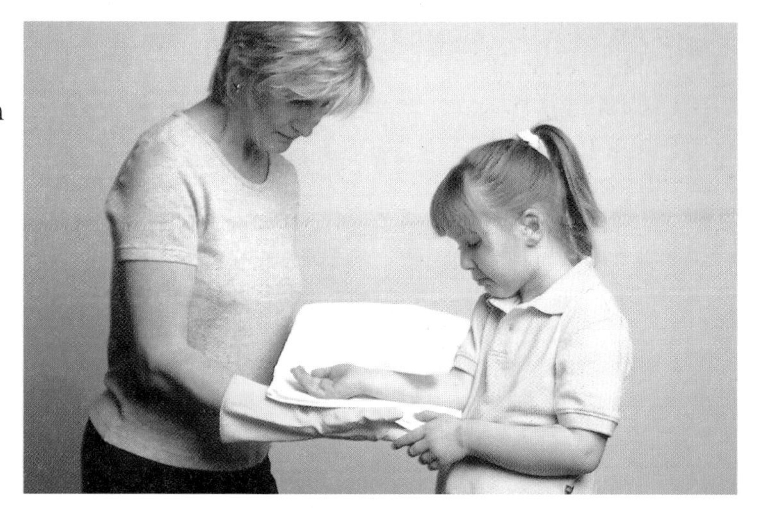

Sprains and strains

Follow the **RICE** procedure:

R Rest the injured part

I Apply ice or a cold compress

C Compress the injury

E Elevate the injured part.

1. Rest, steady and support the injured part in the most comfortable position for the child.
2. Cool the area by applying an ice pack or a cold compress. (This could be a pack of frozen peas wrapped in cloth.)
3. Apply gentle, even pressure by surrounding the area with a thick layer of foam or cotton wool, secured with a bandage.
4. Raise and support the injured limb, to reduce blood flow to the injury and to minimise bruising.

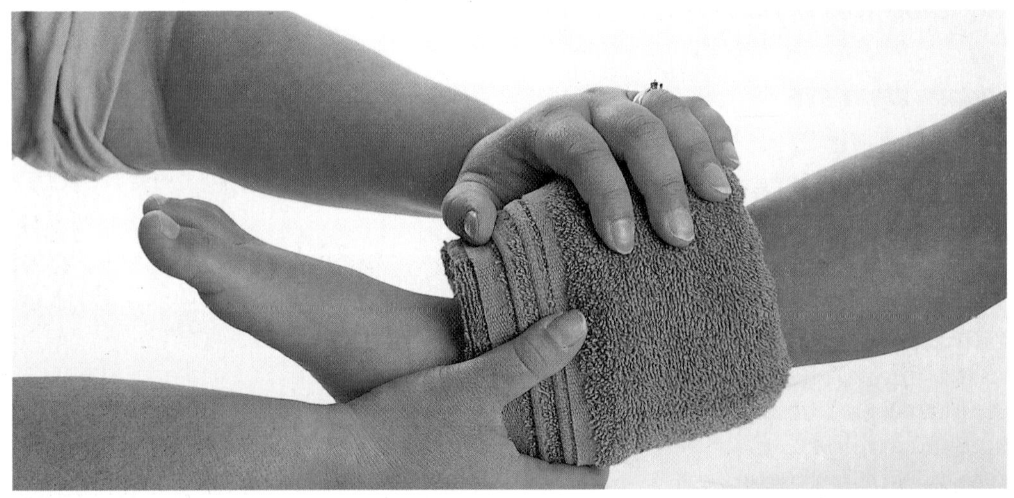

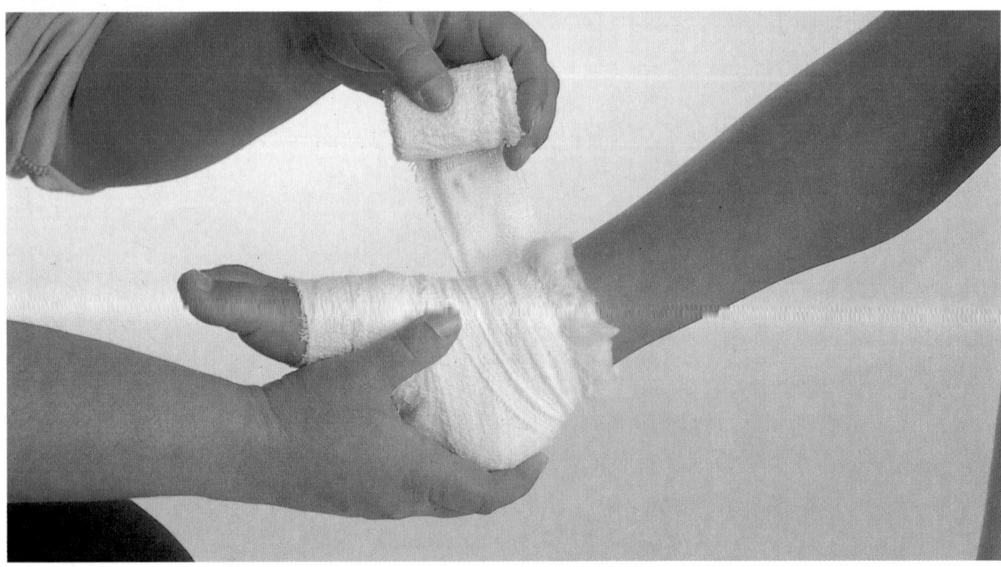

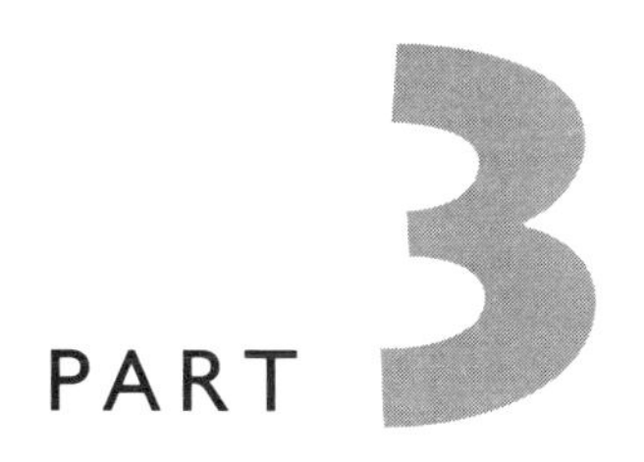

PART 3

Working with sick children

Chapter 8: Caring for sick children

◆ *The needs of sick children* ◆ *Caring for sick children at home* ◆ *Caring for sick children in early years settings* ◆ *Giving medicines*

The needs of sick children

The needs of children who are sick are:

- **Physical needs**: food and drink, rest and sleep, temperature control, exercise and fresh air, safety, hygiene and medical care.
- **Intellectual and language needs**: stimulation, providing appropriate activities.
- **Emotional and social needs**: love, security, provision of play and contact with others.

The most important part of caring for sick children is to show that you care for them and to respond to all their needs. If a child is going to have to be nursed for some weeks, it is often useful to draw up a plan of care, just as nurses do in hospital. This has the following benefits:

- It helps you to keep a record of any changes in the child's condition and to ask for outside help if necessary.
- It reassures you that you are providing for all the child's needs.
- It enables you to plan a simple programme of activities to keep the child entertained and occupied.
- It enables another family member or colleague to assist in the general care, allowing you a break.

Caring for sick children at home

Wherever possible children should stay at home when ill, within the secure environment of their family and surroundings. The child will want his or her primary carer available at all times. The parents may need advice on how to care for their child and this is provided by the family GP and primary health care team – some health authorities have specialist paediatric nursing visiting services.

Meeting physical needs

Bedrest

Children usually dislike being confined to bed and will only stay there if feeling very unwell. There is no need to keep a child with a fever in bed. Take your lead from the child. Making a bed on a settee in the main living room will save you the expense of extra heating and of tiring trips up and down stairs. The child will also feel more included in family life and less isolated. The room does not have to be particularly hot – just a comfortable temperature for you. If the child *does* stay in bed in his or her own room, remember to visit them often so that they do not feel neglected.

- Use cotton sheets – they are more comfortable for a child with a temperature.
- Change the sheets daily if possible if the child has a fever – clean sheets feel better.
- Leave a box of tissues on a table next to the bed.
- If the child has bouts of vomiting, pillows should be protected and a container should be kept close to the bed, emptied and rinsed with an antiseptic/disinfectant, for example Savlon, after use.
- Wet or soiled bed linen should be changed to prevent discomfort and paper tissues that can be disposed of either by burning or by sealing in disposal bags are useful for minor accidents.
- A plastic mattress cover is useful as a sick child's behaviour may change and cause him or her to wet the bed.

Hygiene

All children benefit from having a routine to meet their hygiene needs, and this need not be drastically altered during illness.

- The child's room should be well-ventilated and uncluttered; open a window to prevent stuffiness but protect the child from draughts.
- Provide a potty to avoid trips to the lavatory.
- Protect the mattress with a rubber or plastic sheet.
- A daily bath or shower is important, but during the acute phase this can be done in the form of a bed bath – an all-over wash in bed – see below.
- Brush hair daily.
- Clean teeth after meals – apply vaseline to sore, cracked lips.
- Keep the child's nails short and clean and prevent scratching of any spots.
- Dress the child in cool, cotton clothing; put a jumper and socks or slippers over pyjamas if the child does not want to stay in bed the whole time.

Giving a bed bath

1 Make sure that the room is warm enough; close the windows to avoid draughts.
2 Collect the things you will need and place on a table next to the bed: a bowl with warm water, soap, flannel or sponge and towels.
3 Remove the child's nightie or pyjamas.
4 Cover the child with a sheet and remove the top bedding.
5 Place a towel under each part of the body as it is washed.
6 Start by washing the face and upper body.
7 Use a separate flannel to wash the bottom and genital area.

Infection

If the illness is infectious, advice may be needed on how it spreads; visits from friends and relatives may have to be reduced. The most infectious time is during the incubation period but the dangers of infecting others remain until the main signs and symptoms, for example a rash, have disappeared. A child attending nursery or school will usually be kept at home until the GP says they are clear of infection.

Temperature control

If the child has a fever, you will need to take the temperature regularly and use tepid sponging to reduce it (see page 81).

Feeding a sick child

Children who are ill often have poor appetites – a few days without food will not harm the child but **fluid intake** should be increased as a general rule.

Providing drinks
Drinks should be offered at frequent intervals to prevent dehydration – the child will not necessarily request drinks.

- Provide a covered jug of fruit juice or water; any fluid is acceptable according to the child's tastes, for example milk, meaty drinks or soups.

  NOTE: If the child has mumps, do not give fruit drinks because the acid causes pain to the tender parotid glands.
- A sick toddler who has recently given up his bottle may regress and only want to drink from a bottle until he is feeling better.
- Try using an interesting curly straw.
- Give the child an 'adult' glass to make them feel special *or* offer drinks in a tiny glass or egg cup, which makes the quantities look smaller.
- Offer fresh fruit juices, such as pear, apple or mango; dilute them with fizzy water to make them more interesting; vary the drinks as much as possible.
- If the child doesn't like milk, add a milk-shake mix or ice cream.

Essential ingredients of food

Zinc-rich foods include: lamb and pork chops, pecan nuts, peas, haddock, potatoes, egg yolk, peanuts, sardines, tuna, garlic, corn, grape juice, olive oil, spinach, lentils, lettuce, cucumber, butter.

Vitamin C rich foods: citrus fruits, berries, new and sweet potatoes, cauliflower, tomatoes, green and leafy vegetables, bean sprouts, jacket potatoes, kale, cantaloupe melon, watercress, cabbage, peppers.

Magnesium rich foods: wheat germ, oat bran, buckwheat, millet, barley, garlic, raisins, jacket potatoes, crab, bananas, broccoli, cauliflower, sweetcorn, sunflower seeds, chicken, apples, cheddar cheese.

Vitamin A rich foods: fish liver oil, carrots, green and yellow vegetables, eggs, milk and dairy foods, yellow and orange fruits.

Iodine-rich foods: shrimps, haddock, halibut, salmon, lambs liver, tuna, eggs, peanuts, wholemeal bread, cheddar cheese, pork lettuce, green peppers,milk, cream, lamb, raisins.

Omega 3 oils: fish oils, flax or linseed, walnut.

Omega 6 oils: sunflower, safflower, Evening Primrose oils.

Vitamin B foods, including: brown rice, whole-wheat, oatmeal, peanuts, pork, lamb, chicken, peas, legumes, potatoes, organic milk, most vegetables, oat bran, beans, fish, lean meat, broccoli, avocados, peas, cantaloupe melon.

Vitamin E rich foods: soya beans, wheat germs, cold pressed vegetable oils, (safflower and sunflower), broccoli, sprouts, green leafy vegetables, spinach, all wholegrain cereals, eggs, rye and wheat crackers, tomatoes, brown rice, roasted peanuts, oatmeal, carrots, olive oil.

Spelt is a medieval wheat grain, which has less gluten than traditional wheat, and is now widely available in large supermarkets and whole-food stores.

Providing food

Most children with a fever don't want to eat, so while you should *offer* food, you should never force a child to eat.

- Allow the child to choose their favourite foods.
- Give the child smaller meals more often than you would normally.
- If the child has a sore throat, give ice cream or an ice lolly made with fruit juice or yoghurt.
- If the child is feeling slightly sick, offer mashed potato.
- Offer snacks regularly and always keep the child company while they eat.
- Most children who are sick don't find ordinary food very appetising, but may be tempted to eat with 'soldiers' of fresh bread and butter, slices of fruit or their favourite yoghurt.

Try to make food as attractive as possible; don't put too much on the plate at once and remember that sick children often cope better with foods that don't require too much chewing, for example egg custard, milk pudding, thick soups, chicken and ice cream.

Feeding a child with a specific condition		
Condition	**Foods to avoid**	**Foods to encourage**
Asthma	Dairy, chocolate, fizzy drinks	Cold pressed oils, goats cheese, soya milk, fresh fruit, vegetables
ADHD	Sugar, wheat	Zinc, Omega 3 and 6 oils, rye, oats, spelt, fruit and vegetables
Bedwetting	Dairy	Corn tortilla, seeds, beans, green vegetables and apricot
Colds	Mucus-forming foods: sugar, dairy, banana, pork	Lots of fresh fruit and vegetables; zinc-rich foods
Colic	Dairy, wheat	Rye, oats, spelt, corn, rice
Constipation	Wheat	Lots of fruit and vegetables, figs and prunes; rye, oats, spelt, corn, rice, buckwheat
Coughs		
– dry	Crumbly foods	Iodine-rich foods: fish, nori seaweed
– mucusy	Dairy, banana, pork	Fresh fruit and vegetables
– whooping cough	Sugars	Fresh fruit and vegetables, foods rich in vitamin A and zinc, fish oils.
Diarrhoea	Dairy foods	Soya milk and cheeses, rice pudding
Earache	Dairy foods	Soya milk and cheeses, rice, goats milk
Eczema	Dairy foods	As above. EPO*, cold-pressed oils, fish oil
Fevers	Plenty of fluids	Foods rich in vitamin C, calcium and magnesium
Glue ear	Dairy foods	Fish oils, goats/ewes, soya milks/cheeses
Hyperactivity	Sugar and wheat	Zinc-rich foods, Omega 3 and 6 oils, fruit and vegetables
Nappy rash		Vitamin A and C and E foods, zinc, Omega 3 and 6 oils
Runny nose	Dairy, pork, bananas	Fruit and vegetables
Sleep problems		Magnesium-rich foods
Teething		Calcium and magnesium-rich foods, Omega 3 and 6 oils as they are anti-inflammatory

**EPO is Evening Primrose oil*

Safety

- Keep all medicines safely locked away in a secure cupboard.
- Supervise the child at all times; watch out for any sudden changes in their condition.
- Be aware of any complications of the child's condition and watch for warning signs.

Meeting intellectual, emotional and social needs

Play and the sick child

Play is an important part of recovery for a sick or convalescent child. Children who are ill often regress and may want to play with toys that they have long since outgrown. While they are ill, children will have a short attention span. You will need to be understanding and tolerant of these changes in behaviour. Never put pressure on a child to take part in an activity they don't want to; sick children often tire quickly, so toys and materials will require frequent changing.

Use protective sheets to protect the bed covers and supply a steady surface such as a tray with legs or a special bean bag tray.

Ideas for activities

- **Jigsaw puzzles**: the child could start with simple puzzles and progress to more challenging ones, perhaps with family help.
- **Board games**, such as Lotto, Ludo and Halma.
- **Card games**, such as Uno, Snap and Happy Families.
- **Making a scrapbook**: provide magazines, photos, flowers, scissors and glue to make a personal record.
- **Drawing and painting**: provide poster paints, lining paper and a protective plastic apron; children also love to paint with water in 'magic' painting books.
- **Play dough**: either bought or home-made from flour, oil, water and food colouring; playing with dough is creative and provides an outlet for feelings of frustration.
- **Making models** with duplo or lego.
- **Playing with small world objects**, such as toy farms, zoos and Playmobil.
- **French knitting or sewing cards** can be used with older children.
- **Crayons and felt tip pens and a pad of paper**.
- **Books** to be read alone or with an adult.
- **Audio tapes** of songs, rhymes and favourite stories.
- **Videos, cartoons**, and **computer games**.
- If a child is ill for some time, toys and games can be borrowed from a local toy library.
- Encourage other children and adults to visit once the child is over the infectious stage.

Caring for sick children in early years settings

Children who are sick should not be at school or nursery. Playgroups and schools are not appropriate places in which to care for sick children. However, it is often at a day care setting that the child first shows signs and symptoms of an illness. Childminders and nannies working in the family home also need to know how to act to safeguard children's health.

Nannies and childminders should always contact the child's parents directly in case of accident or illness.

In schools or nurseries, you should notify a senior member of staff if you notice that a child is unwell; that person will then decide if and when to contact the child's parents.

Keeping records

Every child's record should contain the following information:

- Child's full name.
- Date of Birth.
- Names and addresses of child's primary carers.
- Address and telephone number of child's home.

▶

ACTIVITY

Caring for Thomas

Thomas is five years old and in his first term at school. He was really enjoying all the preparations for Christmas when he, and two of his friends, developed an itchy rash and were diagnosed with chickenpox. Thomas has all the usual symptoms of the illness – a fever, headache and extremely itchy spots.

1 Read through the section on **chickenpox** and make notes to help you find out about Thomas's needs and possible medical treatment.
2 Using the categories of need outlined above, plan a **daily care routine** for Thomas. The care plan could be used for five days, so try to think of a variety of activities that could be used with the child, both in bed and in the family room. The timetable below gives an idea of what a plan could look like, although only two of the boxes are completed.

When	Physical needs	Emotional, intellectual and social needs
Early morning	Wash or bed-bath, skin care, breakfast, medicines etc	
Late morning		
Early afternoon		Short nap, play Ludo,
Late afternoon		
Notes:	Temp: 37.9	

- Address and telephone number of parent/carer's place(s) of work.
- Additional emergency contact telephone number – possibly a relative.
- Address and telephone number of child's GP and health visitor.

Records of a child's illness should be kept so that the child's parents and doctor can be informed; as with the Accident Report Book (see page 234) these records should include:

- When the child first showed signs of illness.
- The signs and symptoms.
- Any action taken, for example taking the temperature.
- Progress of the illness since first noticing it, for example are there any further symptoms?

Helping a child who becomes unwell

Staff in schools and nurseries should offer support and reassurance to a child who may have to wait a while to be taken home.

- Any incident of vomiting or diarrhoea should be dealt with swiftly and sympathetically to minimise the child's distress and to preserve their dignity.
- A member of staff should remain with the child at all times and keep them as comfortable as possible.
- All early years settings should have a written policy on when to exclude children for childhood infections:

Guide to exclusion periods relating to childhood illnesses		
Illness and incubation period	**Periods when infectious**	**Minimum period of exclusion**
Chickenpox 11–21 days	1 day before to 6 days after appearance of rash	6 days from onset of rash
Rubella (German measles) 14–21 days	Few days before to 4 days after onset of rash	4 days from onset of rash (avoid contact or warn women who are under 14 weeks pregnant)
Measles 10–15 days	Few days before to subsidence of rash	7 days from onset of rash
Mumps 12–26 (commonly 18) days	Few days before to 5 days after onset of swelling	Until swelling has gone
Whooping cough About 7 days	From 7 days after exposure to 21 days after onset of the bouts of coughing	21 days from onset of the bouts of coughing

Giving medicines in an early years setting

Children may have a condition which requires medication, yet still be perfectly well enough to attend nursery or school; examples include asthma, eczema and glue ear. Prescribed medicines and paracetamol may be given to these children only after the parent's or carer's written consent is obtained. The consent should be on a form which includes the following details:

- The child's name.
- The name of the medicine to be given.
- The precise dose to be given.
- The time it should be given *or* if given irregularly, parents must detail the precise circumstances or symptoms that would mean the medicine should be given.
- How it should be given, i.e. oral medicine, eye drops, inhaler, etc.
- Parent's name and signature.

Keeping medicine safe

- Keep medicines in a locked cupboard, except for inhalers which must be easily available for the child at all times.
- Make sure that the medicine is for the particular child; always check the label for the child's name before giving it.
- Keep a written record of medicines given, including the child's name, date, time, the medicine and dose, any problems with giving it.

Giving medicines

Here is a list of essential points when medicines are prescribed for a child:

□ Store all medicines out of reach of children and in child-proof containers.	□ Store medicines at the correct temperature – i.e. in the fridge or away from direct heat if that is the direction on the bottle.
□ Ask the doctor for as much information as possible about the medicines, e.g. if there are likely to be side-effects, if certain foods should be avoided.	□ Make sure you understand the instructions for giving the medicine before leaving the chemist, e.g. how much, how often and when. Check whether it should be given before or after meals.
□ Measure doses of medicine accurately, using a marked medicine spoon for liquid; teaspoons are *not* equivalent to a 5 ml spoon.	□ Make sure that all the medicine is swallowed – this can be difficult with babies – see tips below.
□ Always follow instructions carefully.	□ Throw away prescribed medicines on completion of treatment.

▶

Medicines

Every home should have a properly stocked medicine cabinet, preferably locked but *always* out of reach to children. The cabinet should contain:

- ☐ Children's paracetamol. Paracetamol elixir and junior paracetamol tablets. The doses for children of different ages should be on the bottles.
- ☐ Crepe bandages, open weave bandage and triangular bandage.
- ☐ Mercury thermometer or digital thermometer and a fever strip.
- ☐ A pack of assorted fabric plasters and one of hypo-allergenic plasters.
- ☐ Blunt-edge tweezers, safety pins and scissors.
- ☐ Wound dressings – cotton wool and gauze pad already attached to a bandage.
- ☐ A small packet of cotton wool.
- ☐ Packet of skin closures.
- ☐ A hot-water bottle – when wrapped in a towel it can relieve the pain of an aching abdomen or bruised joint.
- ☐ Surgical tape.
- ☐ Calamine lotion – for soothing itchy spots and rashes.
- ☐ Zinc and castor oil cream – for nappy rashes.
- ☐ A small bottle of liquid antiseptic or mild antiseptic cream.
- ☐ A measuring spoon, dropper or small glass for liquid medicines.

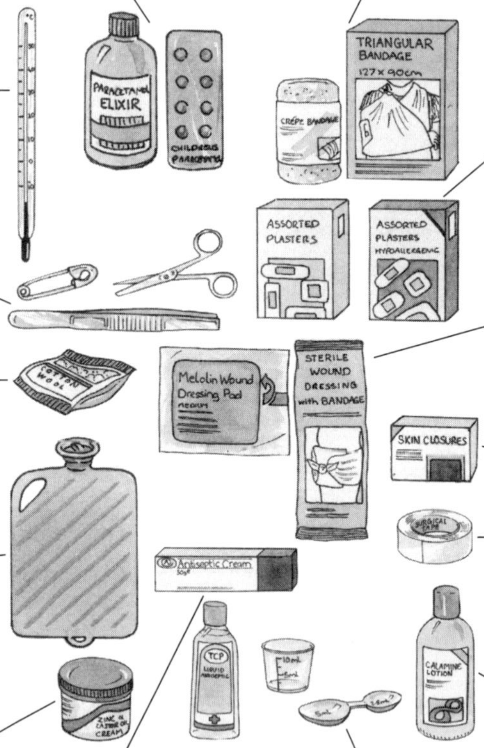

Before stocking the medicine cabinet, discard all the half-empty, improperly labelled bottles and any medicines that are over six months old. Keep down costs by buying non-branded products.

□ Most medicines for young children are made up in a sweetened syrup to make them more palatable.	□ If a child needs to take medicine contained in syrup regularly, remember to brush their teeth afterwards to prevent tooth decay.
□ Remember that your attitude is important – if you show anxiety when giving medicine to a child, they will be anxious too.	□ Never put medicines into a child's drink or food as the child may not take it all. If necessary, tablets can be crushed and added to a teaspoon of jam or honey followed by a drink.
□ **DO NOT give aspirin to any child under the age of 10, because of the risk of Reye's syndrome.**	
□ **Always obtain written consent from the child's parents before giving any medicines.**	

Oral medicines

Most medicines for children are given as sweetened syrups or elixirs. They can be given with a spoon, tube or dropper.

Before giving any medicine:

1 Wash your hands.
2 Always check the label on the bottle and the instructions. If it has been prescribed by the doctor, check that it is for your child and follow the instructions exactly; for example, some medicines have to be taken with or after food – although generally oral medicines are best given before meals as they enter the bloodstream quickly.
3 Shake the bottle before measuring the dose. Always pour any medicine bottle with the label uppermost so that the instructions remain legible if the medicine runs down the side of the bottle.
4 Some medicines don't taste good, for example iron preparations. Always be truthful when the child asks, 'Does it taste bad?' Answer 'The medicine doesn't taste good, but I'll give you some juice as soon as you've swallowed it.'
5 If the child is reluctant, you should adopt a no-nonsense approach and be prepared to resort to bribery if necessary, for example offer to tell them a favourite story or to give them a chocolate. Never punish or threaten a child who refuses to take medicine.

Giving medicines to a baby or young child

- If possible, get someone to help you in case the baby wriggles.
- Cradle the baby comfortably on your lap, in the crook of your arm, so that he or she is slightly raised with the head tilted back. (Never lay a baby down flat while giving medicine because of the risk of inhalation.)
- Put a bib on the baby and have some baby wipes or a flannel close at hand to wipe clean.

Giving medicines

Using a spoon

1 If the baby is very young, sterilise the spoon by boiling it or placing in sterilising solution. Gently pull down the baby's chin if he or she will not open their mouth – or get someone else to do this.

2 Place the spoon on the baby's lower lip, raise the angle of the spoon and let the liquid run into the baby's mouth.

Using a dropper

1 Take up the required amount of medicine into the glass tube.

2 Place the dropper in the corner of the baby's mouth and release the medicine gently.

Using a tube or syringe

1 **Tube.** Pour the required dose into the tube

2 **Syringe.** Fix the special adapter to the bottle and withdraw the required dose.

3 **Tube.** Place the mouthpiece on the baby's lower lip and let the medicine run gently into the mouth

4 **Syringe.** Place the end of the syringe in the child's mouth, pointing towards the cheek and slowly squeeze in the dose.

- If you are on your own, wrap a blanket around the baby's arms so that you can stop him or her wriggling.
- Only put a little of the medicine in the mouth at a time.

Giving medicines and tablets to older children

Older children don't seem to mind taking medicine, and often want to pour it out for themselves. Always supervise children and make sure that they take the medicine exactly as prescribed. After giving any medicine to a child, write down the time and the dosage.

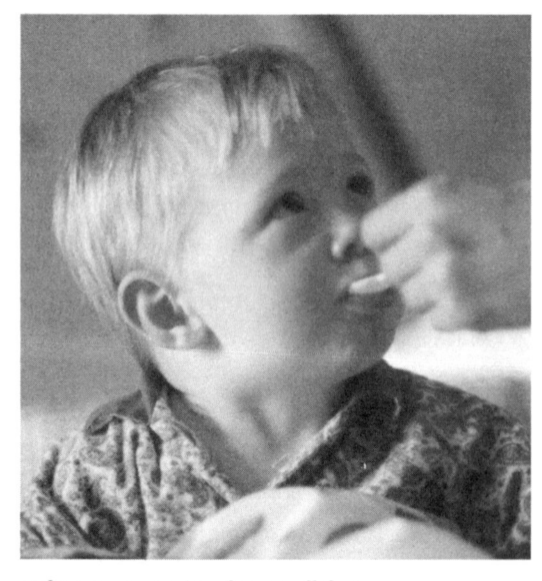

Using a spoon to give medicine

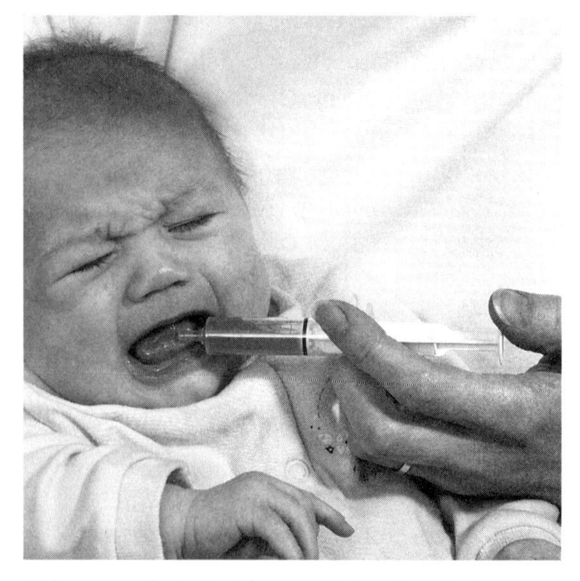

Using a syringe to give medicine to a baby

How to give eye drops or eye ointment

An important part of the healing process after an eye operation or an injury to the eye is the instillation of the prescribed eye drops and/or ointment. This is often a new experience for most children and their parents or carers, and the following guide may be useful.

Preparation

- □ A simple and honest explanation of what you are about to do, and perhaps a demonstration on the child's favourite doll or teddy, will help.
- □ It may be easier for you if the child lies flat, on a bed or settee, with the head tilted back.
- □ Babies and young children may wriggle and put their hands up to their face – try wrapping them in a blanket so that they feel secure and their arms are tucked out of the way.
- □ Try to distract the child afterwards. This will reinforce the idea that having eye drops put in is quick and easy, and there is nothing for them to be afraid of.

General directions

- □ Read the label on the bottle/tube for directions.
- □ Wash your hands.
- □ Position the child.
- □ Gently pull down the lower lid with one finger and squeeze one drop into the eye. If using ointment, squeeze about half an inch of ointment into the lower surface of the inside of the lower eyelid.
- □ Try not to allow the bottle/tube end to touch the child's eye.
- □ Replace the top of the bottle/tube immediately after use.
- □ Discard the bottle/tube once treatment is completed, otherwise use a fresh bottle/tube every 4 weeks.
- □ Do not save it or use it for anyone else.

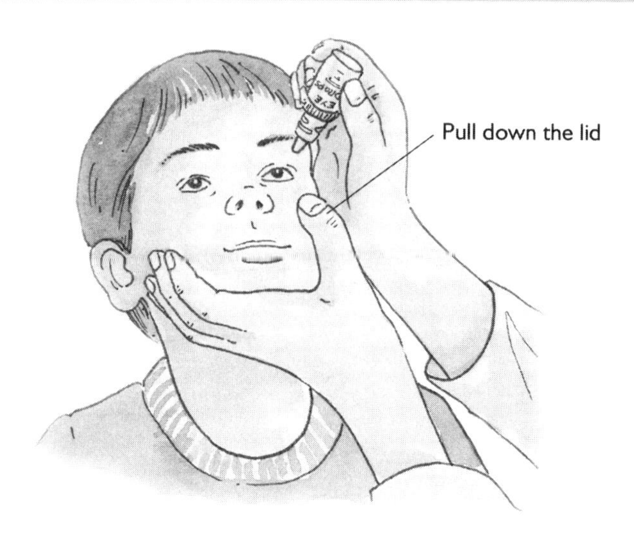

Giving eye drops

How to give ear drops

The child should lie down on one side – on a bed or on your lap – with the affected ear uppermost. Place a pillow under the child's head to keep it steady and comfortable.

- □ Pull the pinna (the top of the outer ear) gently backwards towards the back of the head; this straightens out the ear canal.
- □ Hold the filled dropper just above the canal entrance. (Many ear drops are supplied in plastic bottles with pointed nozzles – invert the bottle and squeeze gently to release the required number of drops).
- □ Release the required number of ear drops into the ear.
- □ Gently massage the base of the ear to help disperse the liquid.
- □ Encourage the child to remain lying down in the same position for a few minutes.
- □ Put a piece of cotton wool loosely in the outer ear to prevent any leakage; don't pack it in too tightly as it may cause harm and be difficult to remove.

How to give nose drops

To a baby:

- □ Put the baby on a flat surface before you begin and get someone to help you if possible.
- □ Tilt the baby's head backwards slightly and gently drop liquid into each nostril.
- □ Count the number of drops as you put them in; 2 or 3 drops are normally sufficient – any more will run down the throat and cause the baby to cough and splutter.
- □ Keep the baby lying flat for 1 or 2 minutes.

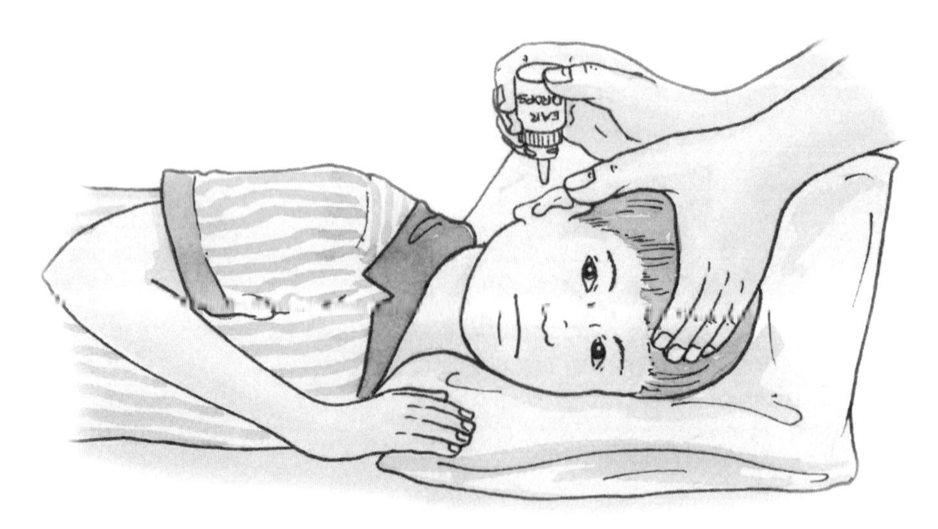

Giving ear drops

To an older child:

- □ Ask the child to blow their nose and to lie down on a comfortable surface with their head tilted slightly backwards.
- □ Gently release the prescribed number of drops into each nostril. Encourage the child to stay lying down for 1 or 2 minutes.
- □ Both ear drops and nose drops can be warmed to make them more comfortable; stand the bottle in warm, *not hot*, water for a few minutes.
- □ Don't let the dropper touch the child's eye, ear or nose, or you will transfer the germs back to the bottle. If the dropper does touch the child, wash it thoroughly before replacing it in the bottle.

Revision questions

1. Why should aspirin never be given to a child under 10 years?
2. Why is it important to keep written records about any child who becomes ill when in your care?
3. List the details which should be included on a parental consent form for giving prescribed medicines to a child in an early years setting.
4. How would you care for a child who is taken ill in an early years setting and whose parents/carers cannot be located?
5. Why is play important for a sick child who is being cared for at home?

Chapter 9: Caring for children in hospital and with chronic illness

◆ *Children in hospital* ◆ *Play in hospital* ◆ *Caring for children in hospital* ◆ *The effects of chronic illness on the family* ◆ *Supporting the family of a child with chronic or life-threatening illness* ◆ *Terminal care* ◆ *The child's perception of death*

Children in hospital

Most children will have had some experience of going to hospital before they are eight years old. Some will have been taken to the accident and emergency department or to a specialist outpatient department. One in every four children has had a hospital stay by the age of five. How a child reacts to a hospital stay will depend on many factors, in particular on:

- ◆ The child's age.
- ◆ Personality.
- ◆ The reason for being in hospital.
- ◆ The admission process.

- Any previous experience of hospitals – even visiting relatives.
- The investigations and treatment needed.
- The attitude and manner of the hospital staff.
- The atmosphere in the ward.
- The way their parents react to the stay, for example they may transmit their anxiety to their child.

The children's charter

Under the extension to the patient's charter, 'Services for children and young people', issued by the NHS in 1996, parents can expect:

□ Their child to be cared for in a children's ward under the supervision of a consultant paediatrician.	□ Their child to have a qualified, named children's nurse responsible for his or her nursing care.
□ To be able to stay in the hospital with their child.	□ If their child is having an operation, and where circumstances permit, they can expect to accompany them into the anaesthetic room and be present until they go to sleep.
□ To be told what pain relief will be given to their child.	□ The NHS to respect their child's privacy, dignity and religious or cultural beliefs.
□ Their child to be offered a choice of children's menus.	□ To have facilities to breastfeed their child.
□ Their child to wear his or her own clothes, and have personal possessions.	□ The hospital to be clean, safe and suitably furnished for children and young people.
□ That all the staff they meet will wear name badges, so that they know who everyone is, and for security.	□ Their child to have the opportunity for play and to meet other children.
□ Their child has the right to receive suitable education.	

Hospitals have changed a great deal over the last thirty years in their provision for children. At the very least parents should be able to stay with their child as much as possible (this is Department of Health policy).

- The hospital may provide a chair, mattress or folding bed for a parent to sleep on. This may not necessarily be next to the child's bed.
- Most hospitals do not have strictly enforced visiting hours for parents, and parents should be able to give their child his or her meals, bath, etc.

- ◆ There should be access for parents to washing facilities, use of a sitting room, kitchen, toilets, telephone and restaurant.
- ◆ Children's ward kitchens often have supplies of breakfast cereals, baked beans, etc. for children who do not like hospital food.
- ◆ There should be provision for children from ethnic minorities who have preferences in relation to food, washing and bathing and clothing.
- ◆ There should also be every encouragement for mothers to breastfeed their baby and space to do so in privacy.
- ◆ If parents are not able to be with their child as much as they would like, they can tell the ward sister about any food fads, comfort habits, special words, etc. that their child has.
- ◆ Most hospitals allow children to wear their own clothes as much as possible, and also to bring in their own toys.

Reasons for admissions to hospital

There are two main types of admission to hospital:

1 Emergency admissions
Children may be admitted to hospital after visiting the hospital's accident and emergency department. There will have been no opportunity to prepare the child or the parents for the experience, so the family will need a great deal of support and understanding.

Examples of emergency admissions include:

Accidental injuries □ Road traffic accidents □ Burns and scalds □ Poisoning □ Falls □ Foreign bodies – inhaled or swallowed	**Infections** □ Meningitis □ Gastro-enteritis □ Bronchitis □ Pneumonia
Acute abdominal pain □ Appendicitis □ Urinary tract infection	**Diabetic coma** □ Diabetes
Breathing difficulties □ Asthma attack □ Epiglottitis	**Convulsions** □ Febrile convulsions □ Epilepsy

2 Planned admissions
In planned or routine admissions, children and their families may have visited the hospital previously – for example, to an outpatient department. They will have been given a period of notice and a date for the planned admission. Some children may have been on a waiting list for routine surgery. Most hospitals run special pre-admission programmes to help prepare children for their stay. Examples of planned admissions include:

Routine (not emergency) surgery	Investigations and treatment
□ Removal of tonsils (tonsillectomy) □ Removal of adenoids (adenoidectomy) □ Repair of hernia	□ Cystic fibrosis □ Diabetes □ Spina bifida/hydrocephalus
Cancer treatment	**Respite care**
□ Leukaemia □ Other malignancies	□ Children with a chronic illness for review of their care and to give their main carers a break

The needs of children in hospital

In recent years health care professionals and parents have come to understand that a child's life really is turned upside-down when they go into hospital. Only 20 years ago people knew very little about how much a hospital stay may affect a child's development and well-being. Usually, children were alone during their stay. At one stage parents were even told that it would be better if they did not come to visit their child. This was to prevent children from troubling the staff on the ward with their crying.

James and Joyce Robertson made a series of films in the 1950s that showed how children reacted to being separated from their parents during a brief stay in hospital. The research showed that when small children were suddenly separated from their parents, they experienced feelings of **loss and grief**, which went through certain stages:

- They reacted strongly at first. They cried and looked for their parents, but at first were able to be comforted.
- Then they despaired about what was happening; they acted as if they were numb to any feelings or interest in life.
- Later, when the longed-for parents had still not returned, the children became passive and apathetic.

This behaviour used to be interpreted as a sign that a child had accepted the situation. They were considered 'easy' children by the staff. The problem is that these children were being harmed by their experience. They felt their parents had let them down. In some cases – as adults – they had a hard time committing themselves emotionally to other people. Now we have come to understand these psychological mechanisms better and parents are encouraged to stay with their child in hospital to make the difficult experience as normal as possible.

There are a lot of other things that could upset a child in hospital:

- Lots of new, strange people suddenly coming into his or her life.
- Eating new, unfamiliar food.
- New smells.
- Strange sounds.
- Different routines.

Some children may feel they are punished for being naughty and therefore are being sent away. Each child reacts differently to being in hospital. Their reaction depends to a large extent on how painful the stay is. Some children feel safe and secure as long as their parents are there, but some react very badly to a stay in a hospital. A child may:

- Suffer nightmares.
- Cry a lot.
- Throw tantrums.
- Return to earlier stages of their development and start sucking their thumb or bedwetting.
- Refuse to eat.
- Become withdrawn, refusing to have anything to do with the adults.

Preparing a child for hospital

For many children the idea of going to hospital for the first time can be very frightening. They are likely to be worried about having to stay away from home, and may be very afraid of what will happen to them in hospital. Parents and carers can help children to avoid much of this distress by preparing them for their hospital stay in advance. There are many reasons why this is helpful:

- To help the child cope with the change in routine.
- To help the child feel less frightened.
- To help the child understand why they are going to hospital.
- To correct any wrong ideas the child may have about hospital.

Children who have not been in a hospital before will not know what to expect, what will happen to them once they are there, or how they will be treated. If possible, try to arrange a visit to the children's ward before admission. This can help both the child and the parent or carer to feel more relaxed about the experience. Many hospitals now have pre-admission units where children can go a few days before admission to be examined and to become familiar with the hospital environment. Common questions children in hospital ask are:

- Will I get better?
- What will the doctors and nurses do to me?
- Will I be blamed – or laughed at?
- Can I go home?

Guidelines for preparing a child for a hospital stay

The best way to prepare a child is by giving them information – but not to overload them.

1 Tell the child a few days before that he or she is going to hospital – if possible, arrange to visit the ward and speak to the nurses, or attend a pre-admission unit.

2 Explain truthfully and simply why the child is coming into hospital. There are many books that will help to give a young child some idea of what to expect – see book list below.

3 If the child is having an operation, explain that they will have a special hospital 'sleep' which will stop them from feeling any pain. Following the operation they may feel a little sore but the nurses will give them something to take the pain away.

Activities that may help prepare a child

There are many ways in which you can help a child prepare for a hospital stay, whether at home or in a nursery or school setting:

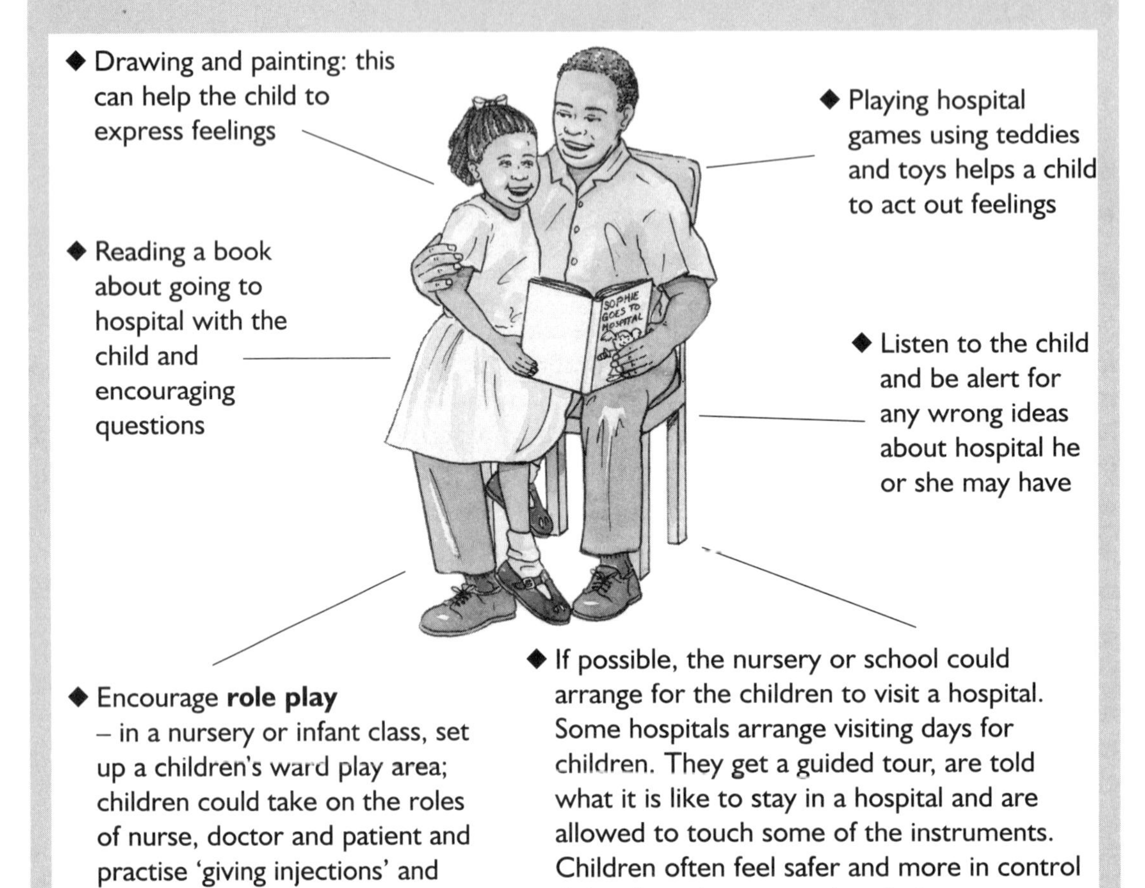

Books for young children about hospital

For children aged 2–4 years

Miffy in Hospital, Dick Bruna (Egmont). A reassuring, simple picture book featuring the white rabbit Miffy's visit to hospital to have her tonsils removed.

For children aged 3–7 years

Topsy and Tim Go To The Hospital, Jean and Gareth Adamson (Ladybird Books). Explains what happens when Tim has to go into hospital after falling out of a tree and bumping his head – he has an X-ray and has to stay in hospital for two nights.

I Don't Want To Go To Hospital, Tony Ross (Andersen Press). The Little Princess is adamant that she won't go into hospital to have a lump removed from her nose, but when she does go, she is reluctant to leave as everyone treats her like a princess.

For children aged 5 years and over

Hospital, Carol Watson (Franklin Watts). From the Busy Places series, this book charts 24 hours during a typical day at a hospital, focusing on staff, patients and visitors.

4 Don't let the child see your own anxieties, as this will only make them feel frightened.
5 Unless you are going to stay with the child, explain to them that you will not be there all the time, but tell them when you will be visiting.
6 **Always tell the child the truth**. Don't lie by saying, for example, that something will not hurt when it might. This will destroy their trust in adults.
7 Make sure that the child realises that he or she will be coming home as soon as they are well enough (although it is important not to promise an actual day).
8 Encourage the child to express his or her feelings – so that you know how to help in the most appropriate way.

The day before admission

Depending on the age of the child, you can involve them in packing the things they need to take with them:

- Comfort blanket or special cuddly toy, if used; plus a spare if possible.
- Some toys and books: children usually regress when they are feeling ill, so choose toys and books that are on the young side.
- Pyjamas or nightie.
- Wash-bag, with soap, flannel, toothbrush and paste, brush and comb.
- Photograph of family.
- Dressing gown and slippers.
- Favourite fruit drink.
- Parent-held child health record.

Staying in hospital

On arrival at the children's ward, a named nurse will show the child around and help them to settle in. If the parent is staying too, the child will be shown where he or she will be sleeping. The child will be encouraged to unpack their belongings into their own bedside locker. On admission, the nurse will obtain general information – name, age, date of birth, next-of-kin, family details and religion, etc. – if not already known from a pre-admission programme. The nurse will also find out any allergies and the medication the child is taking and will ask about the child's **normal routine**.

What the hospital needs to know	
□ **Communication** What is the child's level of understanding and language development. Does the child need a hearing aid or glasses?	□ **Hygiene** What is the child's usual routine for bathing, washing and cleaning teeth?
□ **Rest and sleep** What is the child's usual pattern of naps and bedtime sleep? What is their usual sleeping position?	□ **Food and drink** If a baby, is the baby bottle fed, breastfed or weaned? Are there any dietary restrictions? Can an older child feed themself?

▶

□ **Play** Does the child have any favourite games or toys? What sort of play does the child enjoy?	□ **Comfort** Does the child have any comfort habits, e.g. thumb-sucking or holding a comfort blanket or teddy?
□ **Toilet habits** Does the child wear nappies? How independent is the child in going to the toilet? What are the normal bowel movements?	

The care plan

The nurse will work with the parents to write an individual care plan for their child, which will cover all the categories of need mentioned above. The role of the parents will be discussed and arrangements made for them to stay with their child, if at all possible.

Having an operation

If the child is going to have an operation, a **hospital play specialist** or **nursery nurse** will prepare them for the event and parents are encouraged to accompany their child to the anaesthetic room and stay until they are 'asleep'. When the operation is over, the parent is invited to collect their child from theatre with the ward nurse.

How you can support a child in hospital

Stay close to the child at all times so that they feel safe. The closeness, along with talking and explaining things, will create a feeling of security. Let them know that there is at least one stable and predictable element in their life. Don't expect the child to 'behave' when they go into hospital, and never lose your temper and yell at them. Often the child may not be able to control their feelings:

- If the child cries, let them express their fear. It is also important to stay with the child. Tell them that you understand and that you are not going to leave. Hold the child in your arms or hold his or her hand. Touch is very soothing.
- If the child has a temper tantrum, it is important that you try to stay calm, even though it will be hard. Talk quietly to the child. Cuddle them if that is possible. It is fear of the unknown that makes a child react like this. Never tell the child off but try to calm them down instead.
- Explain to the child what is going on. Ask the hospital staff to explain what they are going to do to the child before they do it. It is important to let the child know the truth. If you do they will know they can trust you. It is not a good idea to tell the child that something is not going to hurt, if it is.
- If a child sucks their thumb or wets the bed, it is because they are scared and this is perfectly natural. Don't tell the child off or tell them they are too big to be wetting the bed – doing that will just create more anxiety. The child needs security, closeness and the certainty that he or she is not going to be left alone.
- If the child appears withdrawn it is very important that they experience a lot of positive contact. Talk to them, cuddle them, sing to them, tickle them, play with them; do anything you can think of that might help to bring them out of their shell.

Things to do with a child in hospital

Play activities may be provided by trained play staff – see below. You can help by providing activities that don't require too much concentration. These could include:

- Reading stories.
- Simple board games, colouring books, or paper and crayons.
- A portable cassette player and some tapes of the child's favourite nursery rhymes, pop songs or stories.
- Hand-held electronic games.
- A tray that the child can use for different activities such as jigsaws, using play dough, or playing card games.
- Old magazines or catalogues for the child to cut up if old enough to handle scissors safely.
- For an older child, renting a video or bringing in some computer games might be a good idea. It will give the child something to do. Don't leave the child alone with the TV or the computer. Watch a video or play a game together.

Day care surgery

Children who are having a minor operation are often treated in day care units. Having been examined beforehand, they are admitted to the unit a few hours before the operation, and can be taken home the same day – as soon as they have recovered sufficiently. This reduces the stress of separation caused by hospital admission and prevents the disruption of family routines, especially when parents have to arrange child care for their other children.

The multidisciplinary team in hospital

The professionals who care for children in hospital are part of a **multidisciplinary team**. This includes:

- **Doctors**: Paediatricians and other specialist consultants, registrars and house officers.
- **Nurses**: The head of nursing on a particular ward is a sister (or charge nurse if a man). Sisters are now sometimes called ward managers. Under her there will be other registered nurses as well as student nurses. There will also be nursing auxiliaries, who are not qualified nurses, who help with duties such as bathing and meals. During their education all nurses gain some experience on children's (paediatric) wards, but some receive additional specialist training to become **registered sick children's nurses**.
- **Hospital play specialists**: Some hospitals have hospital play specialists who play with children on the wards, and also help prepare them for admission or for medical procedures.
- **Play leaders and nursery nurses**: General hospitals often have trained nursery nurses and play leaders who work in different areas of the hospital, such as outpatient clinics, children's units and adolescent wards.
- **Teachers**: Hospital-based teachers provide lessons for children of school age who are in hospital for longer than a week. This may be in consultation with the child's school.

Other staff who may help the child in hospital include physiotherapists, occupational therapists (OTs), speech and language therapists, medical social workers and dieticians.

Play in hospital

For children, play is at the very centre of their lives. From the earliest age, playing helps children to learn, to relate to others and to have fun. Play can make a real difference to children in hospital, as they are at their most vulnerable – ill, separated from their friends and family surroundings. Play in hospital is important because it:

- creates an environment where stress and anxiety are lessened
- helps the child to regain self-confidence and esteem
- provides an outlet for feelings of frustration and anger
- helps the child understand what is going to happen to them – hospital procedures and treatments
- helps in assessment and diagnosis
- speeds recovery and rehabilitation.

The role of the hospital play specialist

The title hospital play specialist (HPS) was coined in the 1970s to describe the role of staff who used play in the hospital setting. They are not the same as play therapists or play leaders, although they do use play as a therapeutic tool. Children's hospitals in the UK have large play departments employing hospital play specialists, play leaders and nursery nurses. In general hospitals, small teams of play staff work in different areas of the hospital, such as outpatients clinics, children's wards and adolescent units.

Hospital play specialists work as part of a multi-disciplinary team; their role is to:

- organise daily play and art activities in the playroom or at the bedside
- provide play to achieve developmental goals
- help children to cope with anxieties and feelings
- use play to prepare children for hospital procedures
- support families and siblings
- contribute to clinical judgements and diagnoses through their play-based observations
- act as the child's advocate
- teach the value of play for the sick child
- encourage peer group friendships to develop
- organise parties and special events.

Types of hospital play

Play as preparation for a medical or nursing procedure

During a nursing assessment, a child may have a series of nursing procedures, such as having their temperature taken, blood tests, oxygen levels measured, blood pressure taken or being given medicine for pain relief. Using play as preparation helps by:

- distracting the very young child, as their level of understanding is limited and they may be frightened of unfamiliar investigations
- showing children what will happen to them so that they know what to expect and what is expected of them
- assessing their level of understanding and likes and dislikes and providing appropriate toys and play activities
- listening to children and encouraging them to ask questions about the procedures.

A variety of techniques may be used – always geared to the individual child and their specific needs:

- Bubbles are a very good way of amusing and distracting a young child. They are also a useful assessment tool, for example if medical staff are querying an arm injury, a child will only use the healthy arm to catch the bubbles, leaving the injured arm limp.
- Dolls with injection sites and intravenous infusions which can be used with coloured water.
- Puppets and small world figures can be used to act out certain hospital procedures, such as being wheeled on a trolley to the operating theatre.
- Books, videos, audio tapes and photographs can all help to make the planned procedure less threatening.

Play as therapy after a medical or nursing procedure

After an uncomfortable medical or nursing procedure or after surgery, many children will have no choice but to lie in bed until they are physically recovered. Using play after a procedure helps by:

- reassuring children that life goes on as normal
- assessing their understanding of the treatment and their reaction to it
- encouraging children to play out their experiences and so feel more accepting
- giving children control over what they are doing – the child is in control of the play process.

A variety of techniques may be used:

- Dolls specially adapted to show the specific treatment the child has had – for example the doll may have an intravenous infusion attached to one arm or may have a large bandage covering its head.
- Medical equipment such as stethoscopes and syringes (without needles).
- Books and photos showing children at various stages of recovery.
- Music activities: these can be based around the needs and skills of the parent and the child. Many hospitals will have musical equipment available for family use through music therapy, physiotherapy, occupational therapy, or recreation departments. **Passive music activities** can be performed with little or no active participation on the part of a child who is required to stay quiet –

or a child who is unable to move actively after surgery or procedures. Children could have a tape recorder or walkman to listen to their favourite tapes or radio stations.

- For children unable to leave their hospital rooms, small hand instruments (hand-held drums, tambourines, bells, castanets, maracas, etc.) can be played to music or on their own.
- Basic art supplies (i.e. coloured pencils, crayons or markers and paper) can be used by children to draw while listening to music. This can easily be done in a hospital bed for children unable to move far distances.
- Active musical activities, such as songs that require hand or body movement, can be adapted to various activity levels of children. For all ages, moving to music can provide some gentle exercise. A popular song is 'The wheels on the bus go round and round . . .'

Play therapy

Play in hospital could almost always be described as play therapy, that is, play which enables children to feel more secure in potentially threatening situations. Play therapists may be qualified nursery nurses who have taken a further course in play therapy, psychotherapists or hospital play specialists. Play therapy involves:

- using activities and toys which satisfy the needs of children with fears and anxieties
- enabling children to gain some measure of control over their lives and over what is happening to them
- establishing a good relationship with the children
- providing activities that will promote healthy development.

Toys and activities can often be classed as either *therapeutic* or *diversional*:

- **Therapeutic toys and activities** let children 'play out' their anxieties: for example clay, sand, hammer and peg toys, medical kits, puppets and anatomically correct dolls.
- **Diversional toys and activities** divert children's attention away from their illness or problems by promoting creativity and the enjoyment of developing new skills: for example paper and paint, board games, video games, puppets, mobiles, rattles and musical instruments.

CASE STUDY

Using play in an accident and emergency department

Maria is a two-year-old child who was brought into the accident and emergency department by her mother. She had suffered a burn to her right shoulder from boiling hot water. The skin was very red and had several large blisters. Maria was assessed by the nursing and medical team and given pain relief, then taken to a cubicle. The cubicle is used to provide a private area for the child and parent to relax and play while waiting for the pain relief to take effect.

Armed with lots of noisy toys and a pot of bubbles, the hospital play specialist, Darren, went to see Maria. Sitting on the floor at the child's level, blowing bubbles with laughs and squeals from Maria, Darren started to get to know Maria and her mother better. Maria's mother felt guilty about the accident and found it very useful to talk to Darren during the play session. As the three of them established a good relationship, the HPS learned a lot about Maria's likes and dislikes – information that would be needed during the cleaning and dressing of the burn.

The time came for the dressing of Maria's burn. She sat on her mother's lap for comfort and support. Darren used toys to distract Maria and encouraged the mother to be a part of her daughter's treatment. The procedure is painful and uncomfortable. Maria occasionally protested by crying; this seemed to be partly due to discomfort and partly because no two-year-old likes to sit still for too long. But the dressing was completed without any delays and a calm, relaxed atmosphere was maintained throughout.

Questions

1 List the feelings that both Maria and her mother might be experiencing when they arrived at the accident and emergency department.
2 What specific skills did Darren use to help Maria and her mother?
3 How could you provide play therapy for a six-year-old child who is coming into hospital for an operation to remove his adenoids?

Caring for children in hospital

Some common procedures in hospital

There are many different investigations which a child in hospital will have; some of them are also carried out in doctors' surgeries. Children should always have the procedure explained to them, in words that they can understand.

Common hospital procedures		
Throat swab *What happens?* The child is asked to open the mouth wide. The doctor or nurse presses the tongue down and quickly brushes the back of the throat with a swab. *Why?* To find out what bacteria or virus is causing a throat infection and to give the correct antibiotic treatment.	**Blood tests** *What happens?* The doctor will apply some 'magic' pain numbing cream before inserting a needle into the back of the hand or in the arm to draw a small amount of blood. *Why?* To test blood for type and group, for anaemia, infection, blood gases and other disorders.	**Urine sample** *What happens?* Babies and young children will wear a urine collecting bag until the sample is obtained; older children will be shown how to provide a mid-stream specimen in a sterile container. *Why?* To test for infection, blood or the presence of sugar (in diabetes).
Stool specimen *What happens?* Nurses collect a sample of faeces passed into either a nappy, potty or bedpan and place it in a specimen	**X-ray** *What happens?* You or a nurse will be asked to hold the child firmly in a particular position while the X-ray picture is taken.	**Setting a limb in plaster** *What happens?* This is often applied under anaesthetic when the fractured limb is fixed in position, but children can

▶

pot. *Why?* To find out what is causing digestive tract disorders or infections.	There is no danger of radiation. *Why?* To find out about fractures and other disorders not visible from the outside.	be frightened by the tiny saw used to remove the plaster after healing. *Why?* To set the bones in position and to prevent movement while the fracture mends.

Isolation

Some children in hospital need to be nursed in isolation; this means that they are kept apart from other people, in a separate room. This is to protect them from infection while their immunity is low. Children cared for in an isolation room or cubicle will have certain restrictions; these vary according to their illness and treatment, but often include the following:

- ◆ Their visitors have to follow special rules such as wearing aprons and washing their hands when they enter and leave the room.
- ◆ Restrictions on what the child can eat. For example, they may not be allowed salads, unpeeled fruit, soft cheese, or cream.
- ◆ They may only be allowed one or two visitors a day.
- ◆ Toys, games and clothes cannot freely be taken in or out of the room.

The usual reasons for isolating children are:

- – when their immune system is weakened by any illness
- – when they are having high dose chemotherapy, bone marrow or stem cell transplant, for example children with leukaemia; this makes them vulnerable to infection because of a temporary low white blood cell count.
- – when they have an infection that can easily be passed on to others.

Supporting a child in isolation

Children nursed in isolation need a parent or carer to stay with them to an even greater extent than do children on an open ward, because of the extra strain of loneliness or boredom. Parents and carers also need a lot of sympathetic support from hospital staff, friends and relatives. They are having to cope with a number of very stressful events:

- ◆ The anxiety about their child's illness and treatment.
- ◆ The unnaturalness of being confined with their child for long periods of time.
- ◆ The lack of privacy resulting from the need for continuous observation and care by nursing staff.

Some hospitals provide a sitting room where parents can go and have a cup of tea and share problems with others in similar situations.

The hospital school

Children who are in hospital for longer than a week have the opportunity to attend the hospital school. It is extremely important that whenever the sick child's condition allows, education and school work should continue in hospital. The hospital school:

- provides a valuable link between the past and the future, and introduces a sense of normality to the hospital ward
- involves qualified teachers and nursery nurses, who assess each child's needs and draw up an appropriate teaching programme
- offers intellectual stimulation and occupation
- has special facilities and resources to be able to provide education for children with a wide range of conditions
- provides relief of anxiety for those children who fear they are falling behind their school peers while in hospital
- encourages parental co-operation.

Children who are long-stay patients in hospital

The longer a child has to stay in hospital, the greater the strain placed on the family, and the harder it is for a parent to stay all the time. Many children have to spend several weeks or even months as in-patients. This could be because of fractures, where the child may be in plaster and **traction**, or when a child has to undergo a lengthy treatment for a life-threatening illness. Older children can often be entertained for at least some of the time by stories, television and audio tapes. For children who are confined to bed, mirrors fixed at different angles give children different views; babies can have a variety of interesting mobiles and 'feely' toys around their cot. Some children who are in traction can be nursed at home, if there are adequate support staff in the community.

Returning home after a hospital stay

Some children are unsettled after being in hospital; their life is changing all over again when it's time to go home. When the child is ready to be discharged from hospital, nursing staff will arrange a meeting with the parents to discuss what may happen when the child returns home. As it is well known that we tend not to do all that is said to us when we are under stress, staff will give parents some *written information*, for example instructions for medication and care routines. The parents are alerted to possible behaviour changes in their child after a stay in hospital:

- **Regression**: children may revert to a more babyish way of speaking, may start to wet themselves or want to be cuddled more than usual; this behaviour is usually short-lived and parents are advised that it is normal and to go along with it.
- **Sleep disturbance**: some children have vivid dreams and nightmares; others may not want to sleep in their own room, but want to sleep in the parents' room. This is because children are often anxious after a stay in hospital and need to regain their self-confidence and independence.
- **Aggression**: some children behave in an aggressive way to their parents and siblings; they use their family as a release for all the pent-up frustrations of having been in hospital. This behaviour is usually short-lived.

Some children experience problems in adjusting to their school routine and their teacher should be made aware of any problems the child is having.

The effects of chronic illness on the family

What is chronic illness?

Chronic disorders are usually contrasted with acute conditions – those of sudden onset and of short duration. A child with a chronic illness shows little change in symptoms from day to day and may still be able to carry out normal daily activities – although there may be some difficulty. Chronic illness can be defined as:

- a chronic condition that has lasted or is expected to last more than three months
- a condition that requires more than the average medical attention for a child of the same age
- a continuous disease process, with progressive deterioration, often in spite of treatment.

Many children have more than one significant health problem or complex condition. When a child has a chronic condition, it affects **all areas of his or her life**, including social and educational development. Many children with a chronic illness require care that is comprehensive, family centred and co-ordinated. This helps the child to reach his or her potential with minimum interference from their illness. Children may also experience acute exacerbations – or flare-ups – of their symptoms.

Examples of chronic illness in children include:

- Juvenile chronic arthritis (see page 183).
- Cystic fibrosis (see page 154).
- Eczema (see page 209).
- Sickle cell anaemia (see page 159).
- Asthma (see page 193).
- Chronic renal failure.
- Psoriasis – a skin disorder (see page 219).
- Diabetes (see page 121).
- Thalassaemia (see page 159).

How families react to chronic illness and life-threatening illness

Every parent expecting a baby hopes that the baby will be perfect, and if the baby is disabled in any way, this will have a profound effect on the family and on the way it functions. Each family is unique in the way that it will react initially and adjust in the long term. Parents whose baby or child develops a chronic or life-threatening illness may react in the following ways, which are part of what is known as the grieving process:

- **Disbelief, numbness, shock and pain.** Even when parents suspect that there is something seriously wrong with their child, actually having their suspicions confirmed may still produce feelings of shock and panic. Explanations from doctors and nurses may be impossible to fully comprehend and they may feel numb and withdraw initially from others while they try to take in what has happened.
- **Despair and anger**. There may be powerful feelings of resentment and anger: 'Why is this happening to us?', and some of their anger may be directed towards professionals who are responsible both for breaking the bad news and for providing treatment and care.

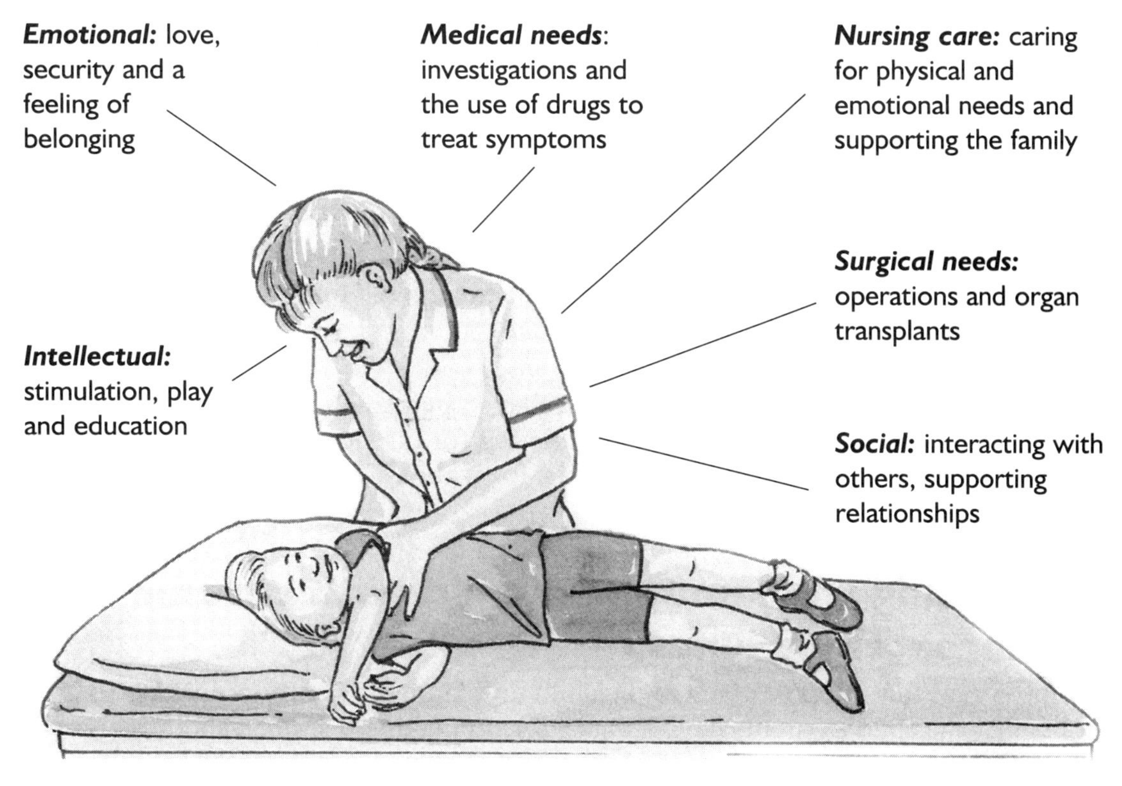

The various needs of a child with chronic illness

- **Guilt**. Parents may feel that the child's illness or disability could have been prevented by them. 'If only we had noticed sooner that something was wrong earlier . . .' is a common reaction as parents struggle to come to terms with a child's life-threatening illness.
- **Confusion**. Parents may be unable to understand what is happening and begin to question their ability to be good parents and to worry about how they will cope in the future.
- **Isolation and feeling a loss of control**. Parents may feel an increasing sense of isolation and feel that they have no control over events. They may feel that nobody else can appreciate what they are feeling and nothing can take away their pain.

The reactions of brothers and sisters

Just as there are variations in the way parents react to a child's illness, the way in which the sick child's brothers and sisters react will differ greatly. Their reaction will depend upon their age and stage of development – and particularly on their level of understanding. Common reactions include:

- **Jealousy**. Children may feel jealous of all the attention the sick child is getting. Parents and other relatives appear to be focusing all their attention on the ill child, with disruption of previous routines. Some children regress and develop attention-seeking behaviour in an effort to claim more of their parents' time.

- **Guilt and fear**. Siblings may feel guilty that they are well and able to play and do things that their sick brother or sister can't. They may be frightened at the strength and power of their parents' feelings of sadness and may even be afraid that they too could develop the same illness.
- **Grief**. Children may go through a similar grieving process as do adults. They may feel overpowering feelings of sadness and loss; these feelings can result in:
  - loss of appetite and lack of energy
  - mood swings – one minute seeming full of energy and optimism, and the next seeming withdrawn and uncommunicative
  - sleeping problems.
- **Neglect**. Siblings can feel unloved and neglected by parents and others, whose loving attention may seem exclusively reserved for the sick child. They feel somehow very different from their friends, for whom life seems to go on as normal.

Supporting the family of a child with chronic or life-threatening illness

It is important that support given to the child and family is **family-centred**. This means that the child's parents have a major role in making decisions about the sort of care their child receives, where the care takes place and how they can establish networks of support.

Professional carers, such as doctors, nurses, social workers and early years workers should recognise the needs of the child and the whole family and aim to meet those needs in an honest, caring and supportive manner:

- Parents should be involved in every aspect of their child's illness and be encouraged to make decisions about the care their child will receive, for example how much they will be involved in practical care. Parents should never feel pressurised to undertake nursing tasks, such as changing dressings, unless they feel comfortable about them.
- Information about the child's illness and the care and treatment involved must be given in a way that is easy to understand, and professionals should operate an 'open door' policy which encourages parents to ask about any aspect of care they are unsure about.
- Care plans should be drawn up *with* the parents' involvement, and should take account of the physical, emotional and social needs of the whole family.
- Parents who are caring for a sick child at home may feel isolated, and many parents will experience stress and tension within their marital relationships. Support groups can help enormously, by putting parents in touch with others who are going through the same difficulties.
- Financial help should be available for all parents caring for a chronically ill child at home or in hospital. Extra costs incurred as a direct result of their circumstances include:
  - Transport costs to get to the hospital or assessment centre.
  - Increased household bills for heating, lighting and laundry.

- One parent having to give up work to look after the sick child.
- Increased telephone bills as parents have to keep in touch with hospital staff, family and friends.

The Benefits Agency can advise parents about the different allowances payable in individual circumstances.

Providing support in the early years setting

Whether you are working in the family home as a nanny, in a nursery or in a school, you will need to keep well-informed about the family's situation and to offer appropriate support. You will need to be aware of:

- The child's needs and their stage of development.
- How they may be feeling.
- Any behaviour changes.

How you can help

You need to offer practical and emotional support to the child and to his or her family:

- **Key workers** can develop a strong emotional bond with the child and provide a safe, trusting relationship which will help the child and the parents; there should always be a back-up person to help when the child's key worker is away.
- Always find time to listen to the child.
- Observe the child closely and try to see if there are any areas of difficulty the child is experiencing.
- Allow the child to express their feelings; encourage children to use play as a form of therapy to release feelings of tension, frustration and sadness; you could offer activities such as playing with dough, bubble-blowing, water play, small world play and home corner play.
- Reassure them that they are very much loved by their family and their carers.

CASE STUDY

Hayley

Hayley is the second child of healthy parents. She appeared to be a healthy baby until she was six months old, when she caught a cold from her brother, Jason, who is three years older. Her cough rapidly worsened, and after episodes of high fever and vomiting every feed, **pneumonia** was diagnosed and Hayley was rushed into hospital. She responded well to treatment and intravenous feeding, but X-ray pictures revealed an abnormality of the bronchial tubes. Pancreatic enzyme tests confirmed the diagnosis as **cystic fibrosis**.

Hayley's parents began the daily routine, so familiar to anyone coping with cystic fibrosis, of physiotherapy (postural drainage and coughing to clear the lungs) and antibiotic medicine, vitamin supplements and vital pancreatic enzymes. Recurrent chest infections meant that Hayley received the different drugs via a nebuliser worked by a compressor; this delivers mist containing tiny droplets of the drugs which can get right down into the lungs where they are needed. Hayley progressed normally until she was in her first year at infant school. Then she began to complain of colicky pain and had bouts of vomiting and constipation – this was diagnosed as meconium ileus equivalent, which is a type of intestinal obstruction.

Hayley was admitted to hospital for intravenous fluids, pain-relieving medicine and special enemas given under X-ray control. Hayley had not been a hospital patient before, apart from when she had two severe bouts of pneumonia which needed hospital care.

Hayley is now a cheerful, optimistic seven-year-old, who enjoys dancing and PE; although she is small for her age, she can mostly keep up with her peers, apart from a tendency to wheeze with any strenuous exertion. Hayley's parents share her care and try to make sure that family life doesn't revolve around Hayley's condition.

Questions

1 Make a list of Hayley's needs.
2 How are these needs met, and who is responsible for Hayley's care?
3 Find out about the Cystic Fibrosis Research Trust; how could the Trust help Hayley and her family?
4 One in 20 of the UK population are carriers of the cystic fibrosis gene; the chance of two carriers becoming partners is 1 in 400. What is the chance of a child of two carriers having cystic fibrosis? Should Jason, Hayley's brother, be worried that he may be a carrier, and can he be genetically tested?

Terminal care

A terminal illness is one where treatment no longer has any prospect of curing the illness, and death will ultimately result. There are various reasons why a child may die:

◆ As a result of a congenital defect that is incompatible with life – e.g. **anencephaly**.	◆ Unexpectedly, e.g. as a result of a cot death (**sudden infant death syndrome**).
◆ Suddenly, after an accident, e.g. a road traffic accident or a **head injury**.	◆ As a result of an acute illness, e.g. **meningitis**.
◆ As a result of a life-threatening illness, e.g. **cancer**.	

Children with a terminal illness may be cared for:

– at home, with support from professionals
– in hospital
– in a children's hospice.

The death of a child is always hard to bear; we certainly don't expect to outlive our own children. Death in childhood was not so unusual one hundred years ago, when life expectancy was short and thousands of children died from diseases such as diphtheria and tuberculosis. Now, however, we have come to expect that modern technology and advanced medical techniques will solve most health problems.

Many conditions which the children have deteriorate slowly over a number of years, placing an enormous strain on family life. Although families willingly invest their total love, energy and attention in the care of their sick children, their lives become ruled by the relentless timetable of nursing and medical tasks. Holidays, family activities, and outings are denied; parents rarely have a normal mealtime, a full night's sleep or any time to themselves. Healthy brothers and sisters often feel left out as attention focuses on the sick child.

Caring for the child at home

The majority of children with terminal illness die at home, as home is felt by most parents to be the most comfortable place for them. The family is supported in caring for the ill child by the primary care team and the community paediatric nurse team, which oversees the daily care and supports the family. Respite care is provided when needed, either in the hospital where the child has been treated or in a children's hospice.

Caring for the child in a hospice

There are very few children's hospices in the UK, but the number is steadily growing as they offer such a wide range of services for the dying child and the family. A children's hospice supports children and young people who are expected to die in childhood, together with their family and friends. The children either have life-shortening conditions, such as Duchenne muscular dystrophy, or life-threatening conditions, such as cancer or heart disease. Due to the hereditary nature of some of the illnesses, some families have two or more affected children. Medical treatment may have been tried, but not achieved a cure, or, as in most of the cases, there is no treatment available.

A children's hospice aims to:

- Help families with caring for their child, enabling them to enjoy quality time with their child, siblings or on their own.
- Offer a 'home from home', providing a relaxed atmosphere in an informal and comfortable setting.
- Tailor their care to the families' needs and wishes.
- Offer bereavement counselling and support, working with groups as well as working with brothers and sisters.
- Offer a system of 'contacts', who befriend named children and their families and ensure support is continued between visits.
- Provide flexible, family-centred care, support and friendship throughout the course of a child's illness and continuing after their death.
- Employ staff who are specially chosen for their personal qualities and/or qualifications which will enhance the care and support offered to children and families. The care teams at all children's hospices are led by a qualified children's nurse.
- Provide specialist respite, emergency, palliative and terminal care, either within the hospice or in the family home.
- Information, advice and practical assistance and 24-hour telephone support.

The child's perception of death

Long before we realise it, children become aware of death. They see dead birds, insects, and animals lying by the road. They may see death at least once a day on television. They hear about it in fairy tales and act it out in their play. Death is a part of life, and children, at some level, are aware of it. Studies show that children go through a series of stages in their understanding of death:

1 **Nursery age children (aged $2\frac{1}{2}$ to 5 years).** Children usually see death as reversible, temporary, and impersonal. They watch cartoon characters on television who miraculously rise up whole again – even when they've been crushed or blown apart, which tends to reinforce this belief.
2 **Between the ages of 5 and 9 years.** Most children are beginning to realise that death is final and that all living things die, but still they do not see death as *personal*. They harbour the idea that somehow they can escape through their own ingenuity and efforts. During this stage, children also tend to ***personify*** death, that is, they make the idea of death into a person; they may associate death with a skeleton or the angel of death, and some children have nightmares about them.
3 **From nine or ten and through to adolescence.** Children begin to comprehend fully that death is irreversible, that all living things die, and that they too will die some day. Some begin to work on developing philosophical views of life and death. Teenagers, especially, often become intrigued with seeking the meaning of life.

Talking to children about death

Many of us are inclined not to talk about things that upset us. We try to put a lid on our feelings and hope that saying nothing will be for the best. But even though we are not talking about something doesn't mean that we are not communicating. Children are good observers; they read messages on our faces and in the way we walk or hold our hands. When we avoid talking about something that is obviously upsetting, children often hesitate to bring up the subject or ask questions about it. To a child, this avoidance can be a message – 'If Mummy and Daddy can't talk about it, it really must be bad, so I'd better not talk about it either.' In effect, instead of protecting children by avoiding talk, we sometimes cause them *more* worry and also keep them from telling us how *they* feel.

On the other hand, it is not a good idea to confront children with information that they may not yet understand or want to know. As with any sensitive subject, we need to strike a balance between avoidance and confrontation. This involves:

- being sensitive to their need to communicate when they are ready
- trying not to put up barriers that may inhibit their attempts to communicate
- offering them honest explanations when we are obviously upset
- listening to and accepting their feelings
- not putting off their questions by telling them they are too young
- trying to find brief and simple answers that are appropriate to their questions; answers that they can understand and that do not overwhelm them with too many words.

Perhaps most difficult of all, it involves examining our own feelings and beliefs so that we can talk to children about death and dying as naturally as possible – when the opportunities arise.

CASE STUDY

Saying Goodbye to Ben

The following article was written by a mother whose son died aged three years and nine months.

It is now over four years since Ben was born, and I have lost all sense of time in relation to events. Sometimes it seems only a few weeks since his birth and only yesterday that we were told he wouldn't live to be a year old. Ben had been born with hypertrophic obstructive cardiomyopathy, a heart-muscle disease very rare in children, but inoperable.

Our lives were full of hospital after that, lots of clinic visits, admissions and a long stay for **open heart surgery**. The hospital became like a second home – except it was a home you don't want to go to. The nurses and doctors became good friends – but they were friends you would rather not have to make. One of the most consoling aspects of our stays in hospital was the contact we made with other parents; you form your own support groups, which are very important. Most sick children need to have their mother or father with them for reassurance. Nowadays, most hospitals encourage parents to stay, but it can be exhausting to be there without a break. You long for the day you can leave, but when you are told you can go home, it suddenly seems too soon. You aren't ready to carry the whole responsibility. And when you get home, where is everybody? You have lost not only the nurses and doctors and the support of other hospital parents, but most of your friends and neighbours, it seems.

People avoid you because they do not know what to say. If only they would simply put their arms around you without saying anything. Instead, parents find themselves landed with the extra burden of having to make it easier for other people, jollying along an awkward phone conversation. You find yourself consoling people who should be consoling you, and who might like to, if they knew how.

One of the hardest things about the whole gruelling business is balancing your life between the child in crisis and the others who need you too. Ben was our fourth child and, though the three others could be amazingly understanding for children of primary school age, they are nevertheless only human and were understandably resentful at times, although they wouldn't have parted with their fragile little brother for anything in the world.

After 19 months of living with Ben and his disease and coping with the trauma of open heart surgery, we had to face the fact that he had deteriorated so much that he now needed a heart transplant. We were lucky; many children never get the chance they deserve, and die while on the waiting list. We will always hold a special place in our hearts for a very brave family in France who thought of others in the midst of their tragedy. After the transplant, we had real hope. Ben had a new, healthy heart and was growing and developing normally, though he had to take powerful medicines to prevent rejection.

Then, one Thursday in June, 18 months after the operation, Ben became ill. He was admitted to Birmingham Children's Hospital the same evening and transferred to the intensive care unit and put on a ventilator the next day. Although Ben had been very close to death in the past, I had never before experienced the feelings I did now. The memory of that terror and helplessness will never leave me.

He just lay there, the ventilator tube protruding from his nose, wires and tubes connected to his beautiful, perfect little body. Tony and I sat by him, stroking him, holding his hands and kissing his downy skin. I felt as if part of me was being torn away, and I could do nothing but watch and wait. I talked to Ben, though I didn't think he could hear me.

The consultant was with Ben all day and all night and at one point we told him that if Ben were to die, we wanted to donate any of his organs which could be used.

At 4.10 a.m. on Saturday 9 June, our fourth child, Benjamin, died. Less than 48 hours after appearing well and healthy, our precious, beautiful child was gone. All the struggles, research, appointments, treatments, hospital stays – everything concerned with Ben and the fight to prolong his life was over.

Together, Tony and I gently wrapped Ben in a blanket and wept. I remember crying his name over and over, telling him how much we loved him, how special he was, that we didn't want him to leave us. I wanted to hold him and never let him go.

Devastating and terrible though Ben's dying was, it was made more bearable by the loving way in which the staff treated him, and the support we had from Acorns – one of the very few children's hospices in the country, which offers support to families who have children with life-threatening conditions. Acorns is close to the hospital and our other children stayed there the night, so we could be with Ben. Now the social worker, Steve, brought them to see him for the last time. After we had washed and dressed Ben, we laid him in a cot with his sheepskin fleece – he had slept on it ever since he was a new-born baby – placing his cuddly toys around him, just as he always had them in his cot at home. Then we went out to see Lucy, Matthew and Thomas. I have a memory of their sleepy, worried faces and then their sadness and tears. They wanted to see him and it seemed the most natural thing they should do. They had always visited him in hospital and were completely involved in his life. Now they needed to be part of his death.

Ben's short life made an impact on many people, as we know from the hundreds of messages we received. It has changed me too. I used to think ahead, working myself up about tomorrow and next month and next year. Ben taught me to live for today. Despite the tragedy of Ben's death, I haven't been destroyed. I am stronger, more independent. I don't worry about ridiculous things. The people nothing ever happens to are the ones who worry. They carry on about a scratch on the car or someone forgetting their birthday. When I have a bad day and the children are yelling, I am reminded that they are here, and I am glad to hear them.

I feel now I can talk to anyone, argue with experts and do anything for my family. I am no better or stronger than any other parent but I have something to offer, because of what I have been through. Ben will always belong to the five of us and all who cared for him. There is a sense in which we can never be separated.

Sue Pasternak has set up a support group for families whose children have heart and heart and lung transplants. She also raises funds for the hospice Acorns – a registered charity.

ACTIVITY

Task 1

Read through the moving story – 'Saying Goodbye to Ben' – and then answer the following questions. This could be done as a small group discussion and then the answers fed back into the whole group:

1 Why did Ben's mother find it hard to return home after being with her son in hospital?
2 How did friends and neighbours react to Ben's family? Why do you think they reacted this way?
3 What effect did Ben's chronic illness have on his three siblings?
4 What support did Ben's family receive after Ben had died?

Task 2

Find out about the various support groups for children who are dying and their families and put the information into a booklet that can be used by all students. Examples include:

- CRUSE
- The Compassionate Friends
- SANDS (Stillbirth and Neonatal Death Society)
- The Child Bereavement Trust
- Dial–A–Dream.

Respect for other beliefs

It may help to tell children that different people believe different things and that not everyone believes as we do, for example some people believe in an afterlife; some do not. By indicating our acceptance and respect for others' beliefs, we may make it easier for children to choose beliefs different from our own but more comforting to them.

Books to read with children about life-threatening illness

Kathy's Hats: A Story of Hope, Trudy Krisher (Albert Whitman and Company). A story of a child with cancer and the hats she wears.

On The Wings Of A Butterfly: A Story About Life and Death, Marilyn Maple. A story of a child with cancer.

I Have Cancer, Althea. A story of a child with cancer.

Books to read with children about dying and bereavement

For very young children:

Everett Anderson's Goodbye, Lucille Clifton (Henry Holt – An Owlet book). This little picture book goes through the stages of grief in very few words and big pictures

Badger's Parting Gift, Susan Varley (Mulberry Books). Old Badger gives parting gifts to his friends.

For older children:

Remember the Secret, Elisabeth Kubler-Ross (Celestial Arts). A book about death and grief with a more religious background and message.

I'll Always Love You, Hans Wilhelm (Crown Publishers – A Dragonfly Book). A boy's dog dies and the boy realises that you never stop loving your dog, or anyone, even when they die.

The Tenth Good Thing About Barney, Judith Viorst (Aladdin Paperbacks). A very good book about death and the sad feelings of a little girl coming to terms with the death of her cat with the help of her father.

When Dinosaurs Die: a Guide to Understanding Death, Laurie Krasny Brown and Marc Brown (Little Brown). A multicultural look at dying and the customs that surround it.

The Cemetery Quilt, Kent and Alice Ross (Houghton Mifflin). A wise story of a girl who goes to her grandfather's funeral and talks to her grandmother about death and how she feels about it.

Revision questions

1 How could you help to prepare a young child for a planned admission to hospital?
2 How can an early years worker or a hospital play specialist prepare a child who is going to have an operation?
3 What are the benefits to a child in hospital of:
   a role-play
   b small world play
   c diversion or distraction techniques?
4 List three behaviour changes that children might display after being discharged home from hospital.
5 What are the aims of hospice care for children?

Chapter 10: Child health surveillance and screening

◆ *Child health surveillance* ◆ *Screening* ◆ *Your role in child health screening and surveillance* ◆ *Health education* ◆ *Your role in child health education* ◆ *The role of professionals in promoting and maintaining child health*

Child health surveillance

Child health surveillance is a programme of care provided by professionals, with the aim of preventing illness and promoting good health and development. Its primary purpose is to detect any abnormality in development so that the child can be offered treatment as early as possible, for example early detection of a hearing impairment gives a young child a better chance of receiving appropriate treatment and special education. Most surveillance is carried out in child health clinics and, from the age of five onwards, in schools. Child health surveillance includes regular assessment, through **screening** and through observations by parents, teachers and other child care and education workers. The areas covered are:

- Growth
- Illness
- Child abuse
- Health education programmes
- All-round or holistic development
- Behaviour
- Immunisation

The inverse care law

The families who are most in need of health surveillance are often those who are least likely to make use of the services provided in child health clinics. Although children in the UK enjoy better health than at any other time, the provisions of a National Health Service have not led to equality of health experience. The following are seen as *priority* groups by health visitors and the primary care team when organising caseloads and targeting resources:

- Very young and unsupported parents, particularly those with their first baby.
- Parents thought to be at particular risk of abusing their children.
- Parents who are socially isolated, due to mental health problems or language or cultural barriers.
- Families living in poor housing, including B&B accommodation, or housing where there is overcrowding.
- Parents with poor self-esteem or a lack of confidence.
- Parents with unrealistic expectations about their child, or with a poor understanding of the child's needs.
- Parents/children experiencing significant bereavement (including as a result of a recent divorce).
- Previous cot death in the family.

Delivering health care to families in such circumstances is difficult and often involves close liaison with other community services, such as social service departments or housing departments.

Screening

The aim of a screening programme is to examine all children at risk from a certain condition; the term screening refers to the examination of apparently healthy children to distinguish those who probably have a condition from those who probably do not. Hearing defects are often detected in this way at one of the routine checks carried out at the child health (or surveillance) clinic.

Screening is part of the child health surveillance programme. Screening:

- is carried out by health care professionals – health visitors, midwives, doctors and school nurses
- involves checking all children at specific ages to monitor health and development
- is available to all families in the UK
- mainly focuses on four areas: all-round development, vision, hearing, specific medical conditions
- offers the opportunity for valuable health education and advice to be given to parents.

Skin – vernix and lanugo may still be present; milia may show on the baby's nose; black babies appear lighter in the first week of life as the pigment, melanin, is not yet at full concentration

Spine is checked for any evidence of spina bifida

Face is examined for: cleft palate – a gap in the roof of the mouth; facial paralysis – temporary paralysis after compression of the facial nerve, usually after forceps delivery

Feet are checked for webbing and talipes (club foot), which needs early treatment

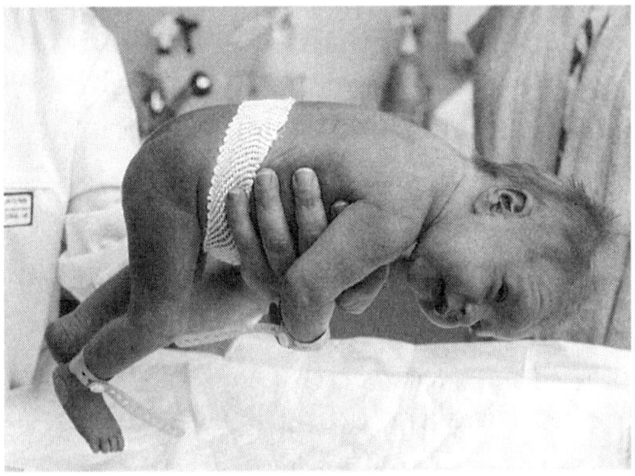

Head is checked for size and shape: any marks from forceps delivery are noted

Genitalia and **anus** are checked for any malformation

Eyes are checked for cataract – a cloudiness of the lens

Hips are tested for congenital dislocation

Neck is examined for any obvious injury to the neck muscles after a difficult delivery

Abdomen is checked for any abnormality, e.g. pyloric stenosis, where there may be obstruction of the passage of food from the stomach; the **umbilical cord** is checked for infection

Heart and **lungs** are checked using a stethoscope; any abnormal findings will be investigated

Hands are checked for webbing (fingers are joined together at the base) and creases – a single unbroken crease from one side of the palm to the other is a feature of Down's syndrome

Examination of new-born baby by paediatrican

Screening tests in pregnancy

During pregnancy women have routine examinations and investigations, including blood and urine tests. The aim is to detect any abnormalities in the foetus and to check on its health. Some women request certain screening tests or are advised to have specific tests by their doctor.

Screening tests and developmental reviews

Shortly after birth, the newborn baby is examined by the paediatrician or family doctor. Specific checks are made to assess the health and development of the baby. The baby's weight and head circumference are also measured and recorded. Many

Table 10.1 Screening tests in pregnancy

Name	Procedure	When	Procedure performed to assess	Comments
Chorionic villus sampling (CVS)	A small piece of the placenta is removed via the cervix (neck of the womb) and the cells examined	At about 8–11 weeks	◆ the risk of Down's syndrome, haemophilia, cystic fibrosis, thalassaemia, sickle cell disease or other genetic disorders	An early test with results available after only 7–10 days Risk of miscarriage is higher than with amniocentesis
Amniocentesis	After an ultrasound scan a hollow needle is inserted through the abdomen to draw off a sample of amniotic fluid from inside the uterus. Foetal cells are cultured for 3–5 weeks and then examined under a microscope	Between 14 and 18 weeks	◆ the presence of an extra chromosome, i.e. Down's syndrome ◆ any missing or damaged chromosomes ◆ missing or defective enzymes which cause metabolic disorders ◆ if the baby is receiving enough oxygen ◆ the baby's sex: important in identifying babies at risk of genetically linked disorders such as muscular dystrophy or haemophilia	May be offered to any woman over 35 or 38 (in some hospitals) when the risk of chromosomal abnormalities is greater to any woman with a history of sex-life disorders The risk of miscarriage is estimated to be increased by 0.5–1% over the existing risk of miscarriage at this stage of pregnancy
***Maternal serum screening test* (Bart's test)**	A blood test which measures the levels of AFP (alpha-fetoprotein) and three hormones – oestriol and two types of human chorionic gonadotrophin	At about 16 weeks	◆ the risk factor for neural tube defects, e.g. anencephaly and spina bifida ◆ the risk factor for Down's syndrome	A non-invasive test useful for women considering invasive tests such as amniocentesis; it does not make a diagnosis of these conditions but indicates the level of risk involved
Triple plus test	A blood test which measures levels of AFP,oestriol and human gonadotrophin, and also NAP (neutrophil alkaline phosphatase).	At about 13–16 weeks	◆ the risk factor for neural tube defects, e.g. anencephaly and spina bifida ◆ the risk factor for Down's syndrome	This test is not routinely available on the NHS, but has a higher detection rate for Down's syndrome than the Barts test. When only the mother's age is used as a determining risk factor, the detection rate is 30%, whereas the Triple Plus test offers an above 80% detection rate
Ultrasound scan	Ultrasound (sound at higher frequency than can be heard by the human ear) is used to produce pictures of the foetus in the uterus	At any stage, but usually between 16 and 18 weeks	◆ the size, age and position of the foetus ◆ the position of the placenta ◆ if there is more than one baby ◆ if the foetus is developing normally ◆ if there are fibroids in the womb ◆ if the pregnancy is in the right place or ectopic	New research indicates that Down's syndrome can be detected using ultrasound. The mother would then be offered amniocentesis

hospitals have abandoned the routine task of measuring the length of the baby as it was found to be inaccurate.

The Apgar score

This is a standard method of evaluating the condition of a new-born baby by checking five vital signs.

The Apgar score

Signs	0	1	2
Heartbeat	absent	slow below 100	fast over 100
Breathing	absent	slow irregular	good; crying
Muscle tone	limp	some limb movement	active movement
Reflex response (to simulation of foot or nostril)	absent	grimace	cry, cough, sneeze
Colour	blue pale	body oxygenated, hands and feet blue	well-oxygenated

The Apgar score is assessed at 1 minute and 5 minutes after birth; it may be repeated at 5-minute intervals if there is cause for concern.

Interpreting the score:

10 The baby is in the best possible condition
8–9 The baby is in good condition
5–7 The baby has mild asphyxia and may need treatment
3–4 The baby has moderate asphyxia and will need treatment
0–2 The baby has severe asphyxia and needs urgent resuscitation

Most healthy babies have an Apgar score of 9, losing one point for having blue extremities – this often persists for a few hours after birth. A low score at 5 minutes is more serious than a low score at 1 minute. In hospital, the paediatrician will be notified if the score is 6 or under at 5 minutes.

A few hospitals also check for **hearing**, using the cradle response test – see page 285.

Other medical checks include listening to the heart and lungs to detect any abnormality, and examining the anus and genitalia for any malformation.

Parent-held records

In most clinics now parents are given a personal child health record or parent-held record for their baby. This is a way of keeping track of the child's progress. Records are kept about the child's:

- Height and weight.
- Immunisations.
- Childhood illness and accidents.

Development reviews

Regular development reviews are carried out in child health clinics and at the child's home by general practitioners, health visitors and school nurses. If a child has a developmental delay, parents will want to know about the problem as soon as possible; it is easier to come to terms with a serious problem in a young baby than in an older child. Health professionals should always take parental concerns seriously and never assume that parents are fussy, neurotic or over-anxious.

If the child's first language is not English, development reviews can be carried out with the help of someone who can speak the child's language. After the age of five years, the **school health service** takes over the assessments (see page 294).

A REVIEW FOR YOU AND YOUR BABY 8 MONTHS AFTER THE BIRTH

This review is done with your health visitor.

Before you see your health visitor, you may wish to write down some of the things you want to discuss – there are spaces provided below. However, if you are worried about the baby's health, growth or development, you can contact your health visitor or doctor at any time.

	YES	NO	COMMENTS
Do you feel well yourself?	☐	☐	....
Do you have any worries bout your baby's health?	☐	☐	....
Does your baby put its hand around a cup or bottle?	☐	☐	....
Do you have any worries about your baby's development?	☐	☐	....
Is your baby interested and curious about its world?	☐	☐	....
Are you happy that your baby is growing well?	☐	☐	....
Does your baby: **Crawl?**	Yes ☐	No ☐	**Roll?** Yes ☐ No ☐
Is your baby sitting alone?	☐	☐	....
Does your baby need support to sit alone?	☐	☐	....
Does your baby babble tunefully, ga ga/ba ba, etc?	☐	☐	....
Does your baby listen to conversation?	☐	☐	....
Have you any worries about your baby's eyesight?	☐	☐	....
Does you baby pick up tiny objects with fingers and thumb?	☐	☐	....
Have you noticed a squint? (Eyes not moving together)	☐	☐	....
Does your baby look for fallen objects?	☐	☐	....
Do you think your baby can hear you?	☐	☐	....
Does your baby use voice to attract attention?	☐	☐	....
Are all immunisations up-to-date?	☐	☐	....
Have you checked your home and car for safety?	☐	☐	....

Do you have fire guards to stop your child touching heaters and open fires?

Sample page from a personal health record

Children's holistic development is reviewed, using these headings:

- **Fine motor skills**: handling toys, stacking bricks, doing up buttons and tying shoelaces (gross and fine manipulative skills).
- **Gross motor skills**: sitting, standing, walking, running.
- **Social behaviour**.
- **Speech and language**: including **hearing**.
- **Vision**.

Reviews give parents an opportunity to say what they have noticed about their child. They can also discuss anything that concerns them about their child's health and behaviour.

Assessment at 6 to 8 weeks

Developmental reviews from 6 weeks onwards are conducted under the headings: Discussion, Observation, Measurement, Examination.

Discussion

Parents are asked generally if they have any concerns about their baby, in particular about:

- feeding
- sleeping
- bowel actions and passing urine.

They are also asked if they think that the baby can:

- hear (e.g. does the baby 'startle' to a sudden noise?), and
- see (e.g. does the baby turn her head to follow the parent or carer?).

Observation of the baby

While the parent (or carer) is undressing the baby for examination, the doctor will look out for:

- the responsiveness of the baby – smiles, eye contact, attentiveness to parent's voice, etc.
- any difficulties the parent has with holding the baby – for example a depressed mother will lack visual attention and may not give a good upporting hold
- signs of jaundice or anaemia.

This is also an opportunity to provide help and support to the parents.

Measurement of the baby

- The baby is weighed naked and the weight plotted on a growth (centile) chart.
- The head circumference is measured and plotted on the growth chart.

Examination of the baby

- The **general appearance** of the baby will give an indication of the general health of the baby and whether he or she is well nourished.
- The **eyes** are inspected using a light – babies will turn their head and follow a small light beam.
- The heart and hips are checked again.

- The baby is placed in the **prone** position and will turn his or her head to one side; hands are held with the thumbs inwards and with the fingers wrapped around them.
- The **posterior fontanelle** is usually closed now; the **anterior fontanelle** does not close until around 18 months.

Health education points

- □ **Nutrition**: breastfeeding, preparation of formula feeds, specific feeding difficulties.
- □ **Immunisation**: discuss any concerns and initiate vaccination programme.
- □ **Passive smoking**: babies are at risk here of respiratory infections.
- □ **Illness in babies**: how to recognise symptoms.
- □ **Crying**: coping with frustration and tiredness.
- □ **Reducing the risk of cot death**.
- □ **Accident prevention**: see Chapter 7.

Assessment at 6 to 9 months

Discussion

Parents are asked if they have any concerns about the baby's health and development.

Observation of the baby

- **Socialisation** and **attachment** behaviour is noted; how the baby interacts with her main carer is observed. Most babies are clingy at this age.
- **Communication**: sounds, expression and gestures.
- **Motor development**: sitting, balance, use of hands, any abnormal movement patterns.
- **Muscle tone** is observed while the baby is sitting on the carer's lap.

Measurement of the baby

- Head circumference and weight are measured and plotted on the growth chart.

Examination of the baby

- **Hips** – manipulation of the hips is carried out.
- The **heart** is listened to.
- The **testes** are checked in boys.
- **Visual behaviour**: the baby's vision will be checked for signs of a **squint**.
- **Grasping**: the baby is offered a toy which is usually taken with one hand and passed to the other. The baby is observed for equal use of both hands and accuracy of grasping and passing.
- **Pincer grasp**: some babies can use a pincer grasp to pick up tiny 'hundreds and thousands' sweets. These are usually taken straight to the mouth where they can be safely eaten.
- **Hearing** may be tested; if any abnormality is detected the baby will be referred to an audiologist (a hearing specialist).

Health education points

- ☐ **Nutrition**: weaning, control of sugar intake.
- ☐ **Immunisation**: check it is up to date.
- ☐ **Teeth**: regular brushing once teeth appear.
- ☐ **The need for play and language stimulation**.
- ☐ **Accident prevention**: see Chapter 7.

Assessment at 18 to 24 months

Discussion

The parent or carer is asked if there are any general concerns about their child's development, and particularly with their **vision**, **speech** and **hearing**. They may then be referred to a specialist.

- Behaviour: any problems with temper tantrums, sleep disturbance, poor appetite or food fads.
- Iron deficiency is sometimes a problem at this age and may be a cause of irritability and behavioural problems, as well as anaemia.
- In boys, the carer is asked if the testes are present in the scrotal sac. If not present, the doctor will examine the child and refer him or her to a specialist.

Observation of the child

The child is observed walking to check whether the gait is normal.

Measurement of the child

- Height is measured if the child is cooperative.
- Weight is only measured if there is a cause for concern.

Examination of the child

- **Manipulation skills**: building a tower of six or seven cubes; holding a pencil using a thumb and two fingers; turning the pages of a book singly.

Health education points

- ☐ **Nutrition and dental care**: refer to the dentist if teeth are obviously decayed.
- ☐ **Immunisation**: check it is up to date.
- ☐ **Common behavioural problems**: temper tantrums, sleep disturbances, toilet training.
- ☐ **Social behaviour**: learning to play with other children; sharing possessions.
- ☐ **Accident prevention**: see Chapter 7.

Assessment at 4 to 5 years old (before or just after the child starts school)

Discussion

- Any general concerns about the child's development or emotional or behaviour problems.
- The child's ability to concentrate, to play with others and to separate from their main carer without distress.

Observation of the child
- **Motor skills**: can the child walk, run and climb stairs? Does the child tire more quickly compared with other children?
- **Fine manipulative skills**: can the child control pencils and paintbrushes? Can the child draw a cross?
- **Vision, language and hearing**: observation and discussion with the parent will determine any problems needing specialist assessment.

Measurement of the child
- Height and weight are measured and plotted on the growth chart.

Examination of the child
Other checks will depend on any concerns that the parent or the doctor may have. For example, if the child has asthma an examination of the lungs may take place.

NOTE: In some parts of the country, the age that children are reviewed may vary slightly to those given above, especially after the age of three.

Health education points
- ☐ **Immunisation**: pre-school booster.
- ☐ **Dental care**: diet, danger of sweets and snacks, brushing teeth, dental decay, use of fluoride, visits to the dentist.
- ☐ The child's need for play, conversation and social learning.
- ☐ The recognition and management of minor ailments.
- ☐ **Accident prevention**: see Chapter 7.

For screening carried out in schools, see pages 294–297.

Children's hearing and speech tests

Most children still have their hearing checked by the **infant distraction test**, carried out by health visitors on babies between 6 and 9 months; although still used in many health districts, some are reviewing their use of this test. It tests the ability of babies to turn towards noises, but its detection rate is poor. The test often 'fails' babies with normal hearing, causing unnecessary anxiety in parents, yet profoundly deaf babies may 'pass' easily. Studies show that this test fails to pick up most permanent hearing problems.

Another test, carried out within days of birth, can detect virtually all permanent hearing loss and allows earlier help to be given. This is the **transient evoked otoacoustic emissions (TEOAE) test** or **cradle response test**.

The cradle response test

This hearing test involves:

1. inserting a small sponge probe in the baby's ear
2. stimulating the ear with sound
3. measuring an 'echo'.

The echo response is found in all normal-hearing individuals, so its absence may indicate a hearing loss and the need for further testing.

Parents are usually the first to notice that their child has a problem with hearing, but occasionally a nursery or school teacher will pick up the problem during class activities.

Sweep audiometry test

All school entrants have their hearing tested using the sweep audiometry test. This test involves the child wearing a pair of earphones and listening for tones produced by an audiometer. The tones cover the range of tones needed for speech and each ear is tested separately.

Parents who are concerned that their child is not hearing properly should have access to hearing testing. This is particularly important if:

- the child has had meningitis
- the child has had measles or mumps
- the child has recurrent infections or glue ear.

Speech discrimination test

Any child who is suspected of having a hearing loss, or whose language development is delayed may have the speech discrimination test. This involves using a set of toys, each with a single-syllable name, for example dog, horse, key, tree, spoon, house, cup, etc., which will test the child's ability to hear different consonants like d, g, p, m, s, f and b. The child is gently encouraged to co-operate with the tester and together they name the toys using a normal voice. The child is then asked to find the toys with decreasing voice intensity, for example 'Show me the house', 'Put the duck in the box', etc. Each ear is tested through the complete range of sounds.

CASE STUDY

Mark and Tracey have one child, Jodie, aged $3\frac{1}{2}$, who has been diagnosed as having moderate to severe hearing loss; in other words, Jodie is 'deaf'.

When Mark and Tracey went to Portugal for a holiday with another family, they found themselves in the middle of a nightmare. By the end of the flight from England, Mark had blood running down his neck where Jodie had torn at him with her nails. During the holiday, Jodie had not only pushed another child into the deep end of a swimming pool, where he had to be rescued by lifeguards, but she had also shoved an entire restaurant table into the harbour.

For Mark and Tracey it was the last straw. They had been concerned for some time that Jodie's development was slow, her hearing variable and her speech poor. But whenever they raised their anxieties with health professionals they were told not to worry. Even though Jodie failed her hearing test at nine months, they felt reassured when she sailed through the re-test weeks later and passed a further test for speech at 18 months.

After the disastrous holiday, Mark and Tracey were so desperate that they consulted a child psychologist, who recommended simply ignoring Jodie for two hours every time she misbehaved. After a few weeks, Jodie was transformed into a calm, compliant child.

Now Tracey believes it was the cruellest thing she has ever done and is wracked with guilt about the whole episode.

What Mark and Tracey now know is that Jodie is deaf. In fact, she was born deaf. But even after numerous tests, Jodie's deafness was not diagnosed until she was nearly four years old. Jodie had somehow taught herself how to lip-read. Tracey and Mark began to do their own hearing tests on Jodie; when they hid from her while speaking, they realised that she failed to respond – it was obvious that she couldn't hear them.

Jodie was just about to start infant school at four when she was diagnosed as having a moderate to severe hearing loss – after a thorough hospital hearing check. She was fitted with hearing aids. Mark remembers the moment well: 'She smiled the most enormous smile of her whole life', he says. Now eight years old, Jodie is still struggling to catch up with her 'normal hearing' peers. Mark and Tracey just wish they had known what to look out for in those early years.

Questions

1 How did Jodie fail – and then pass – the hearing tests when she was a baby?

2 Why did the advice from the child psychologist result in such an improvement in Jodie's behaviour?

3 What test could have been used to diagnose Jodie's deafness and why is it not universally available?

4 Find out how children's hearing is routinely tested in your health authority and write a brief description of the method used.

Some facts

- About 840 children are born each year in the UK with permanent deafness, mainly due to genetic damage to the cochlea or to the auditory nerve.
- More than half of all children born deaf are still undiagnosed at 18 months, and a quarter of them are not diagnosed until more than $3\frac{1}{2}$, according to the National Deaf Children's Society.

Your role in child health screening and surveillance

During your training, you will have learnt about child development and about what children are expected to achieve at each stage of their development. When working with children, you can use your knowledge and powers of skilled observation to detect any developmental or health problems. Many trained child care workers are increasingly being employed in child health clinics to help doctors and health visitors to carry out routine screening tests and to offer information and advice on all aspects of child health and development.

Health education

Health education is a method of self-empowerment; it enables people to take more control over their own health and that of their children. The aims of health education are:

- To provide information and to raise awareness.
- To change people's behaviour and attitudes.
- To meet national and local health targets, for example promoting self-examination of the breasts to aid in the early detection of breast cancer.

The areas of health education relevant to children are:

- Good nutrition, i.e. eating a healthy, balanced diet.
- Prevention of tooth decay.
- Immunisation.
- Prevention of childhood accidents, including road safety and sunburn.
- Prevention of emotional and behavioural problems.
- Basic hygiene.

The Health Education Authority runs regular campaigns on a variety of health issues:

- **The folic acid campaign**: to increase awareness among pregnant women of the need to eat a diet rich in folic acid; this helps to prevent neural tube defects forming in the unborn baby, for example spina bifida.
- **The sun safety know-how programme**: to encourage parents to keep children safe in the sun; this campaign was backed up by a range of special sun-protective clothing being made available to children.
- **The National Healthy Schools Initiative:** to encourage schools to raise standards of health among school pupils and staff.

Non-government campaigns are often run by voluntary organisations; one example is the British Heart Foundation's campaign for looking after your heart. This uses a cartoon heart called Artie Beat and gives useful advice on choosing a healthier lifestyle to protect your heart (see the example below).

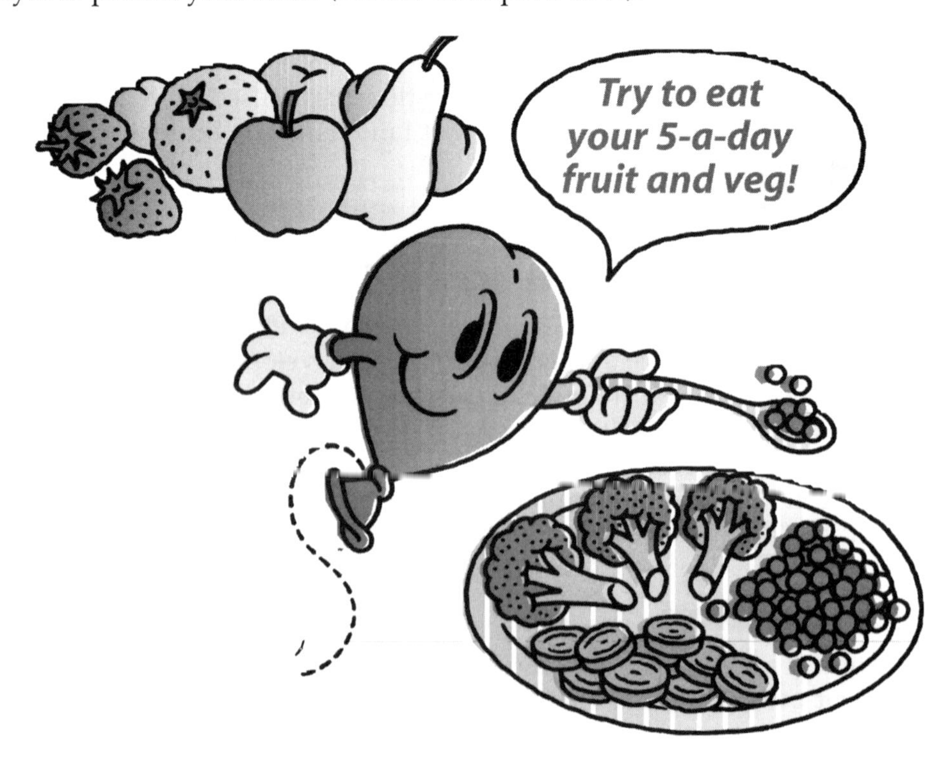

Your role in child health education

There are many ways in which the early years worker can contribute to health education programmes in child care settings. The most important part of your role is to be a good role model for children. Opportunities for teaching children about health and safety include:

- Providing healthy meals and snacks.
- Practising good hygiene routines, such as hand washing and teeth brushing.
- Welcoming visitors to talk about their work in health care – for example inviting a dentist or health visitor to explain the importance of good hygiene routines.
- Choosing books, displays and interest tables which reinforce healthy living practices.
- Using drama and music sessions to encourage children to express their feelings in a safe environment.
- Creating interesting board games with a 'healthy' theme, for example how to avoid accidents when playing outside.
- Demonstrating safety and hygiene routines; for example, a road safety officer can visit the setting to teach children how to cross the road safely.
- Making the home corner into a hospital ward and encouraging role play as patients, nurses and doctors.

ACTIVITY

A health awareness activity

In groups, plan an activity to use with a group of nursery or school-age children. Choose from the following topics:

- Accident prevention
- Healthy eating
- Dental care

Follow these guidelines when planning your activity:

1. Decide how many children will be involved, their ages and stage of development.
2. Choose an appropriate activity, e.g. a story-telling session, a puppet show, a board game, role play session or creative activity.
3. Think about your aims and be specific, e.g. 'My activity aims to help children understand the importance of eating fresh fruit and vegetables'.
4. Design your activity and arrange to implement it with a group of children in your early years setting.
5. After the activity, evaluate its success and suggest ways you could improve it in future.

The role of professionals in promoting and maintaining child health

There is a great deal of overlap between the health professionals who care for children in the community and those who work primarily in hospitals. Each professional works as part of a **multidisciplinary team**.

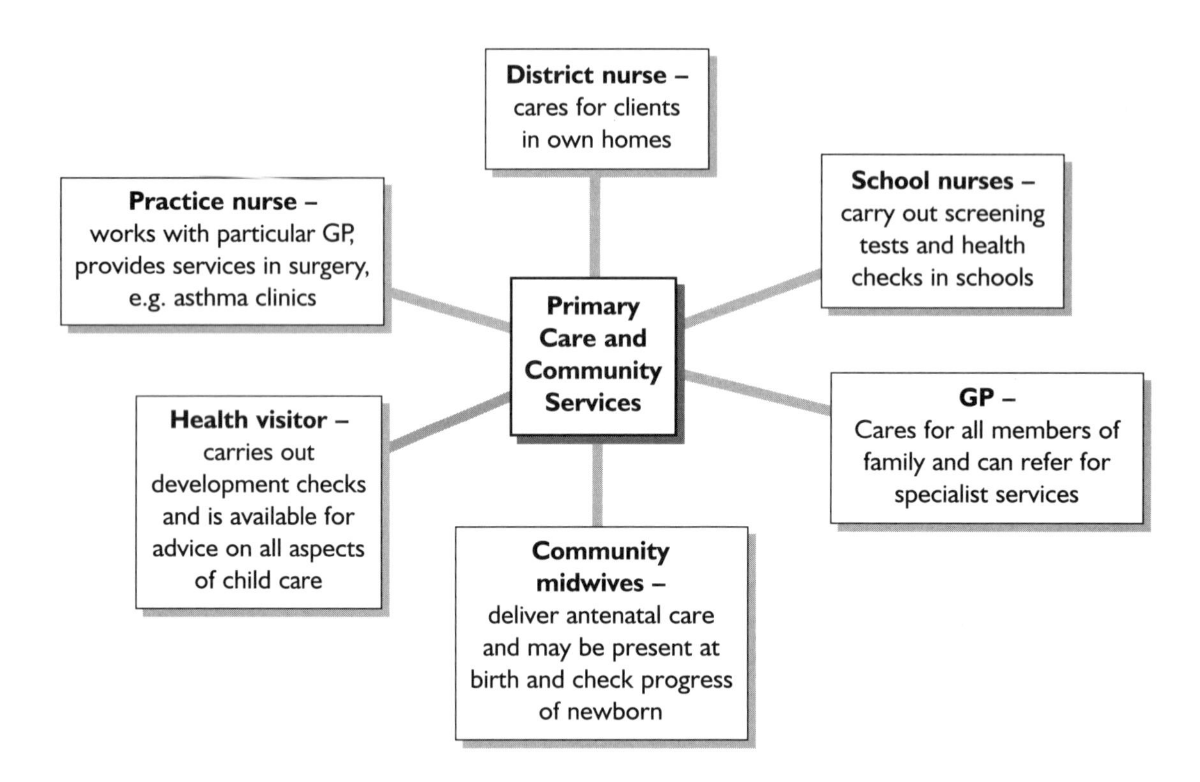

The primary health care team

The primary care health team (PHCT) is made up of a team of professionals which generally includes one or more of the following: general practitioner, practice nurse, health visitor, district nurse, psychiatric nurse, chiropodist and other health professionals:

- **General practitioner (GP) or family doctor**. This is a qualified doctor who has taken further training in general practice. Many GP group practices also have a doctor who has taken further training in obstetrics. GPs are doctors who are often the first port of call for health services. They are responsible for the general health of all children and their families. The general practice records are the only medical records which follow a person throughout life, so it is very important for other professionals to keep the GP well-informed. The GP is responsible for:
  - Diagnosing and treating conditions.
  - Organising other members of the PHCT to become involved in patient care.
  - Referring patients for specialist treatment.
  - Liaising with other agencies – for example social services or the education department.
  - Health promotion within the community.
- **Health visitor**. Health visitors are registered general nurses with an academic qualification in social health. They are trained to work with all ages, from birth to the very elderly. Their key objectives are primary health care education, health promotion and disease prevention. They offer screening services, assessing a child's development, providing support, etc. They have the facility to refer to other agencies whether voluntary or statutory. The major part of the health visitor's role

is spent helping and advising parents with children under five years of age on issues such as feeding, growth and development, immunisations and child protection.

Their role in the community includes:

- Taking over from the community midwife in visiting all new babies 10 days after the birth; this is a statutory obligation to try to visit, but they do not have the right of entry into a home as do social workers.
- Offering advice on all aspects of child care and development until the child is five years of age.
- Conducting child health clinics: monitoring the weight and development of babies; offering advice on general development, behaviour and toilet training, safety issues, nutrition, immunisation.
- Performing developmental assessments in the clinic or at home.
- Conducting hearing tests.
- Supporting families during times of crisis.
- Monitoring cases of suspected child abuse and neglect.

◆ **Practice nurse**. Practice nurses are qualified nurses who support the team's work in health promotion and prevention of ill-health. Some practice nurses take further training to become **nurse practitioners**, who are able to prescribe treatments and medicines for minor ailments. The practice nurse's work includes:

- Practical treatments such as treating minor injuries, changing dressings and doing cervical smears and ear syringing.
- Immunisation programmes.
- Monitoring children and adults with conditions such as asthma and diabetes.
- Family planning advice and counselling.

◆ **District nurse**. A district nurse is a registered general nurse who also has a qualification in community nursing. They are attached to GP practices, but also work in clinics and health centres. Their role is to provide nursing care at home to clients who may have recently been discharged from hospital, but still need some nursing care; or those who are disabled or terminally ill who want to remain at home. The GP, social worker or the hospital can refer a client to a district nurse. Patients can also refer themselves.

◆ **Community paediatric nurse**. A few health authorities employ district nurses with special training in paediatrics to care for sick children at home. Children are best cared for at home, if such specialist help is available. Their work includes caring for:

- children with acute (short-term) illnesses
- children who require long-term treatments or therapies – for example children with cystic fibrosis or any form of cancer
- children who have a chronic illness or disability
- children who are terminally ill and whose parents wish to care for them at home.

Community paediatric nurses also provide support for parents looking after sick children and liaise with other staff in the community, for example health visitors, district nurses, GPs, teachers and social workers.

- **Community midwife**. Community midwives are trained to care for pregnant women, delivering their babies and supporting parents in caring for their new-born babies at post-natal clinics and check-ups. They are practitioners in their own right and need only refer to a doctor if a pregnancy or labour is not progressing normally. Most routine antenatal care is carried out by midwives and a midwife delivers most babies born in the UK – in hospitals, GP units and at home. In the community, midwives have a statutory responsibility to care for both mother and baby for 10 days after delivery.

Health education in pregnancy

The midwife, doctor and health visitor are available throughout pregnancy to give advice on diet, rest, exercise or any issue causing concern; they can also offer advice on the current maternity benefits and how to apply for them.

The **inverse care law** operates in this area of health. The women most at risk of developing complications during pregnancy are those in poor housing, on a poor diet or whose attendance at antenatal clinics is poor or non-existent. The midwife and health visitor will be aware of the risks such factors pose for both mother and baby and will target such individuals to ensure that preventive health care, such as surveillance and immunisation, reaches them.

Parentcraft classes

Childbirth preparation classes are held in hospitals, health centres, community halls or private homes. They usually welcome couples to attend from about the 28th week of pregnancy and aim to cover:

- All aspects of pregnancy: diet and exercise; sexual activity; how to cope with problems such as nausea, tiredness and heartburn.
- Labour: pain control methods, breathing and relaxation exercises.
- Birth: what happens at each stage and the different methods of delivery.

The classes usually include a tour of the maternity unit at the hospital where delivery will take place. They are also valuable meeting-places for discussion with other parents-to-be about all the emotional changes involved in becoming a parent. Classes may also be held for women with special needs – expectant mothers who are schoolgirls, or in one-parent families, or whose first language is not English. Some areas provide classes earlier in pregnancy (from 8 to 20 weeks) or **aquanatal** classes where women can practise special exercises standing in shoulder-high water.

Some organisations, for example National Childbirth Trust (NCT), also offer parent education classes; these are usually held in small groups in the tutor's home. Fees vary according to circumstances.

Services offered by the primary health care team

The services offered by the primary health care team will include some or all of the following:

- Child health clinics (see page 294).
- Antenatal clinics.
- Immunisation clinics.

- Specialist clinics – for example, for asthma, diabetes, etc.
- Family planning clinics.

The health centre

The primary health care team are based in a health centre, which may also offer the following services:

- **Speech and language therapy**. Speech and language therapists are expert in the development of language and communication. They can help to promote language and communication in people with developmental disabilities and hearing problems. They normally work in clinics, health centres, schools and hospitals as part of a multidisciplinary team. Where a child is experiencing severe difficulty in expressing themselves, a speech and language therapist may introduce a communication aid that can either extend or replace speech.
- **Community dietician**. Dieticians provide advice, information and teaching on nutrition and diets. They work with parents, professionals and the general public. Children may be referred to the dietician if they have feeding difficulties, an eating disorder or any condition that requires a special diet. They also have an important role in health promotion, for example advising families on low incomes how best to ensure they have a balanced diet.
- **Community physiotherapists**. Physiotherapy is the treatment of disorders of movement and function in the human body caused by problems in the muscles, bones or nervous system. Physiotherapists assess and treat these disorders by natural methods such as exercise, manipulation, heat, as well as electrical or ultrasonic procedures. They may teach a series of exercises that can be carried out regularly at home. Physiotherapists work in hospitals, schools, child development centres and in the community – visiting patients in their homes.
- **Community occupational therapists**. Occupational therapists (OTs) are expert in understanding how chronic illness and developmental disorders can affect activities of daily living. They give practical advice to parents and carers about how to reduce everyday problems faced by children and their families. Within local authority social services departments, occupational therapists are responsible for the assessment and provision of suitable equipment and for major adaptations to an existing or new environment at home, school or work to enable a child to function as independently as possible.
- **Community paediatrician**. Community paediatricians are doctors expert in the health and development of children, particularly children with developmental disorders and chronic illnesses. They are also expert in physical examination and investigation and know when and how to refer to other specialists.
- **Clinical medical officer (CMO)**. The CMO is a doctor who is present at child health clinics and who carries out school medicals. In areas where there is not a community paediatrician available, the CMO will co-ordinate services. They can initiate the statementing process.
- **Community dental service**. Community dentists carry our screening dental examinations in schools and health centres – usually when the child is aged 4–5 years, 8–9 years and twice more at secondary school age. If a problem is found on screening, the child is referred for dental treatment.

Child health clinics

Child health clinics are often held at the health centre or in a purpose-built centre. In rural areas, the clinic may take turns with other community groups in village halls or community centres. Depending on the population served, clinics may be weekly or fortnightly and are run by health visitors, health care assistants and nursery nurses. A doctor or community paediatrician is usually present at specified times. Services provided at a child health clinic include:

- Routine developmental surveillance (see pages 281–285).
- Medical examinations.
- Immunisations.
- Health promotion advice.
- Antenatal and mothercraft classes.

All child health clinics should have a room where parents can meet and get to know one another. There should also be a notice board where parents and carers of children can access information about a wide range of health services in their local area. In addition, there should be:

- An area where babies can be changed – with changing mats, bins for soiled nappies, a basin, etc.
- A weighing area with scales.
- A safe play area for babies and older children, with a variety of toys and play equipment.
- A place for parents to park prams and pushchairs.
- A toy library where toys can be borrowed and exchanged regularly.
- A private room where parents can talk in confidence to the health visitor.
- A consultation room where the doctor can carry out physical examinations and discuss health issues in confidence.
- A comfortable waiting area for parents and provision for breastfeeding.

Parents are invited to the child health clinic to:

- have their babies weighed: details are entered on the child health record
- discuss any problems such as feeding, sleeping or toilet-training difficulties
- have their child assessed – for example hearing tests and developmental assessments
- discuss and receive immunisations for their child.

Often, child health clinics operate an appointment system; others see parents within clinic opening times. For many parents the clinic offers a welcome opportunity to meet other parents and children and to make new friends.

The school health service

The school health service is part of the community child health service and has direct links with those who carry out health checks on children before they start school. The aims of the school health service are to:

- ensure that children are physically and emotionally fit so that they can benefit fully from their education and achieve their potential

- prepare children for adult life and to help them achieve the best possible health during the school years and beyond.

Many different services are provided:

- **Routine testing for vision, hearing or speech**: to discover which children may need further tests or treatment. If treatment is thought to be required, the child's parents will be informed and consent requested.
- The **school nurse**: the school nurse may work with one or more schools, and provides an important link between the school and health services. School nurses provide the following services:
  - Growth measurements – height and weight.
  - Advice on management of health conditions; for example, if a child has a long-term illness or special need, they will discuss possible strategies with the child's teacher.
  - Enuresis (bedwetting) support and advice, including providing an enuresis alarm.
  - Immunisation.
  - Give advice on health and hygiene, sometimes running workshops or similar sessions for parents on specific health issues, for example treating head lice or coping with asthma.
  - Test eyesight from time to time.
  - Work with the **school doctor**.

The attention of the school doctor is drawn to any possible problems, and parents and the GP or family doctor are informed if any further action is considered necessary. The health visitor and school nurse also act as an important link between home and school.

- The **school doctor** visits the school regularly and meets with the school nurse (or health visitor) and with teachers to find out whether any pupils need medical attention. In addition, the doctor reviews the medical notes of all children in Year 1 and of all new pupils transferring to the school. The staff involved work closely with parents and with others who are caring for children, both at school and in other branches of the health service.
- Parents are usually asked to complete a **health questionnaire** (see pages 296–297) about their child at certain stages and asked if they would like their child to have a full medical examination. In addition, the school doctor may ask for parental consent to examine a child if his or her medical records are incomplete or if the doctor particularly wishes to check on the child's progress. Parents are invited to be present at any medical examination and kept informed if the school doctor wishes to see their child again or thinks that they should be seen by the family doctor or a specialist.
- The **audiometry team** checks children's hearing on a number of occasions before the age of 13 or 14 years. The school doctor will be told if a child seems to have a hearing problem. The doctor will then examine the child and let the family doctor know the result.
- The **speech and language therapist** can provide assessment and, if necessary, treatment if the parent, a teacher or the school doctor feels that a child may have a speech or language problem.

Westbury NHS Trust
COMMUNITY HEALTH SERVICES
CONFIDENTIAL HEALTH QUESTIONNAIRE

Please complete this and return it to the school in a sealed envelope, addressed to the school nurse. The information may be discussed by her with the school doctor.

CHILD'S NAME .... DATE OF BIRTH ....

OTHER NAMES ....

BOY/GIRL

.... POST CODE ....

TEL. No.: (home) ....TEL. No.: (work) ....

FAMILY DOCTOR .... HEALTH VISITOR ....

NAME AND ADDRESS OF CLINIC ATTENDED ....

....

....

SCHOOL ....

(1) **MEDICAL HISTORY**

Has your child ever had:–

Whooping cough	Yes/No
Measles	Yes/No
Mumps	Yes/No
Chickenpox	Yes/No
German measles (Rubella)	Yes/No

(2) Has your child ever had any serious illness? Yes/No
If yes, please give details:

(3) Has your child ever attended hospital? Yes/No
If yes, please give details, the age of the child and the name of the hospital:

(4) Did your child have a developmental check between the ages of 3 and 4 years? Yes/No/Don't know

FAMILY HISTORY

Does any member of your family have a disability or suffer from ill health?
e.g. visual or hearing problems, heart disease, diabetes, epilepsy, etc. Yes/No
If so, please give details:

CURRENT MEDICAL INFORMATION

(1) Does your child suffer from:

Bronchitis	Yes/No
Asthma	Yes/No
Wheezing cough with colds	Yes/No
Ear trouble or poor hearing	Yes/No
Eye trouble (squint, lazy eye, needs glasses)	Yes/No
Fits, faints or blackouts	Yes/No
Allergies, e.g. hay fever	Yes/No
Skin problems, e.g. eczema	Yes/No

(2) Does your child receive speech therapy? Yes/No
Has he/she ever had speech therapy? Yes/No

(3) Does your child take any pills, tablets, drugs, medicines, inhalers, require injections or special health care? Yes/No
If so, please give details.

(4) Do you have any worries about any of the following?

Speech	Yes/No
Hearing	Yes/No
Eyesight	Yes/No
Growth	Yes/No
Weight	Yes/No
Eating	Yes/No
Sleeping	Yes/No
Behaviour	Yes/No
Bed wetting	Yes/No
Soiling	Yes/No
Learning	Yes/No
Clumsiness	Yes/No

(5) Does your child have any other illness, medical or other problems?
Please describe.

IMMUNISATION

It is very important that these are up-to-date. You can find out which immunisations your child has had or still needs by looking in your child's health book or by checking with the clinic, GP or health visitor.

Your child should have had:

Three injections (in the first year) against diphtheria, whooping cough, tetanus, usually given at the same time as polio vaccine (drops). Sometimes, for medical reasons, the whooping cough is not given.

One injection against measles (usually between 1 and 2 years of age), or MMR (measles, mumps and rubella) all in one dose (between 1 and 2 years of age, or when starting school).

A booster against diphtheria, tetanus and polio before starting school at 5 years old.

IMMUNISATION HISTORY

Has your child been immunised against? *Please give dates*

	1st dose	2nd dose	3rd dose
Diptheria and tetanus			
Whooping cough			
Polio (drops)			

Measles, one dose	YES/NO	DATE ......
Measles, mumps, rubella (MMR) one dose	YES/NO	DATE ......
Pre-school booster, one dose	YES/NO	DATE ......

For older children:–

Rubella (German measles)	YES/NO	DATE ......
BCG (against TB) sometimes given at birth	YES/NO	DATE ......
Tetanus and polio booster (15–18)	YES/NO	DATE ......

Special educational needs co-ordinators

Special educational needs co-ordinators liaise with colleagues in **special schools** and with the parents of children with special needs. They are responsible for co-ordinating provision for children with special educational needs, keeping the school's special educational needs (SEN) register and working with external agencies, for example the educational psychology service.

Educational psychologists

Educational psychologists are primarily involved in the educational assessment of children with learning difficulties and in preparing the **statement of special educational needs**. They are *dual* professionals, that is, they are both psychologists as well as qualified and experienced teachers. They conduct evaluations of children's educational, psychological and emotional needs, offer therapy and contribute psychological expertise to the process of assessment. Parents need to give their consent before an educational psychologist is involved.

Special needs teachers

Special needs teachers are qualified teachers with additional training and experience in teaching children with special needs. They are supported by special needs support teachers, who are often peripatetic; this means that they visit disabled children in different schools. Sometimes they specialise in a particular disorder, for example visual impairment.

Special needs support assistants may be qualified nursery nurses and often work with individual children under the direction of the specialist teacher.

Child psychiatrist

Child psychiatrists are doctors who are expert in understanding how illness and developmental disorders can affect children's behaviour, emotional adjustment and social relationships. They are often called upon to diagnose specific developmental and behavioural disorders, such as autism, and usually work in close contact with the child's parents to provide a framework for therapy.

The child development team

The child development team (CDT) is a group of medical and non-medical professionals expert in child development, often co-ordinated by a community paediatrician and based at a **child development centre**. Team members typically include community paediatricians, educational psychologists, speech and language therapists and occupational therapists. A main job of the CDT is to produce a comprehensive assessment of development which will help to plan treatment, education and other arrangements. The team works with the parents to plan the most appropriate treatment to enable each child to reach his or her full potential. Their aims are to:

- reach a diagnosis of the child's condition and to determine the likely outcome
- assess the need for special adaptations to the home to make life easier, for example bath rails and ramps in doorways
- provide access to wheelchairs or other aids to mobility
- provide access to special equipment, for example communication aids or computers

- decide on the most appropriate education for the child
- plan the treatment and therapy that the child may need
- advise the family about any financial benefits they may be entitled to receive
- provide and arrange **respite care** when needed.

Each child and family is allocated a link worker who is available to translate if the first language is not English and to advise the team about relevant cultural factors.

The learning disabilities service

That is a team of professionals who are expert in helping parents and carers to manage behavioural problems and mental illness in people with developmental disorders. Team members may include psychiatrists, clinical psychologists, nurses and occupational therapists. They provide understanding and advice, and medical treatment when necessary.

Portage worker

Portage workers may work with the learning disabilities service, or with CDTs, and will have particular expertise in working with parents of pre-school children, helping them with developmental difficulties using a home-teaching method devised in Portage, Wisconsin, in the United States.

The education welfare service

The educational welfare service is a specialised department run by the local education authority. Its prime aim is to improve and maintain attendance where this has fallen below 85 per cent. This involves a close partnership between home and school, working with families and pastoral staff. **Education social workers** use a variety of strategies to help improve attendance. Such strategies include:

- home visiting
- seeing young people in school
- monitoring report card systems
- doing in-depth group work with small groups of young people.

However, when necessary, it may be appropriate to involve legal proceedings, as parents have a legal obligation to educate their children – usually at full-time school. Education social workers need to have a clear knowledge and understanding of other areas of work which may have a direct impact on achieving regular and beneficial attendance at school. This includes child protection, exclusions and licensing young people for child employment and performances. The education welfare service also provides practical help in the form of grants for essential school clothing, travel allowances and free school meals for children from low income families.

Hospital services for children

There are many different reasons for a child having to go to hospital. Every year, 1 in 4 children under the age of five years will be examined in an accident and emergency department. Children are admitted as **in-patients** for a variety of reasons. These include:

- Diagnosis and treatment following an acute illness or serious accident, such as pneumonia or head injury.

- Diagnosis and treatment for chronic illnesses, such as diabetes or asthma.
- Diagnosis and treatment for life-threatening illnesses, such as leukaemia or sickle cell anaemia.
- Surgery
  - planned, for example removal of tonsils or adenoids
  - unplanned, for example to remove an appendix or following an accident that has caused internal injuries.

Accident and emergency departments

The child's need for treatment should be assessed immediately on arrival in the accident and emergency department. Many departments operate a system called **triage** which prioritises the most urgent cases. There may be a **triage nurse** who is skilled in this. The majority of children seen in accident and emergency units will go home after treatment; more serious injuries and illness will call for admission as an in-patient. The department to which they are admitted will depend on the type of injuries sustained. Some hospitals have a separate accident and emergency department for children. This makes the experience much less frightening as the unit will be staffed by paediatric nurses and doctors. There are usually also play leaders or hospital play specialists to support sick children and their families.

Outpatients departments

Outpatient departments are usually run within the various branches of specialist medicine, although some hospitals have a separate paediatric clinic for babies and children.

In-patient care

If a child has to be admitted to hospital as an in-patient, it is important that they are prepared as well as possible for the experience.

The following list describes the work done by different departments within a general hospital:

Accident and emergency (A&E)	A special department in a hospital, which deals with accidents and acute illness – sometimes called Casualty.
Cardiology	The study of the structure and function of the heart.
Chemotherapy	The use of specific drugs and chemicals to treat cancer.
Dermatology	The branch of medicine concerned with the skin and the disorders that affect it.
Endocrinology	The study of the endocrine system; any internal organs which produce secretions, such as thyroid and pituitary glands, pancreas, stomach and liver.
ENT	The speciality concerned with disorders of the ear, nose and throat.
Gynaecology	The medical speciality concerned with the female reproductive tract.

Haematology	The study of the nature, functions and disorders of the blood.
Midwifery	The profession concerned with the assistance of women in pregnancy and childbirth.
Neonatology	The study and treatment of the baby in the first month of life.
Neurology	The medical discipline concerned with the study of the nervous system – i.e. the brain, spinal cord and nerves.
Obstetrics	The branch of medicine dealing with pregnancy and labour.
Occupational therapy	Treatment aimed at enabling people disabled by physical illness or serious accident to relearn muscular control and co-ordination.
Oncology	The study of the causes, development and treatment of cancer.
Ophthalmology	The study of the eye and the disorders that affect it.
Orthopaedics	The branch of surgery concerned with disorders of the bones, joints and muscles.
Outpatient treatment	Medical care given to a person on a day basis in a hospital or clinic.
Paediatric intensive care	The constant, close monitoring of seriously ill children, which enables immediate treatment to be given if the child's condition deteriorates.
Paediatrics	The branch of medicine concerned with the growth and development of children, and with the diagnosis, treatment and prevention of childhood diseases.
Pathology	The study of disease, its causes, its mechanisms, and effects on the body.
Physiotherapy	Treatment of muscular and skeletal conditions by natural forces, e.g. massage, exercise, heat, etc.
Psychiatry	The branch of medicine concerned with the study, prevention, and treatment of mental illness and emotional and behavioural problems.
Psychology	The scientific study of mental processes, such as memory, thought, feelings, and perception.
Radiography	The use of X-rays to obtain images of parts of the body.
Radiotherapy	Treatment of cancer, and occasionally other diseases, by X-rays and other sources of radioactivity.
Renal	A medical term meaning related to the kidney.
Rheumatology	The study of joints and muscles.
Special Care Baby Unit (SCBU)	A highly specialised team of trained doctors and nurses working with babies who are premature or who have neonatal problems requiring intensive treatment.

Speech and language therapy	Treatment to help with speech, language and communication disorders.
Urology	The study of disorders of the urinary tract.
X-ray examination	A method which assists in the diagnosis of a disease, disorder or dysfunction in the body. When X-rays are directed onto parts of the body they pass through bone and tissue to different extents to produce an image on a photographic film.

ACTIVITY

1. Write brief explanations of the following terms:
   - ☐ Triage
   - ☐ Portage worker
   - ☐ Respite care.
2. Arrange to visit a local child health clinic and prepare a fact-sheet for parents. Include the following information:
   - ☐ The services available, including the times parents can attend with their children.
   - ☐ A description of the procedures carried out.
   - ☐ The responsibilities of the health care staff.
   - ☐ The advantages of attending the clinic.

Revision questions

1. What is child health surveillance?
2. What is screening, and why is it important?
3. What health education points are discussed during the child's first year?
4. At what age is the MMR immunisation given? Why might parents be reluctant to accept the MMR?
5. Name two recent health education campaigns relevant to baby and child health.
6. List the professionals who make up the primary health care team and briefly describe their roles.
7. Describe the role of the health visitor in promoting health.
8. List the services available at child health clinics.
9. Which screening and surveillance checks are carried out by the school nurse?
10. What is respite care?

Glossary

Acetabulum The cup-shaped cavity on the hip bone, receiving the head of the femur.

Acupuncture An alternative method of treatment which originated in China; it involves the insertion of fine needles at specific points on the skin and has been found to enhance health and the immune system as well as addressing specific symptoms.

Adrenaline A drug used to treat anaphylaxis. (It is very similar to the hormone called adrenaline that is produced naturally in our bodies and is responsible for feelings of excitement and stimulation.)

Allergen The substance causing an allergy.

Allergy A condition in which the immune system responds to a substance inappropriately.

Amenorrhoea The absence of menstrual periods.

Amniocentesis A means of genetic screening of a foetus inside the womb.

Anaemia A condition in which the concentration of the oxygen-carrying pigment, haemoglobin, in the blood is below normal.

Anaphylactic shock A potentially fatal immune response when the body system literally shuts down. The most common causes are a severe allergic reaction to insect stings and certain drugs.

Anaphylaxis A severe allergic reaction that affects the whole body.

Anencephaly Having no brain; a very rare congenital disorder which is incompatible with life.

Anterior fontanelle A diamond-shaped soft area at the front of the head, just above the brow. It is covered by a tough membrane; you can often see the baby's pulse beating there under the skin. The fontanelle closes between 12 and 18 months of age.

Antibodies Substances that are produced by our immune system in order to protect our body from 'intruders' such as bacteria and viruses. Particular kinds of antibodies are also involved in allergic reactions.

Antigen A foreign substance that the body recognises and reacts against.

Antihistamines Medicines that are used to treat allergic reactions. They work by blocking the effect of histamines. Available as creams, tablets and nasal sprays.

Apnoea Cessation of breathing, either temporarily (for a few seconds to a minute or two) or for a prolonged period.

Areola The pigmented ring around the nipple.

Asperger's syndrome A disorder which shares many of the same characteristics as **autism**.

Asthma A disease affecting the ability to breathe easily.

Attachment An enduring emotional bond that an infant forms with a specific person. Usually the first attachment is to the mother, some time between the ages of 6 and 9 months.

Attention deficit (hyperactivity) disorder (ADHD) A behavioural disorder in children.

Autism A disorder which disrupts the development of social and communication skills.

Benign Not cancerous although may be capable of causing problems.

Biopsy The removal of sample of tissue for examination, often by microscopy. It is done to observe any evidence of disease or degeneration so assisting diagnosis and treatment.

Blood transfusion The infusion of large volumes of blood or blood components directly into the bloodstream.

Bonding A term used to denote the feelings of love and responsibility that parents have for their babies.

Breech presentation During labour the baby is lying with bottom or feet downwards. (The normal presentation is **cephalic**, i.e. head downwards.)

Bronchiolitis An acute viral infection of the bronchioles – the smallest airways in the lungs.

Bronchitis Infection of the bronchi – tubes which transfer air to and from the lungs.

Cancer A new growth of tissue caused by the excessive and uncontrolled growth of abnormal cells that have the ability to invade and destroy other tissues.

Caries, dental The medical term for tooth decay.

Carrier A person who is able to pass on a disease without actually suffering from it.

Catheter A tube used either for withdrawing fluid from a body cavity or for introducing fluid to a body cavity.

Central line A central line is a fine plastic tube, which is inserted into a vein in the child's chest. This procedure is carried out under a general anaesthetic. When inserting the line, the surgeon makes a small cut into a vein in the neck and feeds the line down towards the heart. The other end is then tunnelled under the skin to emerge on the front of the chest as an external line. A removable bung is placed on the end of the line, which allows sampling of blood or injection of drugs.

Cervical smear test A test to detect abnormal changes in the cervix (the neck of the womb) and so prevent the development of cervical cancer.

Chickenpox (varicella) A mild viral childhood infection, characterised by a distinctive, itchy rash and a slight fever.

Child development centre A unit which provides specialist multi-professional support for children with special needs and their families.

Chorionic villus sampling A method of collecting the chorion cells from the pregnant mother. Chorion cells are situated on the wall of the uterus (womb). They have the same origin as the foetal cells and can, therefore, be analysed to detect certain foetal abnormalities in the foetus.

Chromosome A thread-like structure in the cell nucleus that carries genetic information in the form of genes.

Cochlea The spiral-shaped organ in the inner ear that transforms sound vibrations into nerve impulses for transmission to the brain.

Coeliac disease A rare disease caused by an extreme sensitivity of the small intestine to a protein (gluten) present in the cereals of wheat, rye, barley and oats.

Colostrum A creamy yellowish fluid produced by the breasts during pregnancy. Low in fat and sugar, it is uniquely designed to feed the newborn baby.

Commensal A usually harmless bacterium or other organism that normally lives in or on the body.

Complementary medicine Treatments or therapies which work alongside conventional medical care, e.g. **homeopathy** and **acupuncture**.

Conception The biological process which involves an egg being fertilised by a sperm so that it then becomes implanted in the lining of the womb.

Congenital Present at birth; a congenital disorder need not be hereditary, though many are.

Conjunctivitis Inflammation of the conjunctiva (the thin transparent membrane which covers the whites of the eyes and lines the eyelids).

Contact dermatitis A type of eczema that occurs when the skin reacts to something it comes in contact with.

Corticosteroid A steroid medicine that is used to treat or prevent allergic reactions by reducing inflammation. Used in preventer medicines for people with asthma and in creams to treat eczema. Severe cases of these and other allergies may also be treated with corticosteroid tablets.

Coryza The medical term for the common cold.

Cranial osteopathy A treatment where the bones of the skull are very gently manipulated and moved into place; it works particularly well on babies and small children, whose bones are more easily modified and may have been affected during a difficult birth.

Croup Inflammation and narrowing of the main airways to the lungs.

Cyanosis Blueness of the skin.

Cystic fibrosis A serious inherited disease which causes recurrent chest infections and inability to absorb nutrients from the intestines.

Cytomegalovirus One of the family of herpes viruses. A pregnant woman can transmit the virus to her unborn child; this may cause malformations and brain damage in the child.

Dander Animal dander includes the tiny particles of skin and dried sweat and saliva that are shed by animals such as cats and dogs. These are a major cause of allergies such as asthma, eczema and allergic rhinitis.

Dermatitis Inflammation of the skin.

Diabetes mellitus A disorder caused by insufficient production of the hormone insulin by the pancreas.

DNA DNA (Deoxyribonucleic acid) is the 'building block' for all genetic material.

Down's syndrome the most common chromosomal abnormality; children with the condition have a characteristic physical appearance combined with slow mental development.

Ectopic pregnancy A pregnancy that develops outside the uterus, most usually in the fallopian tube.

Eczema A group of skin conditions characterised by dry, red, flaky, itchy skin. The most common form of eczema is caused by allergy.

Embryo The unborn child during the first eight weeks of development following conception.

Emollients Special moisturisers – available as bath oils, creams and ointments – that are used to help prevent eczema.

Encopresis Faecal incontinence or soiling not due to organic disease or involuntary loss of control, but resulting from deliberate intent.

Endorphins Chemicals that create a happy feeling in your brain.

Enuresis Bedwetting; the involuntary passage of urine, especially during sleep.

Epidemic Episodes of disease which spread rapidly and affect large numbers of people, e.g. flu.

Erythema Also known as fifth disease, erythema infectiosum is a mildly contagious viral illness which mainly affects children over two years old during the spring months.

Fallopian tube The tube that extends from the uterus to the ovary.

Febrile convulsions Convulsions which mainly occur in young children who have high temperatures.

Fever Known medically as pyrexia, a fever is defined as a body temperature above 37 °C.

Foetal alcohol syndrome A pattern of physical and mental abnormalities due to excessive maternal alcohol intake during pregnancy.

Foetus The unborn child from the end of the eighth week after conception until birth.

Folic acid A vitamin of the B complex. It is involved in the synthesis of amino acids and DNA. Green vegetables, liver and yeast are major sources of folic acid in the diet.

Food intolerance or food sensitivity A sensitivity or bad reaction to certain foods that does not involve the immune system, so is not an allergy.

Forceps Special tongs that fit around the baby's head to form a protective 'cage'; they are used during the delivery of a baby when problems occur, e.g. if the baby is showing signs of foetal distress.

Fragile X syndrome An inherited chromosomal abnormality, which causes learning difficulties.

Gastro-enteritis Inflammation of the stomach and intestines.

Gene Unit of the chromosome containing a code or characteristic pattern which is passed on through generations. Genes influence hair and eye colour and blood types, etc.

Genetic counselling Information and support provided by a specialist doctor, usually a geneticist, to parents who have known conditions in their families or who are concerned about the future possibility of genetically transmitted conditions.

Gingivitis Inflammation of the gums in the mouth.

GUM Genito-urinary medical clinic – often called 'special clinic'.

Haemoglobin Iron-containing pigment in the red blood cells.

Haemolytic disease of the newborn A disease in which there is excessive destruction of the red blood cells in the foetus and the neonate, resulting in jaundice. It is usually caused by Rhesus incompatibility between the infant's blood and the mother's.

Haemophilia A genetic disorder that causes episodes of spontaneous bleeding.

Hay fever An allergy caused by breathing in pollen and by pollen getting in the eyes. Affects the delicate lining of the nose and eyes.

HEAF test A skin scratch test carried out to see if there are any antibodies to TB (tuberculosis).

Hepatitis Inflammation of the liver.

Hernia Protrusion of a part of the intestine through the abdominal wall.

Herpes simplex The virus that causes cold sores.

Histamine A chemical that is released into the body during an allergic reaction and causes inflammation in certain parts of the body.

Hives Another name for urticaria.

Holistic Seeing a child in the round as a whole person, emotionally, intellectually, physically, socially, morally, culturally and spiritually.

Homeopathy Treatments based on using natural substances to treat a wide range of conditions.

Hormone A substance made and secreted by a gland and carried in the bloodstream to parts of the body where it has a specific effect on the way the body works.

Hydrocephalus 'Water on the brain' – an abnormal accumulation of cerebrospinal fluid in and around the brain.

Hyperglycaemia An excess of sugar (glucose) in the blood.

Hypertension Abnormally high blood pressure (the pressure of blood in the main arteries).

Immunotherapy A treatment for certain allergies, such as allergy to bee and wasp stings and severe hay fever. It involves having a course of injections of tiny amounts of the allergen. The treatment should make the person less sensitive to the allergen.

Impetigo A common, highly contagious bacterial skin infection.

Insulin A hormone which enables the body to use and store glucose (sugar).

Intravenous Within a vein; an intravenous infusion is the slow introduction of a volume of fluid into the bloodstream via a vein.

Kawasaki disease A childhood disease that causes fever, swollen lymph nodes and symptoms that affect the skin and mucus membranes.

Koplik's spots Tiny white spots with a red base, which can sometimes be seen on the insides of the cheeks a day or two after the first symptoms of measles appear.

Leukaemia A form of cancer in which the bone marrow produces many abnormal white blood cells.

Lumbar puncture A hollow needle is used to draw out a small amount of cerebrospinal fluid from the spinal canal for examination in the laboratory.

Malignant or cancerous If a tumour is malignant it grows uncontrollably and can travel to other parts of the body.

Marfan's syndrome A rare inherited disorder which results in abnormalities of the skeleton, heart and eyes.

Measles (morbilli) A childhood viral infection that causes fever and a characteristic rash.

Meningitis Inflammation of the meninges (the membranes covering the brain and spinal cord).

Mononucleosis Glandular fever – a viral infection that typically causes a high fever, lack of energy and swollen lymph nodes (glands).

Mumps A mild viral infection that causes fever and swelling of one or both of the parotid (salivary) glands.

Neonate A newly born infant under the age of one month.

Nettle rash Another name for urticaria.

Neural tube defects Defects in the normal development of the embryo's brain and spinal cord.

Nutrients Essential dietary factors, such as carbohydrates, proteins, certain fats, vitamins and minerals.

Occupational therapist (OT) A professional who treats people disabled by injury or illness to regain the use and control of their muscles.

Oedema An abnormal accumulation of fluid in the body tissues. In pregnancy, oedema is often shown as swollen ankles and fingers.

Oncology The study and treatment of cancer.

Ophthalmologist A specialist in the study of the eye and its disorders.

Ophthalmology The study of the eyes.

Oral In the mouth.

Orthopaedics The correction of deformities of the bones and skeleton.

Osteo- To do with the bones.

Osteogenesis imperfecta An inherited condition – children have bones that are very brittle and more susceptible to breaking.

Otitis media Inflammation of the middle ear cavity, between the ear-drum and the inner ear.

Paediatric To do with children.

Paediatric oncologist Doctors who have chosen to specialist in children's cancer.

Paediatrics The medical speciality concerned with the care of children; it deals not only with children's diseases, but covers all aspects of child health and development in the context of the family and the whole environment.

Pertussis The medical term for whooping cough.

Phenylketonuria A rare genetic metabolic disease. Babies are routinely screened for phenylketonuria soon after birth, using the Guthrie blood test.

Phlegm A sticky substance formed by mucus membrane and ejected by coughing.

Placenta The organ that develops in the uterus during pregnancy and links the blood supplies of mother and baby – often referred to as the 'afterbirth'.

Plaque A rough, sticky coating on the teeth that is made up of saliva, bacteria and food debris.

Platelet Blood cell which helps to prevent bleeding.

Play therapist Play therapists are trained to help children cope with the experience of being ill and in hospital by using play.

Pneumonia Inflammation of the lungs – caused by bacteria, viruses – or rarely, a fungal infection.

Pollen The male 'seed' of plants (grasses, flowers, trees) that consists of microscopic dust-like particles. Can cause hay fever and asthma.

Portage A home teaching programme for children with special needs and their parents.

Possetting The regurgitation (or bringing back) of a small amount of milk by infants after they have been fed.

Pre-eclampsia A serious condition in which hypertension, oedema and protein in the urine develop in the latter part of the pregnancy.

Prevalence Something that exists extensively – or is widespread – as in disease.

Preventers Medicines (often based on steroids) that are usually breathed in from inhalers by people with asthma. Help to prevent the disease when taken on a regular basis.

Prognosis The expected outcome of a disease and its treatment.

Psoriasis A skin disease characterised by thickened patches of inflamed, red skin, often covered by silvery scales.

Pyloric stenosis A rare condition in which the outlet of the stomach – the muscle ring known as the pylorus – is abnormally thick, strong and tight. It is corrected by a simple surgical operation.

Pyrexia Fever or above normal body temperature.

Relievers Medicines that are used to treat the symptoms of an asthma attack.

Remission A period of good health when there is no detectable disease.

Renal To do with the kidneys.

Respite care A service provided which offers regular breaks to carers who are looking after sick or disabled children on a long-term basis.

Reyes syndrome This is a *rare* condition, usually preceded by a viral infection such as chickenpox or influenza. It is characterised by inflammation of the brain and liver which can occur if a young child is given aspirin for an infection with fever. It is potentially life-threatening.

Rhinitis Inflammation of the lining of the nose, usually due to an allergic reaction, e.g. hay fever.

Rickets A disorder affecting bone development – caused by a deficiency in vitamin D and calcium.

Roseola (infantum) Sometimes called 'sixth disease', roseola is a fairly common childhood disorder, causing the toddler to feel generally unwell, with fever and a pink rash like that of **rubella**.

Rubella (German measles) A viral infection that infects the respiratory tract and spreads to local lymph nodes, especially those at the back of the neck.

Scarlet fever An infection caused by a species of streptococcus; it causes tonsillitis, fever, abdominal pain and vomiting.

Seborrhoeic dermatitis A minor skin problem affecting very young babies.

Self-esteem The way you feel about yourself – either good or bad – leads to high or low self-esteem.

Septicaemia Blood poisoning.

Sexually transmitted disease (STD) Infection transmitted primarily, but not exclusively, by sexual intercourse.

Shingles An infection of the nerves that supply certain areas of the skin – the medical name is herpes zoter.

Sickle cell disease A serious disorder of the blood in which the normally round blood cells become distorted into a sickle shape.

Sinusitis Inflammation of the mucus membrane linings of one or more bone cavities (sinuses) of the face.

Skin prick test An allergy test that involves putting a small amount of a known allergen on to a scratch in the skin, to see if the body reacts. Used to diagnose a number of allergies, particularly allergy to various pollens, house dust mite droppings and pets.

Statementing An assessment process to determine the specific needs of children with disabilities.

Statutory services Central government services and local government services, e.g. the NHS or social services.

Strabismus Squint. The condition in which only one eye is aligned on the object of interest.

Surgery/surgical The treatment of disease, injury or other disorders by direct physical intervention, usually with instruments.

Thalassaemia A genetic condition which results in abnormal haemoglobin in the red blood cells, causing severe anaemia.

Thrombocytopenia Deficiency of platelets in blood – essential for the clotting mechanism.

Thrush A fungal infection, candidiasis, that occurs in the mouth and nappy area in babies.

Toxoplasmosis An infection caused by the microscopic organism toxoplasma gondii, often acquired before birth, but sometimes passed on by domestic cats or acquired by eating under-cooked meat from infected animals.

Traction The use of pulleys and weights on a long bone to keep it in position after a fracture and to prevent muscle spasm.

Traditional Chinese Medicine A combination of many different therapies, including the use of herbs and **acupuncture**.

Trigger Something that can bring on an allergic reaction but is not necessarily the actual cause of the allergy.

Tumour An abnormal lump of tissue formed by a collection of cells. It may be benign or malignant.

Urticaria A condition characterised by an itchy, pimply rash. Often caused by an allergy. Also called hives or nettle rash.

Uterus Another name for the womb.

Varicella Another name for chickenpox.

Voluntary organisation An association or society which has been created by its members rather than by the state, e.g. a charity.

Weal A blister-like mark on the skin that may indicate an allergy in a skin prick test.

Index

Page numbers in *italics* refer to illustrations or diagrams, those in **bold** to major articles on diseases or disorders.